Exploring
ELECTRONIC HEALTH RECORDS

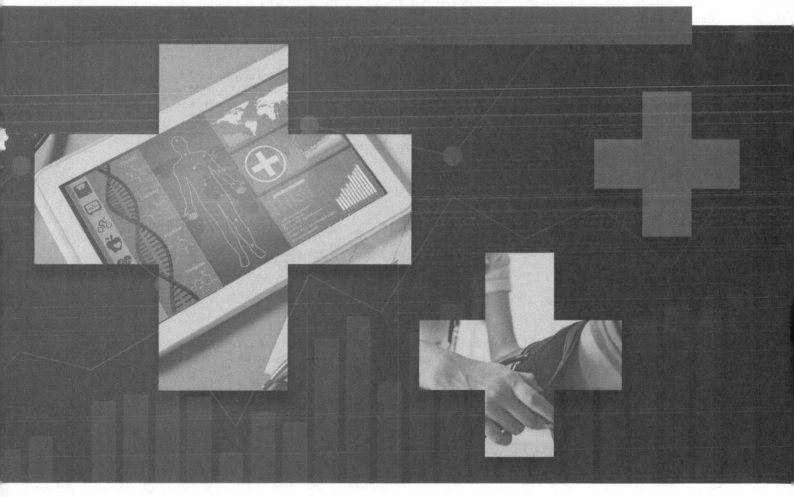

Darline Foltz
University of Cincinnati:
Clermont College

Karen Lankisch
University of Cincinnati:
Clermont College

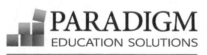

PARADIGM
EDUCATION SOLUTIONS
A DIVISION OF KENDALL HUNT

Minneapolis • Dubuque

Vice President, Paradigm Education Solutions: Linda Ganster
Executive Product Owner: Nancy Roberts
Director of Marketing: Keri Haas
Director of Publishing Services: Wendy S. Jochum
Publishing Specialist Supervisor: Carrie A. Maro
Supervisor of Prepress and Manufacturing: Cari M. Rieckens
Publishing Specialist: Noelle Henneman
Marketing Designer: Baylea Bruce

Cover Photo Credit: *White tablet PC and physician tools on gray surface* © Khakimullin Aleksandr/Shutterstock.com, *Nurse measuring arterial blood pressure of a male patient* © lovelyday12/Shutterstock.com, *Financial chart with uptrend line graph* © Champ008/Shutterstock.com

Interior Photo Credits: Following the index.

ISBN: 978-1-7924-6564-2

© 2022, 2018, 2015 by Paradigm Education Solutions, a division of Kendall Hunt

4050 Westmark Drive
Dubuque, IA 52004-1840
Email: ordernow@kendallhunt.com
Website: ParadigmEducation.com

Brief Contents

Contents

Preface

The role of the electronic health record (EHR) in health care has evolved and expanded rapidly in the last 10 years, and so has the importance of preparing the next generation of students in health information management, health information technology, medical assisting, and allied health. Original textbooks on the subject did not cover the EHR to the extent we needed—they only addressed the physician's office and focused on EHR functions related to insurance and billing. We wanted our students to learn about the EHR in the acute care, outpatient, and long-term care settings, so we decided to write our own textbook. We also wanted a more global representation of the EHR that included clinical and health information functions. To that end, we developed a generic type of EHR software with the functionality needed to teach skills and illustrate concepts that could be applied by any EHR user in any healthcare setting. Thus, the first edition of *Exploring Electronic Health Records* and the generic EHR software were created to provide a hands-on approach to learning the foundational concepts and skills related to EHRs.

The live, web-based application, the EHR Navigator, has allowed thousands of students to explore and develop skills in EHR software from any device with an internet connection. The EHR Navigator gives students experience in multiple healthcare settings, including outpatient, inpatient, and skilled nursing facilities. Due to the success of the program and requests from educators, we expanded the courseware to include a nursing dashboard to give nursing students the opportunity to practice using an EHR system prior to their clinicals. We are proud to share the third edition of *Exploring Electronic Health Records* with colleagues and students to facilitate their preparation to use a live EHR system in their chosen healthcare career.

Teach Me, Show Me, Let Me Try It

Exploring Electronic Health Records, Third Edition, is a current, accurate, and accessible courseware system that introduces students to the concepts and features of EHR systems. The courseware has been designed to help students learn about the functionality of the EHR as it applies to many healthcare careers. Students using this courseware gain an awareness of how the EHR supports efficiencies and accuracy within inpatient, outpatient, and skilled nursing and rehabilitation facilities, and how EHRs contribute to the goals of increased patient safety and security and the provision of high-quality health care.

The online course includes a complete eBook, an interactive glossary, flash cards, activities, and automatically graded quizzes, exams, and assessments. Tutorials and assessments are conducted in the EHR Navigator, which was designed with the best features of many industry EHR systems in mind. The 75 interactive tutorials and their accompanying practice assessments are based on a "teach me, show me, let me try it, and assess my work" educational process. Activities in the EHR Navigator supply ample practice opportunities to ensure that students build skills that are transferable to the many EHR systems they will encounter in their careers. A graded assessment for each tutorial evaluates the student's mastery of the procedure and reports to the grade book.

What's New in the Third Edition?

Exploring Electronic Health Records, Third Edition, and its corresponding courseware have been updated to prepare learners at various levels to step into their new roles and use any EHR system effectively. Enhancements to the core text include:

- **New Chapter 12, Data Analytics**, introduces students to the concept of harnessing clinical data to improve processes and better understand the unique needs of a facility's patient population.
- **New Chapter 14, eHealth and Population Health**, describes the rapidly evolving and expanding field of telemedicine and its role in engaging patients with their personal health record.
- The **EHR for Nursing** chapter, which was previously available as an online-only supplement, has been integrated into the main text and courseware.
- **Updated content** related to policy and industry standards includes coverage of the 21st Century Cures Act and its Final Rule, meaningful use and interoperability, and the ICD-11 code set.
- **Coverage of software and hardware advancements** and technology related to virtual healthcare services is integrated throughout the text and courseware.
- **Enhanced coverage** of Certified Electronic Health Record Specialist (CEHRS) learning objectives is found in Appendix C.

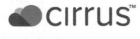

The third edition courseware and the EHR Navigator are powered by Paradigm's Cirrus platform. Cirrus delivers complete course content, including an eBook as well as interactive learning tools, such as case studies, quizzes, critical thinking assignments, exams, a glossary, and flash cards. Additions and expansions to the digital courseware include the following:

- **New Data Analytics and Reporting** modules are explored in a new tutorial and new assessments. Each report module is accompanied by case studies, and the reports can be downloaded for further analysis:
  - **Smoking Cessation**—To study the prevalence of smoking in the community, sort and filter the report by age, gender, and smoking level (frequency).
  - **Immunization Rates**—Review the immunization records for patients, discover the reasons that some patients declined their immunizations, and use the data to develop a strategy for educating the community on the importance of vaccines.
  - **Hospital Readmissions**—Search for readmissions related to heart failure and review the known chronic conditions, current medications, discharge disposition, and length of stay.
- **New Watch and Learn Lessons**: Each chapter is separated into discrete sections and presented in a responsive, web-based format. Visual learners can choose to watch the corresponding Watch and Learn video for the section, a PowerPoint-based presentation of the same chapter content.
- **Streamlined course organization**: Tutorials, practice assessments, and assessments are grouped in a module to help students progress through the EHR Navigator activities.

Additional information on the Cirrus platform can be found in the section "Paradigm's Cirrus Platform."

Chapter Features: A Visual Walk-Through

Each chapter contains features that aid student learning. These features, as outlined below, teach students the fundamentals of EHRs, challenge them to think critically, and give them additional online learning opportunities. The features of each chapter are designed to address different learning styles and stress the importance of professionalism and soft skills.

Engaging **chapter openers** include a **Field Notes** feature in which industry professionals share their insights into the use of EHRs in their field and other related topics.

Learning Objectives establish a clear set of goals for each chapter. The objectives are reviewed and reinforced in the Checkpoint quizzes and again at the end of the chapter.

Key terms are set in bold, contextually defined, and reinforced with flash cards in the online course.

Marginal features include the following:

Expand Your Learning speaks to digitally savvy students and integrates internet resources and online learning opportunities. Web addresses are hyperlinked in the eBook for quick navigation.

On the Job provides insight into soft skills and professionalism.

Why Your Job Matters emphasizes the importance of the roles and responsibilities of professionals in health care.

EXPAND YOUR LEARNING

For more detailed information regarding universal precautions, visit the CDC website at https://EHR3.ParadigmEducation.com/CDC.

ON THE JOB

It is important to keep your voice low when verifying PHI with a patient. While you cannot prevent all information from being overheard, the patient will appreciate the effort and trust that you are making the effort to protect their privacy.

WHY YOUR JOB MATTERS

All healthcare professionals have a responsibility to keep PHI secure and should report any suspicious cyber activity. A data breach for a hospital costs an average of $2.1 million, with the healthcare industry as a whole spending $6 billion every year recovering from cyberattacks.

Feature boxes provide real-life scenarios and give students periodic stopping points to test their learning.

Consider This

A teenage patient brought to the emergency department (ED) of a hospital drifts in and out of consciousness. The ED physician suspects an adverse event from a medication the patient is taking or a possible drug overdose. The ED physician learns that the patient takes medications that have been prescribed by the patient's primary care physician.

Because the patient's EHR is interoperable with the hospital's EHR, the ED physician is able to access the medications prescribed for the patient. How does permitted disclosure of health information in the Privacy Rule allow the patient to receive the necessary care? What could happen if the patient needs to wait while the hospital seeks authorization to release her information?

CHECKPOINT 6.1

1. True/False: A healthcare provider may not release patient health information without a specific authorization or consent signed by the patient.

2. True/False: HIPAA regulations cover only health information documented on paper.

3. The HIPAA Privacy and Security Rules apply only to health plans, healthcare clearinghouses, and healthcare providers who transmit health information in electronic format. What term is used for these plans, clearinghouses, and providers?

_____

Tutorials in the EHR Navigator are called out throughout the chapter to remind students to go to their online course and launch the interactive activities. These tutorials give students hands-on practice in an EHR system.

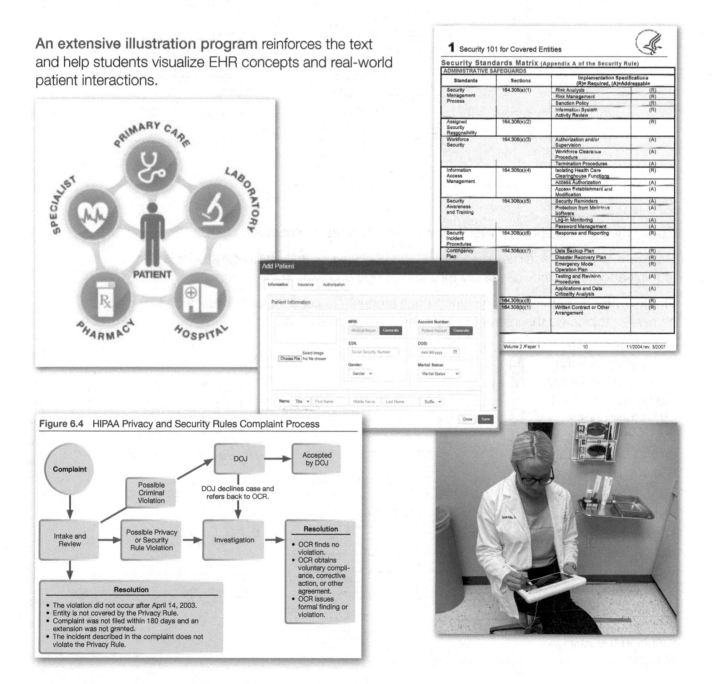

Tutorial 6.1   EHRNAVIGATOR

Releasing Patient Information
Go to the online course to launch Tutorial 6.1. As a Registered Health Information Technician (RHIT), practice releasing patient information using the EHR Navigator.

An extensive illustration program reinforces the text and help students visualize EHR concepts and real-world patient interactions.

Figure 6.4   HIPAA Privacy and Security Rules Complaint Process

The end-of-chapter content includes the following:

The **Chapter Summary** offers an overview of the key points of each chapter.

The **Review and Assessment** section reminds students to complete the review activities and directs them to the online course.

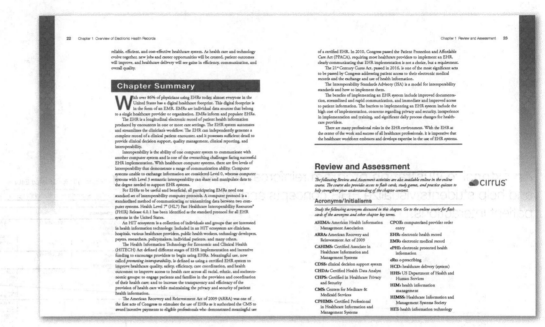

Go on the Record short-answer prompts test students on chapter content.

Navigate the Field activities present real-world scenarios that challenge students to think about how they can apply their knowledge and skills in the workplace.

Think Critically activity prompts encourage students to conduct further research on related topics via the internet or interviews with professionals.

Make Your Case activities require the student to synthesize their knowledge and prove their understanding of a topic through a presentation or other materials.

Explore the Technology activities ask students to conduct research on EHR technology or remind them to complete their practice assessments and assessments in the EHR Navigator.

Appendices

Appendix A contains the answers to chapter Checkpoints. **Appendix B** contains a handwritten medical record that illustrates the components of a typical paper record and is referenced as a learning tool in end-of-chapter and online activities. **Appendix C** is a crosswalk of the domains and topics identified on the National Healthcareer Association's Certified Electronic Health Record Specialist (CEHRS) certification exam and the chapter where the topics are covered in *Exploring Electronic Health Records,* Third Edition.

Paradigm's Cirrus Platform

Exploring Electronic Health Records, Third Edition, powered by the Cirrus platform, integrates seamlessly with Blackboard, Canvas, D2L, and Moodle. Students and educators can access all course materials anytime, anywhere, through a live internet connection. Cirrus delivers students the same learning experience whether they are using a PC, Mac, or Chromebook.

Cirrus courseware provides a complete, digitally delivered training and assessment solution. The courseware includes access to the EHR Navigator tutorials, practice assessments, and final assessments, as well as flash cards, quizzes, and other interactive learning materials from the text. Course content is delivered in a series of scheduled assignments that report to a grade book, thus tracking student progress and achievement.

EHR Navigator

Access to the EHR Navigator app is included as part of the online course. The EHR Navigator is a live program that replicates professional practice and prepares students for today's workplace.

EHRNAVIGATOR

The EHR Navigator provides experience in all areas of EHRs, including adding and scheduling patient appointments, adding clinical data to patient charts, coding, medical billing, managing patient data, e-prescribing, medication administration, nursing and allied health documentation, and data analytics. The EHR Navigator gives students practice in both inpatient and outpatient settings, which include an acute care hospital, a physician's office, and a skilled nursing and rehabilitation facility.

The EHR Navigator's interactive tutorials offer students practice in a format that is easy to navigate, colorful, and user friendly. The interactive tutorials are based on the core content and EHR system principles. The tutorials train students by stepping them through a variety of inpatient, outpatient, and personal health records activities.

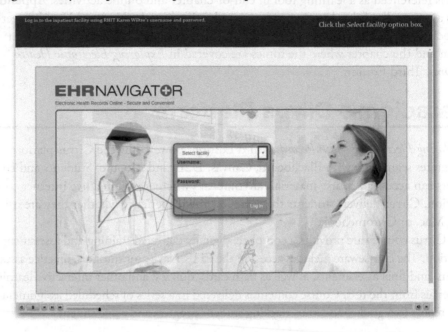

The EHR Navigator also includes assessments that are graded and reported to the instructor. There are multiple practice assessments that correspond to each tutorial, and then a final assessment to test students' understanding of the key concepts and skills.

Instructor Resources

Exploring Electronic Health Records, Third Edition, provides instructors with helpful tools for planning and delivering their courses and assessing student learning. In addition to course planning tools and syllabus models, the *Instructor Resources* provide chapter-specific teaching hints and answers for all end-of-chapter exercises. The *Instructor Resources* also offer ready-to-use chapter tests and PowerPoint presentations.

About the Authors

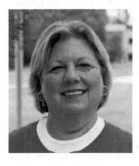

Darline Foltz, RHIA, CHPS, CEHRS

Darline Foltz is an associate professor at the University of Cincinnati–Clermont College. She holds bachelor's degrees in both Health Information Management and Information Processing Systems. Foltz is a Registered Health Information Administrator (RHIA), has more than 40 years of experience in the health information field, and has held multiple hospital management positions. She also holds the Certified in Healthcare Privacy and Security (CHPS) credential and the Certified Electronic Health Record Specialist (CEHRS) credential. As owner and president of Foltz & Associates, Healthcare Consulting Firm, Foltz has provided health information management and information systems consulting services to many clients, including hospitals, long-term care facilities, dialysis clinics, and mental health agencies. Active in professional and community service, she is a former president of the Ohio Health Information Management Association and former chairperson of the long-term care section of the American Health Information Management Association (AHIMA).

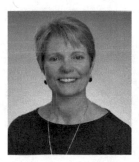

Karen Lankisch, PhD, RHIA, MHI, CHDA, CEHRS, CPPM, CPC

Dr. Karen Lankisch is a professor and program director of Health Information Systems Technology at the University of Cincinnati–Clermont College. Dr. Lankisch also serves as the Director of Online Learning. She is certified through the American Health Information Management Association (AHIMA) as a Registered Health Information Administrator (RHIA) and as a Certified Health Data Analyst (CHDA). She also holds the Certified Electronic Health Record Specialist (CEHRS), Certified Physician Practice Management (CPPM), and Certified Professional Coder (CPC) credentials. Dr. Lankisch has more than ten years of experience in the field of health information.

Dr. Lankisch is a Quality Matters Master Peer Reviewer and has completed reviews both nationally and internationally. She has served on the panel of reviewers for the Commission on Accreditation for Health Informatics and Information Management Education (CAHIIM) since 2016. In addition to being an author, she has served as a national consultant for Paradigm Education Solutions, giving workshops and presentations to instructors on Paradigm's technology learning solutions. Her research interests are emerging technology, online course design, and constructivist approaches to adult education. In 2013, she received the University of Cincinnati Faculty Award for Innovative Use of Technology in the Classroom. In 2016, she was selected for membership to the University of Cincinnati Academy of Fellows for Teaching and Learning. In 2018, she received the University of Cincinnati–Clermont College Faculty Mentoring Award.

Acknowledgments

The quality of this body of work is a testament to the feedback we have received from the many contributors and reviewers who participated in the development of *Exploring Electronic Health Records*, Third Edition.

We would like to thank Stephanie Schempp, the former developmental editor, and the following reviewers who have offered valuable comments and suggestions on the content of this textbook.

Bridgette Stasher Booker, PhD, RHIA, CHTS-IM, MCCT, Alabama State University
John M. Brown III, M.S., M.A, Dallas College, Richland Campus
Kathy Clark, CPC, Guilford Technical Community College
Sherita Y. Freeman, MPhil, MS, Forsyth Tech Community College
Robin J. Maddalena, Tunxis Community College
Chad McKenzie, MBA, Wake Technical Community College
Karen Minchella, Macomb Community College
Donna White, RHIA, CCS, Haywood Community College

Chapter 1 Overview of Electronic Health Records

Field Notes

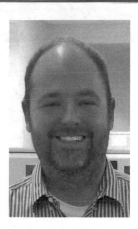

"The adoption and implementation of EHRs in the healthcare field has been the most revolutionary item to impact this sector in over 50 years. EHRs provide improved patient safety, better coordination of care, and even better revenue capture analysis. EHRs can capture anything from patient demographics, diagnoses, accounts receivable, supply inventory, to even clinical documentation. The ability for these sophisticated programs to capture all this data, create new data, and store information related to health care has allowed analysis to be performed at every aspect of a patient's interaction with a medical facility. One such aspect of the EHR's functionality is the ability to capture field notes, or notes a clinician can add about a patient's visit or episode. They provide the clinician the ability to type freely any notes that can help them recall or assess a patient's care at later visits. Such fields can then be analyzed to assist clinicians in providing care, which improve patient safety and overall care. Queries can be built around this field in order to scan through large volumes of text to determine patterns or key words that individually may not be evident, but collectively point to information of value, such as a diagnosis or drug-drug interaction. These free note fields allow for a clinician to record thoughts that may be relevant to the patient's care but not structurally captured by the EHRs predefined fields. These type of fields in EHRs have been and will continue to dynamically change the healthcare landscape for the better."

– Patrick Gruesser, MHI, Senior IT Application Analyst

Learning Objectives

1.1 Define the terms *electronic medical record (EMR)* and *electronic health record (EHR)* and understand their distinctions.

1.2 Explain the concept of interoperability and its importance in the EHR environment.

1.3 Understand the difference between *structural interoperability level* and *semantic interoperability level*.

1.4 Define *computer protocol* and discuss the most common communication protocol, Health Level 7 (HL7).

1.5 Understand the health information technology (IT) ecosystem.

1.6 Describe the Health Information Technology for Economic and Clinical Health Act and the federal incentive program for implementing EHRs.

1.7 Understand the concept of meaningful use and identify the main components of each stage.

1.8 List and discuss the benefits and barriers to implementing EHRs.

1.9 List and discuss the evolving potential roles in the EHR environment.

EXPAND YOUR LEARNING

To find out how access to medical records improves the quality of care received, view the following video:

https://EHR3
.ParadigmEducation
.com/ITVideos.

Most healthcare providers in the United States are required to use electronic health records (EHRs). EHRs replace traditional paper medical records that have been used for centuries, making health information accessible to healthcare providers across the world with only a few keystrokes. This nearly instantaneous access to health information increases facility efficiency, improves patient outcomes, and results in a healthier population.

The concept of computerized patient records may seem new to most people as they have only recently witnessed their healthcare providers adding their visit or hospitalization information into a computer rather than a paper folder. It would probably surprise most patients to learn that the idea of computerizing health records has been around since the 1970s. United States federal regulations and incentives have motivated many hospitals, physicians, dentists, nursing homes, outpatient clinics, and other healthcare providers to implement EHRs, beginning with the **American Recovery and Reinvestment Act of 2009 (ARRA)**. ARRA authorized the Centers for Medicare & Medicaid Services (CMS) to award incentive payments to eligible professionals who demonstrated the appropriate use of a certified EHR. The healthcare providers that participated in EHR implementation in 2011 were eligible for the maximum financial incentives. Financial incentives for healthcare providers continued through 2014. On January 1, 2015, the US government began reducing Medicare payments to healthcare providers without EHR systems that complied

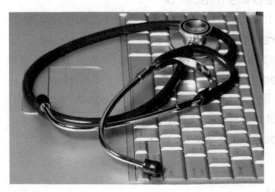

with federal standards. (The specifics of these regulations and the healthcare providers affected will be discussed later in this chapter.)

1.1 EMR versus EHR

The terms *electronic medical record (EMR)* and *electronic health record (EHR)* are often confused with one another and used interchangeably. *EHR* is the term most widely used by professionals and the general population as it encompasses all computerized medical and health records. There is a difference, however, between EMRs and EHRs. EMRs and EHRs are similar in concept but different in both scope and use. The EMR belongs to a single healthcare provider or organization, whereas the EHR integrates EMRs from multiple providers. In other words, EMRs are individual data sources that inform and populate collected patient information to form the global EHR system.

1.2 Electronic Medical Record

An **electronic medical record (EMR)** is an electronic version of patient files within a single organization, and it allows healthcare providers to place orders, document results, and store patient information for one facility, commonly called the **healthcare delivery (HCD) system**. For example, Hope Hospital in Cincinnati, Ohio, might implement an EMR to replace its separate order entry, results reporting, and computerized documentation systems. Implementing a complete EMR will replace the paper medical record and can be used by physicians, nurses, other clinicians, and clerical staff. The EMR becomes the facility's legal record of the course of treatment provided to patients while they are in the care of the facility. The EMR is owned by the HCD system, a concept that is discussed further in Chapter 2. Figure 1.1 represents an EMR and illustrates how each facility's EMR is a separate, stand-alone record.

Figure 1.1   Electronic Medical Records from Different Healthcare Facilities

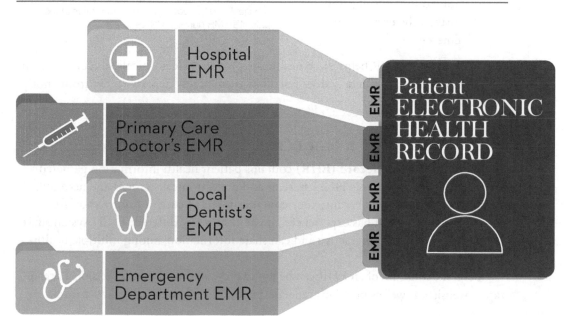

These scenarios indicate possible EMR usage:

- Dr. Iana Schwartz enters an order at the bedside terminal of patient Ellie Smith for a complete blood count laboratory test to rule out anemia.

- Nurse Devon Holloway scans the barcode on patient Susan Miller's identification band followed by the barcode on the medication prior to administering the drug. This procedure helps guarantee the accuracy of the medication's type, dose, and route of administration and helps verify that the patient is not allergic to this medication.

- Admission clerk Shika Nadal registers a patient for admission, creating a new account number that links to the patient's EMR.

- Dental hygienist Sarah Alvaro obtains dental x-rays of patient Lashonda Johnson with a camera that interfaces with the dental office's EMR.

- Dr. Carl Blatt enters his hospital patient visits into his mobile device as he performs patient rounds and then syncs the device with his practice's EMR.

- Linda Agee, practice manager for Cardiology Associates, ensures that all physicians and staff members document services provided and copays collected so that the practice's billing staff can automatically generate accurate bills as a by-product of the data.

- Carol Matta, psychologist for Family Mental Health Associates, Inc., electronically documents her clients' visits after each therapy session so that the records will be available to the on-call psychologists in the event of an emergency.

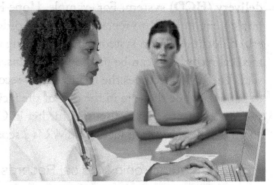
A patient and her doctor review information in the patient's EMR during an office visit.

Although the EMR helps these healthcare providers electronically document their patient encounters, it generally does not allow them access to patient files from another healthcare facility.

Electronic Health Record

The **electronic health record (EHR)** contains patient health information gathered from the EMRs of multiple HCD systems and is electronically stored and accessed. EHRs differ from EMRs because they contain subsets of patient information from each visit that a patient has experienced, possibly at many different HCD systems (see Figure 1.2). EHRs are interactive and can share information among multiple healthcare providers.

Several definitions of an EHR can be found on government and professional organization websites as well as in many academic and healthcare industry–related articles.

Figure 1.2   Clinical, Financial, and Support Uses of the EHR

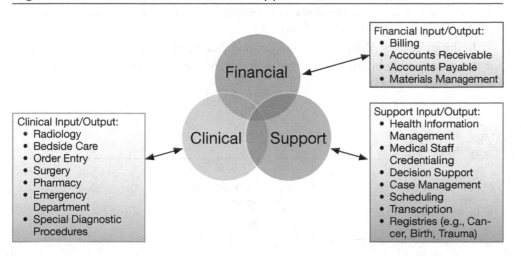

The definition found on HealthIT.gov is, "An electronic health record (EHR) is a digital version of a patient's paper chart. EHRs are real-time, patient-centered records that make information available instantly and securely to authorized users." All the definitions highlight that an EHR is a shift from a paper to electronic record to allow for real-time access as well as the ability to access all of an individual's health records from multiple healthcare providers.

According to the International Social Security Association, "The EHR is a longitudinal electronic record of patient health information generated by one or more encounters in any care delivery setting." The term **longitudinal** indicates that a patient's EHR will continue to develop over the course of care. Every medical event and document can be accessed within the EHR, regardless of facility, country, or time period.

A longitudinal record might contain information from both a cardiologist's office and the emergency department, as described in the example of Kim Singh's EHR below. The patient information can be freely shared among different HCD systems,

Consider This

Kim Singh visits the emergency department of Hope Hospital complaining of chest pain. Kim mentions that she had an echocardiogram and an electro-cardiogram (ECG) performed at the office of cardiologist Dr. Mary Carruthers approximately one month ago. The emergency department physician is able to immediately view Kim's echocardiographic and ECG results.

Kim's health record is located in a central repository of health information in which Hope Hospital, Cincinnati Dental Care, Dr. Carruthers's office, and Happy Knoll Nursing Home all participate. How might Kim's care have differed if the emergency department and the cardiologist did not have EHRs that communicate with one another? How might her care have differed in a paper health record environment?

and the EHR will continue to grow as the patient has additional encounters with providers such as an optometrist, surgeon, outpatient surgery center, nursing home, dental office, or mental health professional.

In the preceding example, the EHR central data repository stores all patient data for the participating healthcare facilities on a privately owned server, which is one method of storing EHRs.

CHECKP✚INT 1.1

1. What is the definition of an *electronic medical record (EMR)?* _____

   _____

   _____

2. What is the definition of an *electronic health record (EHR)?* _____

   _____

   _____

   _____

3. List three major differences between an EMR and an EHR.

   a. _____

   b. _____

   c. _____

1.3 Interoperability

The universal success of the EHR primarily rests on **interoperability**, which is the ability of one information system, computer system, or application to communicate with another information system, computer system, or application. Similar to how individuals must speak the same language to share information and understand what is being communicated, computers must also speak the same language to communicate. Additionally, the EHR systems must be able to operate at a high enough level of interoperability to share and process data.

Levels of Interoperability

With healthcare computer systems, there are five different levels of interoperability that demonstrate a range of communication ability. Computer systems unable to exchange information are considered Level 0, whereas computer systems with Level 3 interoperability can share and manipulate data to the degree needed to support EHR systems. Level 4, the organization level, expands interoperability through the policies and framework of data sharing, both within and between organizations and individuals. See Figure 1.3 for an illustration of the levels of interoperability. Each level is defined as follows:

- **Level 0:** Stand-alone systems have **no interoperability**.

- **Level 1:** This level (also known as **foundational interoperability**) is considered a basic level of communication. This level of communication infrastructure allows systems to securely exchange data without any ability to interpret the shared data.

Figure 1.3   Levels of Conceptual Interoperability Model

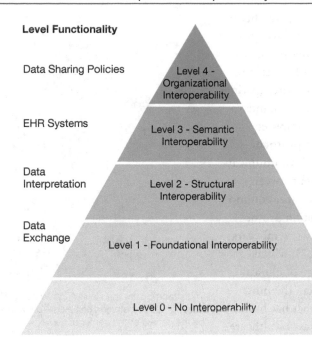

- **Level 2:** This level is called the **structural interoperability level.** It provides a common data format, syntax, and organization for data exchange; the data can be interpreted, but the meaning of the data may not be understood.

- **Level 3:** The **semantic interoperability level** is a high level of interoperability that allows the meaning of the data to be shared. The data and information may also be interpreted, allowing EHR systems to function.

- **Level 4:** The **organization interoperability level** is where the policies of data sharing both within and between organizations and individuals are created and maintained.

The focus when referring to interoperability in relation to the EHR is on structural and semantic interoperability (Levels 2 and 3). A minimally successful EHR system must at least use a common data format that can exchange information, and that format must meet the definition of structural interoperability (Level 2). An ideal EHR system would meet the definition of semantic interoperability (Level 3) so that health information could be understood and interpreted, not merely shared. Level 4 operability allows for open access to and sharing of data among healthcare providers and organizations.

For example, if the EHR of Children's Hospital wants to share data with the EHR of Dr. Wayne Allen, a primary care physician, then both EHR systems must have a common technical foundation and, at the very least, structural interoperability. Structural interoperability facilitates the basic communication and exchange of information between EHRs, enabling the EHR system at Children's Hospital to send the laboratory reports of a patient to Dr. Allen's EHR system. The semantic interoperability of both EHRs allows Dr. Allen to understand the meaning of the laboratory results.

Computer Protocols

The current state of interoperability in the US has been achieved through a combination of computer protocols and public policy. For EHRs to be useful and beneficial, *all* participating EMRs and EHRs need one standard set of interoperability computer protocols. A **computer protocol** is a standardized method of communicating or transmitting data between two computer systems. The most common healthcare communication protocol that has been in use for several years is **Health Level 7 (HL7)**, which focuses on the exchange of clinical and administrative data. The most recent HL7 standard that has been developed is entitled Fast Healthcare Interoperability Resources (FHIR).

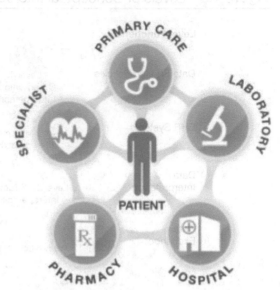

This graphic from the HealthIT.gov website illustrates interoperability between healthcare providers connected by the patient at the center of care.

CMS, in partnership with the Office of the National Coordinator for Health Information Technology, has identified HL7 FHIR Release 4.0.1 as the foundational standard to support data exchange via secure application programming interfaces (APIs). All EHR systems will be required to use HL7 FHIR Release 4.0.1 to support interoperability and ensure the privacy and security of patient information.

A **health IT ecosystem** (illustrated in Figure 1.4) is a collection of individuals and groups that are interested in health information technology (HIT). Included in an HIT ecosystem are clinicians, hospitals, various healthcare providers, public health workers, technology developers, payers, researchers, policy makers, individual patients, and many others. All of these stakeholders in the HIT ecosystem are interested in interoperability. As shown in Figure 1.4, the patient is the starting point of the ecosystem. Health information is accessed and shared for quality and safety in care delivery, population health management, regional information exchange, and analytics for research. Data can then be used to establish or update clinical guidelines to support public health policy and to update clinical decision support systems.

The **Office of the National Coordinator for Health Information Technology (ONC)** is the federal body that recommends policies, procedures, protocols, and standards for interoperability. The ONC is part of the US Department of Health and Human Services (HHS) and was created by the ARRA. The mission of the ONC is "to improve health and health care for all Americans through use of information and technology." In its work to improve health and health care through the use of information and technology, the ONC has been working on interoperability with interested stakeholders of HIT. The ONC published "A 10-Year Vision to Achieve an Interoperable Health IT Infrastructure" that is to be accomplished by achieving the following three goals:

- **2015–2017:** Send, receive, find, and use priority data domains to improve health quality and outcomes.

Figure 1.4   Health Information Technology Ecosystem

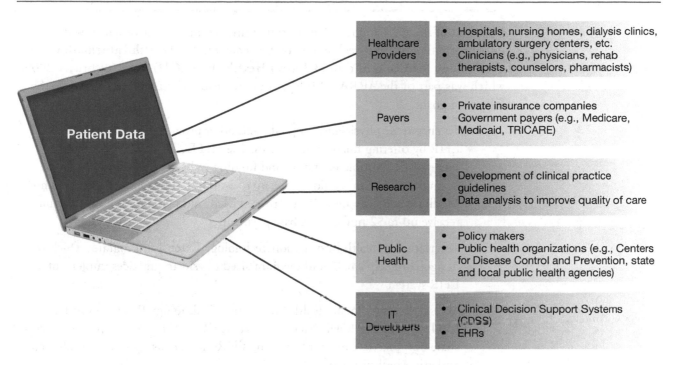

- **2018–2020:** Expand data sources and users in the interoperable HIT ecosystem to improve health and lower costs.

- **2021–2024:** Achieve nationwide interoperability to enable a learning health system in which the patient is at the center of a system that can continuously improve care, public health, and science through real-time data access.

The ONC then developed a Shared Nationwide Interoperability Roadmap to outline the steps needed to be taken to realize the vision, with associated deadlines by which the steps should be completed. The Roadmap was constructed by stakeholders nationwide to coordinate collective efforts around HIT interoperability, and it describes the policy and technical actions needed to realize the vision of a seamless, interoperable electronic health data system.

EXPAND YOUR LEARNING

To learn more about the Shared Nationwide Interoperability Roadmap, see

https://EHR3.Paradigm Education.com/ InteroperabilityRoadmap.

CHECKPOINT 1.2

1. What is the definition of *interoperability*?

2. What level of interoperability is needed for EHRs to interpret data?

3. CMS, in conjunction with the ONC, has identified which computer protocol as the foundational standard to support data exchange via secure application programming interfaces?

1.4 Federal Regulations

Members of the US Congress demonstrated their commitment to nationwide implementation of EHR technology by first enacting the **Health Information Technology for Economic and Clinical Health (HITECH) Act** in February 2009, which was part of the ARRA. This legislation set aside $19.2 billion to achieve the following goals:

- To encourage physicians, hospitals, and other providers to implement the EHR by offering financial incentives. The HITECH Act defined different stages of EHR implementation and funding to healthcare providers. For example, physicians could receive up to $44,000 in incentive payments under Medicare and even more if they treated Medicaid patients. A hospital could receive up to $2 million as a base payment.

- To create the Health Information Technology Extension Program, which was designed to help small- and medium-sized physician practices implement an EHR system

- To establish a national Health Information Technology Research Center (HITRC) and Regional Extension Centers (RECs) to work with each other to share best practices for implementing EHRs and act as resources for physicians and other healthcare providers

Incentive Programs

After a provider implemented an EHR system that met the established government requirements, that provider, upon submission of an application, would receive incentive funds under the Medicare and/or Medicaid programs. Eligible healthcare providers that implemented "meaningful use" (described further in the next section) of a certified EHR received up to $44,000 over five years under the Medicare EHR Incentive Program and up to $63,750 over six years under the Medicaid EHR Incentive Program.

Providers who did not implement an EHR system by January 1, 2015, have been receiving reduced reimbursement from Medicare. For example, physicians who had not adopted certified EHR systems or could not demonstrate meaningful use by the beginning of 2015 saw their Medicare reimbursements reduced by 1%, a rate that was increased to 2% in 2016, 3% in 2017, 4% in 2018, and a maximum reduction of reimbursement of 5% in 2019, which is ongoing until meaningful use is demonstrated. As of 2017, nearly 9 in 10 office-based physicians (86%) had adopted any EHR, and nearly 4 in 5 (80%) had adopted a certified EHR.

Meaningful Use or Promoting Interoperability

Meaningful use is the set of standards defined by the **Centers for Medicare & Medicaid Services (CMS)** Incentive Programs in 2011, that governed the use of EHRs. *Meaningful use* is defined as using certified EHR technology to:

- Improve quality, safety, and efficiency and reduce health disparities

- Engage patients and family

- Improve care coordination and population and public health

- Maintain privacy and security of patient health information

Ultimately, it was hoped that meaningful use compliance would result in:

- Better clinical outcomes

- Improved population health outcomes

- Increased transparency and efficiency

- Empowered individuals

- More robust research data on health systems

Historically, healthcare providers had to prove that they had implemented EHR technology and were therefore eligible for incentive funds by meeting the requirements of meaningful use. Meaningful use is included in the HITECH Act and defines the accepted levels of EHR implementation and qualifications to receive federal incentives. These definitions can be measured in quality and quantity.

Meaningful use requirements evolved in three stages that laid the foundation for electronic capture of data and expanded its use for providers and patients (see Figure 1.5). Stage 1 requirements focused on data capture and sharing. Stage 2 requirements focused on advancing clinical processes, such as medication reconciliation, health information exchange, and patient-specific education. Stage 3 requirements incorporated the same measures as Stages 1 and 2 and outlined advanced coordination of care through patient engagement and participation in a health information exchange and public health reporting. Stage 3 requirements were organized into eight topic areas of objectives in measures:

- Protect electronic protected health information (ePHI)

- e-Prescribing (eRx)

- Clinical decision support systems (CDSS) (provide information regarding a particular diagnosis or treatment to clinicians to enhance decision-making in the clinical workflow of the patient)

- Computerized provider order entry (CPOE) (orders for medications and treatment are entered directly into the EHR)

- Patient electronic access

- Coordination of care (the organization of a patient's healthcare treatment to improve the quality of care and eliminate duplication of tests and procedures)

- Health information exchange

- Public health reporting

In 2018, the federal government required all healthcare providers to participate in Stage 3 meaningful use requirements regardless of their prior participation. The government wanted to move all providers to the same stage of meaningful use to simplify reporting requirements and to have everyone focused on the same objectives and criteria. As part of the changes in 2018, the Meaningful Use Programs were renamed the Promoting Interoperability Programs as the implementation of EHRs had evolved from data collection to the ability to share the data.

Figure 1.5   Stages of Meaningful Use

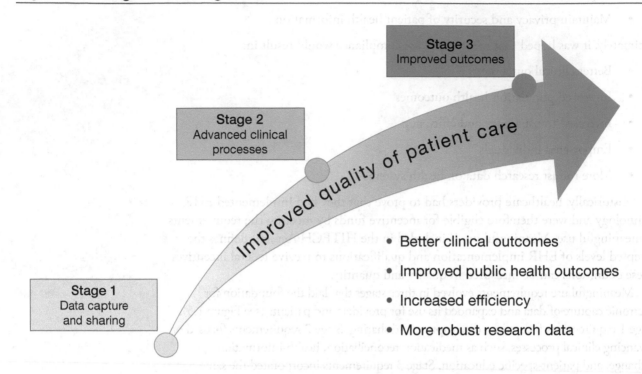

Stage 1
Data capture
and sharing

Stage 2
Advanced clinical
processes

Stage 3
Improved outcomes

Improved quality of patient care

- Better clinical outcomes
- Improved public health outcomes
- Increased efficiency
- More robust research data

21st Century Cures Act

As noted previously in this chapter, the American Recovery and Reinvestment Act of 2009 (ARRA) was one of the first acts of Congress to stimulate the use of EHRs as it authorized CMS to award incentive payments to eligible professionals who demonstrated meaningful use of a certified EHR. While ARRA helped spur the implementation of EHRs, the focus was on encouraging healthcare providers to implement EHRs by offering monetary incentives for doing so. In 2010, Congress passed the Patient Protection and Affordable Care Act (PPACA), requiring most healthcare providers to implement an EHR, clearly communicating that this implementation was not a choice, but a requirement.

In 2011, the ONC reported that only 72% of hospitals and only 9% of non-emergency facilities used certified EHR systems. Then, in 2016, the ONC reported that 9 in 10 hospitals had implemented an EHR along with almost 60% of private practice physicians.

The 21st Century Cures Act, passed in 2016 is one of the most significant acts to be passed by Congress, addressing patient access to their electronic medical records and the exchange and use of health information. You will learn more about this legislation in Chapter 6.

Interoperability Standards Advisory

As you learn about the acts, laws, requirements, and constant changes that are guiding the growth of the EHR, you may wonder how stakeholders (e.g., healthcare providers, HIT companies, health networks) keep up with the interoperability functionality and programming required of the EHR. The ONC maintains the

Interoperability Standards Advisory (ISA), a model for interoperability standards and how to implement them. The ISA is a public list of standards that can be used by stakeholders to determine whether they are meeting federal interoperability requirements and, if not, how to address the issue. Because the ISA is not a law or an enforced standard, it is frequently critiqued and updated by subject matter experts. As EHRs, interoperability, and privacy standards change, the ISA adapts and continues to be of use.

EXPAND YOUR LEARNING

Find out more information about the ISA process at https://EHR3.ParadigmEducation.com/ISA.

1.5 Benefits of EHRs

The transition to EHRs has required and continues to require monumental effort on the part of doctors, healthcare staff, regulators, government officials, and everyone working in the healthcare industry. The final goals of the transition are higher-quality healthcare services, more effective and efficient communication, and healthier patients. Advocates of the transition cite these potential and already realized benefits as reasons to approach this work with excitement and a sense of opportunity. The most obvious benefits (all leading to improved patient care and safety) include:

- Improved documentation

- Streamlined and rapid communication

- Immediate and improved access to patient information

Improved Documentation

A classic complaint about doctors is their terrible handwriting. Many medication errors are the result of illegible and misinterpreted physician notes. Staff members waste time and become frustrated trying to read and interpret clinician notes, and the clinician often needs to be contacted to clarify meaning. Figures 1.6 and 1.7 illustrate the difference between handwritten and electronic progress notes, respectively. Documentation is also improved by reducing the duplication of testing orders and increasing accuracy in patient information.

Figure 1.6   Handwritten Progress Note

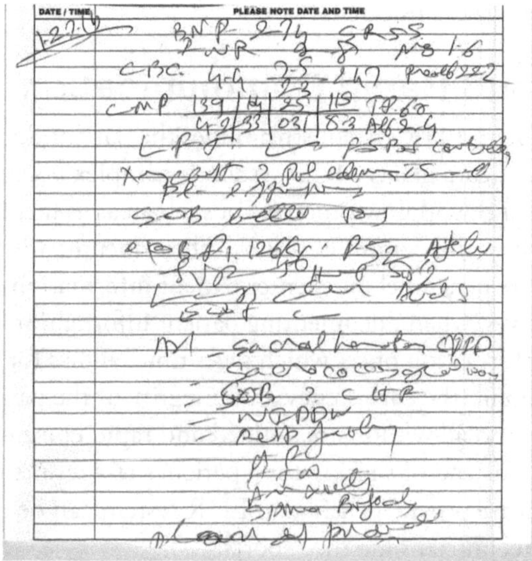

Figure 1.7   Electronic Progress Notes

Progress Note

Patient name:	McDowell, Terrence	Medical Record Number:	585067
Date of Birth:	07/19/58	Patient Number:	1772518
Location:	Northstar Medical Center	Admission Date:	02/18/30
Provider:	Gertz, Lester MD	Room/Bed:	567-1
Date/Time:	02/19/30 14:00		

SUBJECTIVE: Yesterday, this patient was worked up on the ER and subsequently admitted to 567-1 when he was diagnosed with community-acquired pneumonia along with COPD exacerbation. Review of the ER and admission documentation reveals that the patient is a 72-year-old male Caucasian patient with a long-standing history of COPD.

OBJECTIVE:

VITAL SIGNS: The patient's max temperature over the past 24 hours has been 101.3F; his blood pressure at present is 148/90, his pulse is 93. His O2 sats are 95% on 2L via nasal cannula.

HEART: Regular rate and rhythm without murmur, gallop, or rub.

LUNGS: Lungs are very tight. Wheezes bilaterally and rhonchi on the right mid base. Nurses report that he has a productive cough of green purulent sputum.

ABDOMEN: Soft and nontender. Bowel sounds x4 are normoactive.

NEUROLOGIC: Patient is alert and oriented x3. His pupils are equal and reactive.

ASSESSMENT:

1. Chronic COPD with acute exacerbation.
2. Community-acquired pneumonia, awaiting sputum culture report.
3. Generalized weakness and deconditioning secondary to the above.

EHRs use standardized templates and data sets that capture data by typing, scanning, and using drop-down menus, among other features. Physicians can enter complex prescriptions, and typically, patients can electronically fill out forms and questionnaires without incident. A doctor can record patient visit notes directly into the EHR without transcribing tape-recorded or handwritten notes. Not only will daily documentation be more accurate, but medical studies may also be more effectively conducted. For example, a new drug can be closely monitored, and a hospital's effort to track patterns like smoking cessation or overall diet improvement may be much easier. Data can be collected, identified, and sorted within a single database, leading to more accurate and innovative research.

Streamlined and Rapid Communication

The implementation of an EHR system streamlines the patient documentation process. The provision of patient care in any HCD system is complex because of the coordination of staff members and workflow processes in such areas as medications, procedures, testing, decision-making, and communication. When documenting patient care using a paper record, healthcare personnel must enter patient information multiple times on multiple forms. However, when documenting patient information electronically, personnel enter the information once, which saves time, allows for an easy database search, and helps maintain the consistency and integrity of the patient record.

EHR technology also allows for streamlined and rapid communication of information. For example, instead of waiting for a patient's test results to pass among several staff members, healthcare providers using an EHR system can be automatically alerted when the laboratory technicians file the reports.

EHR technology also streamlines the medication-dispensing process and improves medication safety. For example, a patient's paper prescription typically travels from the doctor to the nurse, from the nurse to the clerk, and then from the clerk to the pharmacist. An EHR system allows a physician to use e-prescribing, a process that transmits the prescription directly to the pharmacist. This transmittal process eliminates the need for a nurse or other staff member to enter the medication order into the computer, a clerical step that impedes patient care. e-Prescribing also allows direct communication between the pharmacist and the prescriber to resolve any prescription errors. An EHR system has an automatic feature that alerts prescribers to drug incompatibilities, a step that may take several hours to determine when filling a paper prescription.

Immediate and Improved Access to Patient Information

With a robust, interoperable EHR system, healthcare organizations can nearly instantaneously access a patient's entire health history by viewing a patient's dental records, home healthcare visits, psychiatry records, and any other necessary history. The significance of this ability cannot be overstated. Healthcare staff can spot medical errors and inconsistencies more quickly and can instantly view the results of medical procedures performed across the globe. They can easily track and measure years of patient outcomes without having to search for misplaced records.

Healthcare facilities are not the only ones benefiting from this access. Patients who cannot remember past procedures, diagnoses, or allergies can be protected from hasty and underinformed medical decisions. Patients can monitor personal health goals and even report glucose readings or progress during their exercise routines from home, and patients with an allergic reaction or injury presenting to a different hospital while on vacation will not have to worry. All their health records will be accessible, thus allowing any healthcare provider the ability to make informed and safe choices.

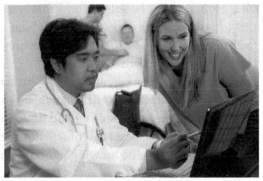

Staff members access a patient's information quickly and efficiently when using an EHR system.

1.6 Barriers to EHR Implementation

With the transition to EHRs, there have been barriers and reservations for healthcare providers, patients, HIT, and business associates. It is important to recognize these reservations and barriers held by some patients, providers, staff, and agencies to better address implementation, policies, procedures, and technologies of EHR systems. Some common criticisms of the EHR system include the following:

- High cost

- Insufficient privacy and security

- Inexperience in implementation and training

- Significant daily process changes

" US expenditures on electronic health records (EHRs) are forecast to total $19.9 billion in 2024. **"**
—Freedonia Group

High Cost

High cost is the most common barrier described by healthcare leadership. Whether the cost is $15,000 to implement an EHR system for a small medical or dental practice or several million dollars for a large hospital, the costs can be a relative burden for most healthcare providers. Although federal financial incentives initially helped offset the costs of implementing EHR systems, healthcare providers did not receive the incentive funds until *after* the systems were implemented and proven to meet US federal standards and those incentives have not been available since 2015. For a small nursing home or mental health center, or even a small hospital, the required large investment in adopting and implementing EHR technology has been a significant barrier.

Some of the financial expenditures that an organization needs to consider for implementing and maintaining an EHR system include:

- Hardware—initial cost and maintenance

- Software-license fees, annual fees for upgrades, support, and customization

- Implementation and training—costs associated with installing, building, testing, and user training

- Staff hires in health informatics and technical support for implementation and maintenance of the EHR system and to provide user support

Insufficient Privacy and Security

One of the biggest benefits to an EHR system—easy access to patients' medical records—is also one of the public's biggest concerns. Unlimited access requires facilities and providers to install secure firewalls (specialized computer programs that prevent unauthorized access) and to implement privacy policies and procedures, access monitoring, and privacy breach enforcement. Violations of online security involving credit card companies, banks, and gaming systems have alerted the public to the risk of storing and distributing personal information online, so the thought of such personal information being only a few clicks away can be troubling, possibly discouraging patients from being honest about their medical histories.

Inexperience in Implementation and Training

US federal regulations requiring HCD systems to implement EHRs have spawned the growth of many EHR systems and vendors. Faced with great variability of products and service levels in the EHR market, physicians, dentists, hospital chief executive officers (CEOs), and others are justifiably reluctant to select an EHR company that may leave its clients with little to no support. Such lack of software support could mean that the healthcare provider would have to implement an entirely new EHR system, resulting in increased costs and disruption of services.

CEOs and office managers are also concerned about hiring the right staff to implement and maintain the EHR. Employers must ensure that new staff members will be qualified to handle the move away from paper records. The US federal government recognized this issue and passed legislation to create certification programs for HIT careers. (This subject is discussed in greater detail later in this chapter.)

Significant Daily Process Changes

Doctors and staff may also be reluctant to embrace a system that requires an overhaul of their daily duties and tasks. A physician might argue that using EHRs will take *longer* to process patients and their information. For example, after a patient checkup, the physician might typically jot down notes or dictate into a tape recorder, then pass that information along to a staff member for transcription. With the EHR, the doctor must log on to the system, locate the patient's chart, enter the information, and then save it to the patient's files. All employees of a healthcare facility will experience similar changes to a system they might have been using for several years or decades. This change in routine could easily feel frustrating and unnecessary, thus creating barriers to change and difficulties in the successful implementation of an EHR system. It may take years for staff members to buy into the new technology. Offices might also see staff turnover because of duty and task changes.

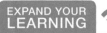

EXPAND YOUR LEARNING

To learn more about topics such as consumer engagement, EHR adoption, health information exchange, the HIT workforce, and more, go to https://EHR3 .ParadigmEducation .com/BuzzBlog, and click the Tag you are interested in reading more about. You will be directed to a government-sponsored site.

CHECKPOINT 1.3

1. List three benefits of implementing an EHR system.

    a. _____

    b. _____

    c. _____

2. List four barriers to successfully implementing an EHR system.

    a. _____

    b. _____

    c. _____

    d. _____

1.7 EHR System Implementation

Implementing an EHR system is a time-consuming, labor-intensive project that, with proper planning, may be implemented with few disruptions. Planning for an EHR implementation is started long before the targeted date of implementation. While most healthcare providers and organizations have already made the switch to EHR systems, it is helpful to understand how that data migrated from paper records to the computer systems we know and use today.

EHR Steering Committee

The planning stages of EHR implementation involve a series of initial steps. The first step is determining a facility's readiness to change from paper records to electronic records. Once that factor is determined, a facility needs to set goals and establish a steering committee to lay the groundwork and move the EHR planning process forward. A typical steering committee is cross-disciplinary and is composed of health-care providers, nurses, health information professionals, administrators, financial staff, information technology staff, and staff from other integral departments. The steering committee establishes a plan that outlines the steps needed for the successful migration from paper records to an EHR system and examines policies and procedures in support of EHR functionality and user support to include implementation and maintenance.

Project Manager

It is recommended that an organization hire or assign a project manager to facilitate the implementation of the EHR system. The project manager works closely with the EHR steering committee, the information technology department, and the vendor implementation team to successfully carry out the implementation plan established by the EHR steering committee.

Workflow Analysis

A **workflow analysis** is an important assessment to conduct in the selection and implementation of an EHR system. A workflow analysis reviews how the organization currently functions and how the paper records are used to care for patients. Workflow analysis should be considered for all back office, front office, health information management, and provider processes.

1.8 Certified EHR

CMS and the ONC have established standards and other criteria for data that EHRs must meet to be considered certified. Certification indicates that an EHR system offers the necessary technological capability, functionality, and security to help providers meet meaningful use criteria. Certification also indicates that the EHR system is secure, maintains confidentiality, and has interoperability.

Healthcare facilities have many choices when selecting an EHR system. They may choose to build their own or use a vendor-purchased system. No matter which option a facility pursues, the organization must select a certified EHR system to comply with federal laws.

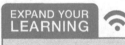

EXPAND YOUR LEARNING

You may view a full list of certified EHR systems on the HealthIT.gov website at https://EHR3 .ParadigmEducation .com/CertifiedList.

Rollout Process

With the EHR system selected, the project manager in place, and the implementation plan created, the **rollout** process can begin. The rollout process occurs in three phases: organizational, training, and operational.

Organizational Phase

The first phase is organizational. The healthcare organization selects a cut-off date, which determines how many years the healthcare organization will go back and convert paper records. For example, the facility may choose to go back five years, and all those records will be digitally converted to the EHR. The remaining records will most likely be scanned and stored electronically. As HCD systems begin the conversion process, there may be portions of patient records on paper and other portions stored electronically. This type of record is known as a *hybrid health record*.

Training Phase

The second phase is training and heavily emphasizes learning, fine tuning, customizing, and testing of the EHR system.

Operational Phase

The rollout process ends with the operational phase, which includes the launch of the EHR system and continual training while maintenance begins. Prior to the "go-live" date, the EHR system must be tested many times, including its hardware, software, backup, networking, connectivity, and recovery components. Most healthcare organizations choose to complete pilots prior to going live. A **pilot** is a test run of the EHR system that identifies issues and problems.

Preparing to Go Live A few weeks prior to the go-live date, staff members should be trained for the required functionalities and assessed for mastery. The healthcare facility should notify its patients that its facility is implementing an EHR system and inform them of the go-live date. This notification prepares patients for upcoming changes, including any potential delays in scheduling, billing, or wait times.

Going Live Healthcare organizations have different approaches to going live. Some facilities choose a phased implementation in which one function of the EHR system is made available at a time. This staggered approach allows for the organization to resolve issues and receive feedback on individual features or applications. Alternatively, an organization can choose a "big bang" approach, making all EHR functions immediately available to all users. This approach speeds up implementation but runs the risk of creating multiple problems or delays.

Consider This

One aspect of EHR implementation is to plan for an IT outage. Boulder Community Hospital in Boulder, Colorado, learned this lesson when it experienced a computer system outage, leaving patients frustrated. To learn more about this incident and the measures taken to rectify the situation, go to https://EHR3.ParadigmEducation.com/Outage.

1.9 Moving Forward

In the same way that building a new subway system or highway is expensive to implement and may cause traffic delays while being built, investment in the EHR is a temporary burden. The savings from replacing inefficient paper medical records will inevitably pay off the initial investment as healthcare providers switch to a more efficient system.

Future Challenges to EHR Implementation

Privacy and security problems are not specific to EHRs; rather, these problems are like those of any company or industry that maintains an online presence. Although efforts must—and will—be made to protect personal health records, the world is just beginning to understand the true risks of managing personal information online. Because of increasing awareness of identity theft, many people have learned not to post the names and birth dates of their children on personal websites, and others have learned not to email credit card and Social Security numbers based on unsolicited requests. In the same way, industries are using significant resources to create security programs and procedures to address past breaches and anticipate future issues. Chapter 6 will discuss privacy and security issues in greater detail.

Interoperability will continue to be a challenge for many years while IT vendors work toward achieving Level 3 (semantic interoperability) and Level 4 (organization interoperability).

Having adequate support for the EHR system, both from the EHR vendor and from qualified staff, will be an important piece of the puzzle for healthcare facilities. Given time, quality EHR vendors are likely to rise to the top, giving healthcare providers confidence in their chosen EHR companies. As the field of HIT grows, more students will graduate with the appropriate knowledge and experience to implement, use, and maintain an EHR system. The inconveniences experienced by doctors and other clinical staff early in the process are essential steps toward the dramatic improvement to the US healthcare system.

Consider This

Dr. Meghana Goyal has worked at University Hospital for 20 years. She takes pride in her excellent memory, rapport with patients, and ability to use small talk and conversation to determine a patient's state of health, especially when working from incomplete medical histories. Dr. Goyal has been successful, but Sean Parker, the hospital administrator, has begun requiring all doctors to be trained on the hospital's new EHR system. Other staff members have received some training, but everyone is still learning, and Dr. Goyal is worried that learning the new system will take time away from her patients. How would you address Dr. Goyal's concerns?

Evolving Roles in the EHR Environment

Managing the transition from paper to electronic records requires individuals with special skills and education. The US Department of Labor, Bureau of Labor Statistics reports that the employment for **health information management (HIM)** professionals is projected to grow 8% from 2019 to 2029, much faster than the average for all occupations, and it acknowledges that the "increasing use of electronic health records will continue to broaden and alter the job responsibilities of health information technicians. For example, with the use of EHRs, technicians must be familiar with EHR computer software, maintaining EHR security, and analyzing electronic data to improve healthcare information." In addition, individuals seeking employment in health care are expected to be familiar with using EHR systems. Curricula in nursing, medical, allied health, and HIT/HIM programs are expected to include the basic, and in some cases advanced, use of EHR software and to understand the importance of the use, privacy, and security of patient information.

The **American Health Information Management Association (AHIMA)** provides many opportunities for credentialing health information professionals interested in implementing and managing EHRs, such as the following:

- **RHIT: registered health information technician (associate degree)** RHITs perform the technical procedures related to the management of health information, frequently working in positions of medical coding, billing, and data management.

- **RHIA: registered health information administrator (bachelor's degree)** The RHIA works as a liaison between healthcare providers, organization staff, payers, and patients. The RHIA is an expert in managing health information and the professionals responsible for managing this information.

- **Certified Health Data Analyst (CHDA®)** is a certification that demonstrates an individual's expertise in data analysis to include acquiring, managing, analyzing, interpreting, and transforming data into accurate, consistent, and timely information while balancing the organization's strategic vision with daily operations.

- **Certified in Healthcare Privacy and Security (CHPS®)** is a certification that identifies an individual's competence in privacy and security protection programs in all types of healthcare organizations. Having this certification denotes competence in designing, implementing, and administering comprehensive privacy and security protection programs in all types of healthcare organizations.

> "Employment in healthcare occupations is projected to grow 15 percent from 2019 to 2029, much faster than the average for all occupations, adding about 2.4 million new jobs. Healthcare occupations are projected to add more jobs than any of the other occupational groups."
> —Bureau of Labor Statistics, US Department of Labor

The **Healthcare Information and Management Systems Society (HIMSS)** is a nonprofit, global organization of information technicians focused on improving health through the improvement of HIT. HIMSS administers two professional certification programs for healthcare information and management systems:

- CAHIMS (Certified Associate in Healthcare Information and Management Systems) is a certification designed for IT professionals new to the health information arena. CAHIMS is designed to be a pathway for careers in HIT.

- CPHIMS (Certified Professional in Healthcare Information and Management Systems) is a professional certification program for experienced healthcare information and management systems professionals.

Employee positions at an HCD provider include chief information officer, systems analyst, systems administrator, database administrator/specialist, EHR project manager, and EHR trainer. These positions are explained in more detail in the student resources and are primarily available at either a healthcare provider or an EHR software vendor. Other health-related entities, such as insurance companies, durable medical equipment companies, and medical billing companies, continue to create positions to work with EHRs for healthcare facility customers. For example, an insurance company adopts policies and procedures for accessing clients' EHRs, so it will need staff to develop and implement these standards.

Creating a national (and international) record-keeping system will not be simple, but this task is a testament to the scope and vision of EHR implementation. Although the current generation may experience struggles as the EHR is implemented, the resulting nationwide EHR system will provide future healthcare providers with a more

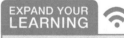

EXPAND YOUR LEARNING

Search the internet for EHR careers and prepare a presentation on different career opportunities.

ON THE JOB

Healthcare professionals should strive to remain positive in their work environments, not only for the sake of their patients but also for coworkers, visitors, and guests.

reliable, efficient, and cost-effective healthcare system. As health care and technology evolve together, new jobs and career opportunities will be created, patient outcomes will improve, and healthcare delivery will see gains in efficiency, communication, and overall quality.

Chapter Summary

With over 86% of physicians using EHRs today, almost everyone in the United States has a digital healthcare footprint. This digital footprint is in the form of an EMR. EMRs are individual data sources that belong to a single healthcare provider or organization. EMRs inform and populate EHRs.

The EHR is a longitudinal electronic record of patient health information produced by encounters in one or more care settings. The EHR system automates and streamlines the clinician's workflow. The EHR can independently generate a complete record of a clinical patient encounter, and it possesses sufficient detail to provide clinical decision support, quality management, clinical reporting, and interoperability.

Interoperability is the ability of one computer system to communicate with another computer system and is one of the overarching challenges facing successful EHR implementation. With healthcare computer systems, there are five levels of interoperability that demonstrate a range of communication ability. Computer systems unable to exchange information are considered Level 0, whereas computer systems with Level 3 semantic interoperability can share and manipulate data to the degree needed to support EHR systems.

For EHRs to be useful and beneficial, all participating EMRs need one standard set of interoperability computer protocols. A computer protocol is a standardized method of communicating or transmitting data between two computer systems. Health Level 7® (HL7) Fast Healthcare Interoperability Resources® (FHIR) Release 4.0.1 has been identified as the standard protocol for all EHR systems in the United States.

An HIT ecosystem is a collection of individuals and groups that are interested in health information technology. Included in an HIT ecosystem are clinicians, hospitals, various healthcare providers, public health workers, technology developers, payers, researchers, policymakers, individual patients, and many others.

The Health Information Technology for Economic and Clinical Health (HITECH) Act defined different stages of EHR implementation and incentive funding to encourage providers to begin using EHRs. Meaningful use, now called *promoting interoperability*, is defined as using a certified EHR system to improve healthcare quality, safety, efficiency, care coordination, and health outcomes; to improve access to health care across all racial, ethnic, and socioeconomic groups; to engage patients and families in the provision and coordination of their health care; and to increase the transparency and efficiency of the provision of health care while maintaining the privacy and security of patient health information.

The American Recovery and Reinvestment Act of 2009 (ARRA) was one of the first acts of Congress to stimulate the use of EHRs as it authorized the CMS to award incentive payments to eligible professionals who demonstrated meaningful use of a certified EHR. In 2010, Congress passed the Patient Protection and Affordable Care Act (PPACA), requiring most healthcare providers to implement an EHR, clearly communicating that EHR implementation is not a choice, but a requirement.

The 21st Century Cures Act, passed in 2016, is one of the most significant acts to be passed by Congress addressing patient access to their electronic medical records and the exchange and use of health information.

The Interoperability Standards Advisory (ISA) is a model for interoperability standards and how to implement them.

The benefits of implementing an EHR system include improved documentation, streamlined and rapid communication, and immediate and improved access to patient information. The barriers to implementing an EHR system include the high cost of implementation, concerns regarding privacy and security, inexperience in implementation and training, and significant daily process changes for healthcare providers.

There are many professional roles in the EHR environment. With the EHR at the center of the work and success of all healthcare professionals, it is imperative that the healthcare workforce embraces and develops expertise in the use of EHR systems.

Review and Assessment

The following Review and Assessment activities are also available online in the online course. The course also provides access to flash cards, study games, and practice quizzes to help strengthen your understanding of the chapter content.

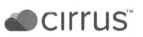

Acronyms/Initialisms

Study the following acronyms discussed in this chapter. Go to the online course for flash cards of the acronyms and other chapter key terms.

AHIMA: American Health Information Management Association

ARRA: American Recovery and Reinvestment Act of 2009

CAHIMS: Certified Associate in Healthcare Information and Management Systems

CDSS: clinical decision support system

CHDA: Certified Health Data Analyst

CHPS: Certified in Healthcare Privacy and Security

CMS: Centers for Medicare & Medicaid Services

CPHIMS: Certified Professional in Healthcare Information and Management Systems

CPOE: computerized provider order entry

EHR: electronic health record

EMR: electronic medical record

ePHI: electronic protected health information

eRx: e-prescribing

HCD: healthcare delivery (system)

HHS: US Department of Health and Human Services

HIM: health information management

HIMSS: Healthcare Information and Management Systems Society

HIT: health information technology

HITECH: Health Information Technology for Economic and Clinical Health

HITRC: Health Information Technology Research Center

HL7: Health Level 7

ISA: Interoperability Standards Advisory

ONC: Office of the National Coordinator for Health Information Technology

PPACA: Patient Protection and Affordable Care Act

REC: Regional Extension Center

RHIA: registered health information administrator

RHIT: registered health information technician

Check Your Understanding

To check your understanding of this chapter's key concepts, answer the following questions.

1. What is the most common communication protocol in health IT?

   a. Structural

   b. Semantic

   c. HL7

   d. NwHIN

2. What is the US federal body that recommends policies, procedures, protocols, and standards for interoperability?

   a. Office of the National Coordinator for Health Information Technology

   b. Centers for Medicare & Medicaid Services

   c. Health Information Technology for Economic and Clinical Health

   d. US Department of Health and Human Services

3. What is an EHR that continues to develop over the course of care?

   a. Vertical EMR

   b. Longitudinal EHR

   c. Personal health record

   d. Interoperable health record

4. Interoperability is

   a. a communication protocol.

   b. the ability of one computer system to communicate with another system.

   c. a longitudinal protocol.

   d. another name for an EMR.

5. The individual data sources that inform and populate the collected patient information of the global EHR are

    a. personal health records.

    b. physician office billing records.

    c. hospital records.

    d. EMRs.

6. The accounting costs of an EHR system may include any of the following *except*

    a. hardware, marketing, vendor support, and software licenses.

    b. software, software customization, implementation, and vendor support.

    c. hardware, software, technical support, and training.

    d. testing and training, implementation, technical support, and software licenses.

7. True/False: The abbreviations *EHR* and *EMR* can be used interchangeably because they represent the same type of electronic record.

8. True/False: Electronic health records (EHRs) are interactive and can share information among multiple healthcare providers.

9. True/False: A workflow analysis reviews how an organization will function in the future and how EHRs are used.

10. True/False: Healthcare providers that did *not* implement an EHR system by 2014 were assessed fines by the US federal government.

Go on the Record

To build on your understanding of the topics in this chapter, complete the following short-answer activities.

1. When members of the US Congress enacted the HITECH Act, they set specific goals the act would accomplish. List and briefly explain these goals.

2. List four of the eight topic areas of the objectives of Stage 3 meaningful use.

3. List the five levels of interoperability.

4. Name two credentials offered by AHIMA for health information professionals.

5. Define *workflow analysis*.

Navigate the Field

To gain practice in handling challenging situations in the workplace, consider the following real-world scenarios and identify how you would respond to each.

1. North City Medical Associates is a physician practice that has struggled over the past 10 years with a tremendous growth in new patients and a lack of

technology to keep up with the additional record keeping, billing, and scheduling. Jackie Lee, office manager at North City Medical Associates, decided to take advantage of incentive funds offered by the US federal government and implemented an EHR system 18 months ago. Jackie now reports that the EHR system has paid for itself several times over through practice efficiency and cost savings. Describe some specific ways in which you believe North City Medical Associates made its practice more efficient and may have experienced cost savings following its implementation of the EHR system.

2. As the health information manager at Wellness Hospital, you have been asked to research what the hospital must prove to meet meaningful use guidelines. Describe what the hospital can do to meet these guidelines.

3. You work for Medical Office Associates. Medical Office Associates implemented the EHR system one year ago. You serve as an EHR and Clinical Documentation Specialist. The providers have submitted their feedback and indicated that the EHR system does not have a Basic SOAP Note template. Research the elements that should be included in a Basic SOAP Note template. Create a memo to the providers describing the elements you would recommend including in the Basic SOAP Note template.

Think Critically

Continue to think critically about challenging concepts and complete the following activities.

1. Interview a health information manager at a hospital regarding the challenges of managing a health information department in a hospital that uses an EHR system.

2. Investigate an entry-level position at https://EHR3.ParadigmEducation.com/EHRCareerAppx.

    a. Select an entry-level position that you might be interested in pursuing.

    b. Describe the position along with the promotional and transitional career pathways.

3. As part of the EHR selection team, you have been given the task to research three certified complete Inpatient EHR Systems. You may use https://EHR3.ParadigmEducation.com/CertifiedList as one source to locate certified EHR systems. Prepare a report comparing and contrasting the three systems. Write a two- to three-page report that would be submitted to the EHR selection committee with a recommendation based on your analysis of the three products.

Make Your Case

Consider the scenario and then complete the following project.

You work at a medium-sized hospital with an attached physician's clinic. Your boss is considering implementing an EHR system. Create a presentation describing the benefits of and barriers to EHR implementation.

Explore the Technology

To expand your mastery of EHRs, explore the technology by completing the following online activities.

1. Perform an internet search and name three EHR software systems commonly used by physician offices.

2. Conduct an internet job search to identify five different types of EHR positions located in your area.

3. Locate a website sponsored by the US federal government that provides information and resources regarding EHRs.

4. Locate two certifications, other than RHIT and RHIA, that can be awarded to individuals in the EHR field.

5. Research the 21st Century Cures Act to determine how it impacts physician practices.

Chapter 2 Content of the Health Record

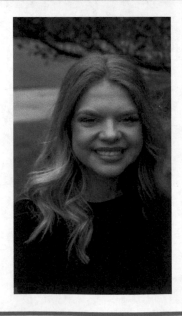

Field Notes

"The electronic health record allows for regulatory requirements to be embedded into standard workflows. As these requirements change, the electronic health record can be edited to meet the needs of the user to document safe care. At times, the electronic health record can be burdensome with duplicative processes; however, the benefit of having an electronic source that provides various stakeholders with information needed from medical records outweighs the burden. The ability to make updates and changes to the EHR to meet the needs of the end users provides a sustainable method to meet regulatory requirements."

– Elizabeth Zimmerly, MSN, RN-BC, Manager of Accreditation and Regulatory Compliance

2.1 Examine the history of the health record.

2.2 Define the term *health record* and its purpose.

2.3 Describe the primary and secondary uses of an electronic health record (EHR) system.

2.4 Differentiate the types of data in the health record.

2.5 Describe the purpose, format, and features of both the paper and electronic health record.

2.6 Explain the importance of proper documentation in the health record.

2.7 Describe the requirements and standards for the health record.

2.8 Explain ownership and stewardship of the health record.

2.9 Describe the transition from the paper health record to the electronic health record.

2.10 Compare and contrast the workflow of the paper health record to that of the electronic health record.

The concept of electronic health records (EHRs) has emerged from the growing partnership between health care and technology. The integration of EHRs in the healthcare practice is built on the foundation of health record content. Health records contain essential elements of clinical, administrative, financial, and legal information that play key roles in a patient's current and future health

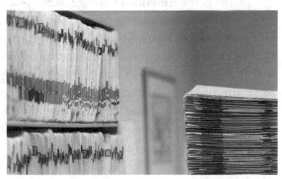

Whether on paper or in an electronic system, health records play key roles in a patient's current and future health care.

care. The healthcare field uses health records to manage and research improvements and innovations. Healthcare settings are required to maintain health records for every patient, and they must all follow licensing, accrediting, and other regulatory body requirements.

2.1 History of the Health Record

According to the US National Library of Medicine, a **healthcare facility** refers to "hospitals, clinics, dental offices, outpatient surgery centers, birthing centers, and nursing homes." Today, each facility creates individual health records for its patients. These records reflect all episodes of care that patients receive. Throughout history, healthcare providers have kept health records for their patients. Although the methods of documentation have changed, the importance of keeping and recording patient information has not.

Early Health Records

Hippocrates, considered one of the most important figures in medical history, and his followers were among the first to describe and document many diseases and medical conditions. However, Chunyu Yi, a famous Chinese physician of the Han dynasty, kept the first known health record (see Figure 2.1). He tracked his patients' names, residences, occupations, disease information, diagnoses, and prognoses. His records provide valuable historic data.

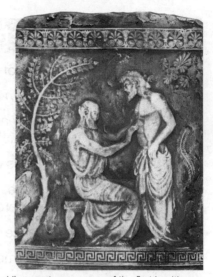

Hippocrates was one of the first healthcare practitioners to document diseases.

Between 1790 and 1821, some of America's earliest hospitals began keeping patient records, including New York Hospital, Pennsylvania Hospital, and Massachusetts General Hospital. Health records, historically restricted by the documentation habits of each individual healthcare provider, began to evolve in the United States during the Civil War. During this time, doctors began to record medical information in an increasingly standardized form, as social and physical mobility meant that they might treat patients they had never seen before. This trend continued as health records were established for immigrants to the United States at the advent of the 20th century.

In 1917, the **American College of Surgeons (ACS)** developed a hospital standardization program that established the **minimum standards**, which identified the elements required for reporting care and treatment. Minimum standards ensured that the health record communicated an accurate account of the healthcare information as well as the status of the patient. Some of the suggested standards for maintaining the patient record included patient identification, personal and family history, the reason for the encounter, a history of the current illness, physical examination, diagnosis, treatment, progress notes, and the patient's condition upon discharge. These standards are still in use over a century later.

Evolution of Electronic Health Records

Beyond traditional shelf filing of handwritten paper records, few advances in medical records storage have been noted. Microfilm was used in the 1950s and optical scanning in the 1980s, but no advancements in actual record keeping were made until the birth of the EHR.

Dr. Lawrence L. Weed is considered to be one of the pioneers in the EHR movement. Dr. Weed, a physician specializing in internal medicine, along with his colleague Jan Schultz developed

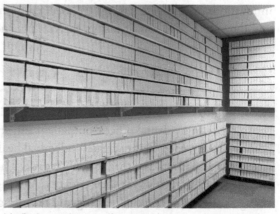

Medical records were often stored on microfilm starting in the 1950s.

Figure 2.1   EHR Timeline

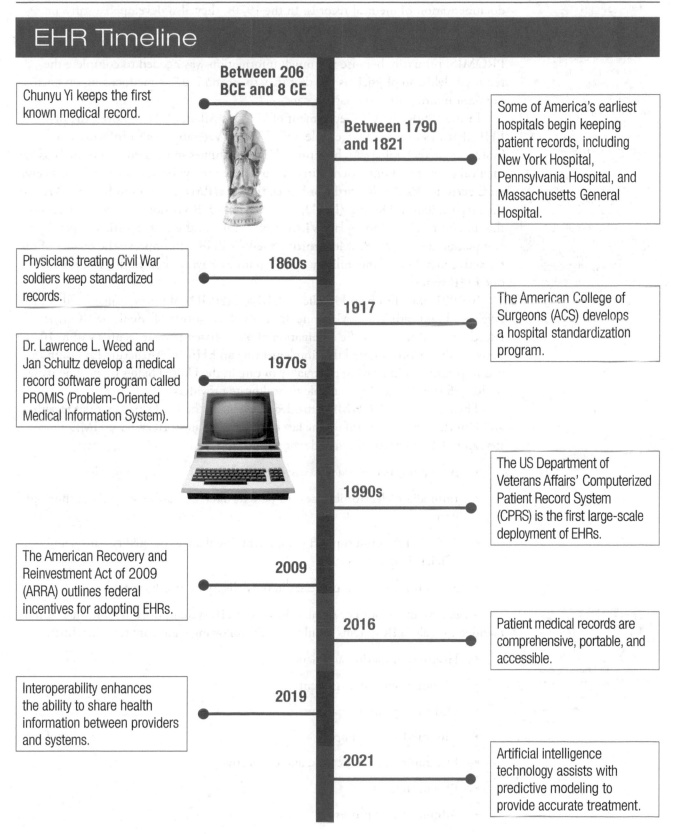

EHR Timeline

Chunyu Yi keeps the first known medical record.

Between 206 BCE and 8 CE

Between 1790 and 1821

Some of America's earliest hospitals begin keeping patient records, including New York Hospital, Pennsylvania Hospital, and Massachusetts General Hospital.

Physicians treating Civil War soldiers keep standardized records.

1860s

1917

The American College of Surgeons (ACS) develops a hospital standardization program.

Dr. Lawrence L. Weed and Jan Schultz develop a medical record software program called PROMIS (Problem-Oriented Medical Information System).

1970s

1990s

The US Department of Veterans Affairs' Computerized Patient Record System (CPRS) is the first large-scale deployment of EHRs.

The American Recovery and Reinvestment Act of 2009 (ARRA) outlines federal incentives for adopting EHRs.

2009

2016

Patient medical records are comprehensive, portable, and accessible.

Interoperability enhances the ability to share health information between providers and systems.

2019

2021

Artificial intelligence technology assists with predictive modeling to provide accurate treatment.

EXPAND YOUR
LEARNING

The National Academy of Sciences was created by President Abraham Lincoln in 1863. The Health and Medicine Division (HMD) is made up of more than 3,000 volunteers who work to provide independent, objective analysis and advice to requestors. To learn more about the National Academy of Sciences and the HMD (formerly the Institute of Medicine), go to https://EHR3 .ParadigmEducation .com/NationalAcademies.

the **problem-oriented medical record (POMR)**, a systematic approach to the documentation of medical records. In the 1970s, they also developed a software program called **Problem-Oriented Medical Information System (PROMIS)** at the University of Vermont under a federal grant. Healthcare providers did not embrace PROMIS, primarily because too much information was needed to complete the required fields, so physicians felt that they spent too much time focusing on documentation rather than on patient care.

In the 1990s, the US Department of Veterans Affairs (VA) deployed the first EHR that was used on a large scale, called VistA (Veterans Health Information Systems and Technology Architecture). VistA continues to be used at hundreds of VA medical centers and outpatient clinics across the country; however, the VA has begun an **Electronic Health Record Modernization (EHRM)** program to have the VA and the Department of Defense (DOD) use the same EHR vendor. Cerner is the vendor that has been selected to replace VistA in all VA medical facilities with a target completion date of 2028. Modernizing the VA's EHR will improve the quality of care for active members of the military and veterans by having their health information in one EHR system.

In 1991, the Health and Medicine Division (HMD) of the National Academies of Sciences, Engineering, and Medicine, formerly the Institute of Medicine (IOM), issued a report calling for the elimination of paper-based patient records within 10 years. In the report, it noted that implementing an EHR infrastructure for health care was imperative to improving the quality of care in the United States by making patient health information readily available to healthcare providers.

Then, in May 2003, HMD provided guidance to the US Department of Health and Human Services (HHS) on the key capabilities of an EHR system. HMD stated that an EHR system should include the following:

- A longitudinal record (discussed in Chapter 1)

- Immediate electronic access to patient data, accessible by only authorized users

- A clinical decision support component to enhance the quality, safety, and efficiency of patient care

- Support for efficient processes in the delivery of health care

To achieve these four key capabilities of an EHR system, the HMD further recommended that all EHR systems should have the following eight core functionalities:

- Health information and data

- Clinical results management

- Order entry and management

- Clinical decision support

- Electronic communication and connectivity

- Patient support

- Administrative processes

- Reporting and population health management

EXPAND YOUR
LEARNING

Read more about the timeline and development of EHRs at https://EHR3 .ParadigmEducation .com/EHRInfographic.

HMD's report provided further detail and specifications of these eight core functionalities by location of the delivery of health care, including hospitals, ambulatory care, nursing homes, and care in the community. HMD also outlined the time period under which these core functionalities should be implemented. The time frames were 2004–2005, 2006–2007, and 2008–2010, resulting in fully functional EHR systems by 2010.

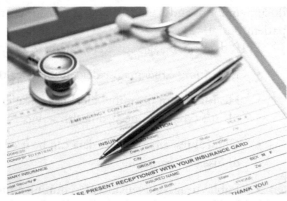
A questionnaire taken by the patient can provide clinical data.

The American Recovery and Reinvestment Act of 2009 (ARRA) outlined federal incentives for adopting EHRs. Included in the ARRA was the Health Information Technology for Economic and Clinical Health (HITECH) Act, which required the timely implementation of EHRs. Without the requirements and incentives of ARRA and the HITECH Act, providers may not have implemented EHRs.

Today, healthcare providers focus on documenting the patient's past and present care. The health record is an essential part of a patient's health care because it helps providers make informed and accurate diagnostic and treatment decisions and it facilitates communication among caregivers.

2.2 Purpose of the Health Record

The **health record** is an accumulation of information about a patient's past and present health. The purpose of the health record, whether recorded electronically or on paper, is to document the health history of the patient. In technical terms, the health record is composed of **data**, which include the descriptive or numeric attributes of one or more variables. Data collected and analyzed becomes **information** organized in a record. A **record** is a collection, usually in writing, of an account or an occurrence.

Documenting in the Health Record

Typically, the health record begins at the first visit or admission. A patient may have different records with each healthcare provider, such as a primary care physician, cardiologist, dermatologist, or dentist. Each provider must accurately enter information in the record, such as who provided the health services; what, when, and why the services were provided; and the outcome. The information in the health record is essential when tracking the patient's illnesses and treatments along with the communication among providers for the continuity of care.

Primary and Secondary Uses of an EHR System

There are five primary uses of an EHR system. As discussed previously, the delivery and the management of patient care are arguably the most important primary uses of the EHR. Other primary uses include financial processes such as billing and reimbursement, administrative processes such as quality improvement and legal documentation, and patient self-management via the personal health record and the patient portal.

EHR data can be aggregated for many secondary uses, such as:

- Education: Students use deidentified health records for study.

- Health system planning: Healthcare leaders and organizations use data to identify trends in needed health services.

- Clinical research: Timely data can be used by researchers in the advancement of disease treatment.

- Public health surveillance: Community and national leaders use health data to identify and manage disease trends.

2.3 Health Record Data

There are four major categories of data in the health record: administrative, clinical, legal, and financial. **Administrative data** includes demographic information about the patient, such as the patient's name, address, date of birth, race, primary language, religion, and marital status. **Clinical data** is information such as admission dates, office visits, laboratory test results, evaluations, and emergency visits. **Legal data** is composed of consents for treatment and authorizations for the release of information. The last category, **financial data**, includes the patient's insurance and payment information for healthcare services (see Figure 2.2).

Figure 2.2 Types of Health Record Data

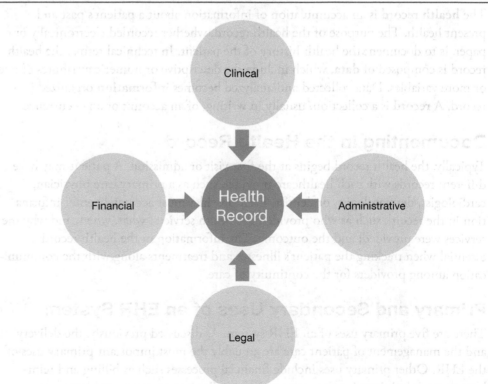

Administrative Data

Administrative data is information that the patient provides or populates in the health record. The administrative information typically found in the health record includes the following:

- Patient's name
- Address
- Telephone number
- Place of birth
- Date of birth
- Age

- Sex
- Marital status
- Ethnic origin
- Emergency contact information
- Primary language
- Religion

The healthcare staff collects administrative information to verify the patient's identity and to help create a patient's demographic profile. See Figure 2.3 for an example of a form used to collect administrative information.

Clinical Data

Clinical data includes the medical information taken and recorded by the healthcare provider. The clinical data should be detailed, complete,

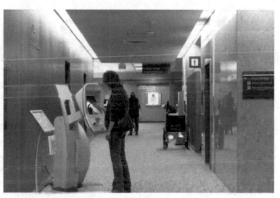

Some facilities, like the Mayo Clinic shown here, allow patients to check in using a kiosk.

Figure 2.3   Admission Face Sheet

Center City Outpatient Program ADMISSION FACE SHEET	

Patient Name: Last _____ First _____ Middle _____

Are you known by a previous name? ❑ No ❑ Yes: _____

Patient Address: _____

Home Phone: _____ Work Phone: _____ Cell Phone: _____

Date of Birth: _____

Sex: ❑ M ❑ F ❑ Non-binary ❑ None, I identify as _____

Occupation: _____

Marital Status: ❑ Single ❑ Married ❑ Separated ❑ Divorced ❑ Widowed ❑ Partner

precise, timely, and accurate, because the information plays a large role in the overall health plan of the patient. The clinical data includes documentation such as the following:

- Pathology and laboratory reports
- History and physical assessments
- Allergies
- X-rays

- List of medications
- Surgeries
- Hospital admissions
- Progress notes

Figure 2.4 provides an example of clinical data.

Figure 2.4 Clinical Data Form

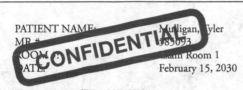

PATIENT NAME: Mulligan, Tyler
MR #:   985093
ROOM: Main Room 1
DATE: February 15, 2030

TREADMILL STRESS TEST

INDICATION
The patient was admitted to Northstar Medical Center complaining of mild chest pains. He is a 26-year-old white male who is actually quite athletic but has been noted on several occasions to have borderline hypertension. He has a family history of coronary artery disease in the father (who, incidentally, was a smoker), who died at the age of 54 secondary to coronary artery disease.

TECHNIQUE
The patient was exercised according to standard Bruce protocol for a total of 9 minutes and 30 seconds, at which time the test was stopped because he had obtained the target heart rate.

FINDINGS
He has a maximal heart rate of 181, which was approximately 93% of the predicted maximum of 195. He developed some clear up-sloping ST- and T-wave segment changes of 1–2 mm, specifically in leads V3, aVF, and anterior leads V3 through V6, but this resolved in the rest period. He developed only a mild blood pressure rise to a maximum of 146/90 at maximal exercise. Blood pressure returned to his resting normal quickly in recovery.

IMPRESSION
Negative treadmill stress test, with negative hypertensive response.

PLAN
Patient was given signs and symptoms of cardiac chest pain, including pressing substernal chest pain, shortness of breath, sweating, nausea or vomiting, or increase of pain with activity.

ADDENDUM
Patient was given extensive cardiovascular precautions, including the possibility of significant cardiac disease despite a seemingly negative treadmill stress test. The patient voiced understanding of this fact and also the need to seek immediate clinical attention should chest pain or other cardiovascular symptoms appear.

_____
Patrick Chaplin, MD

DF/DL
D:
T:

Legal Data

Legal data in the health record may be found on a variety of forms that are also considered legal documents. These documents include the following:

- Release of records: written request to release patient's health information to another healthcare provider or other entity in need of the patient's information

- Health Insurance Portability and Accountability Act (HIPAA) forms: HIPAA notice of privacy authorization

- General consent for care: agreement to general treatment and care

- Informed consent: agreement to a procedure

- Advance directives: written statement describing a patient's wishes regarding medical treatment in the event that the individual is no longer able to make such decisions because of illness or incapacity

Figure 2.5 illustrates an example of a form considered to be a legal document. Chapter 6 explores legal documents in more detail, describing how they are added to and released from the EHR.

Figure 2.5 Legal Data Form

Authorization to Release Medical Records and Billing Information

Name: _____

Address: _____

City: _____ State: _____ ZIP code: _____

Date: _____ (MM/DD/YYYY)

Name of Hospital or Physician: _____

Address: _____

City: _____ State: _____ ZIP code: _____

I, _____, hereby authorize _____ (hospital or physician name) to release to _____ (name of person to receive records) any information in my personal medical records, including all x-rays, computed tomography scans, and any other information pertinent to my treatment, along with all billing information while under the care of _____ during the time period from _____ to _____. I give my permission for this medical information to be used for insurance claim purposes. I do not, however, give permission for any other use or for any redisclosure of this information.

Signature: _____

Patient Name (Printed): _____

Date: _____

This authorization will expire one year from the date of the signature above. I understand that I can revoke this authorization at any time by writing to the healthcare provider, but that revoking this authorization will not affect disclosures made or actions taken before the revocation is received.

I also understand that:

—I am not required to sign this authorization, and my health care or payment for care will not be affected by my refusal.

—Federal privacy regulations will no longer apply to the information disclosed, and the entity receiving the records may not be subject to patient privacy laws and may redisclose the records.

—I am entitled to receive a copy of this authorization.

—A copy of this authorization may be utilized with the same effectiveness as an original.

Consider This

The health record, whether paper or electronic, is the legal record for a healthcare organization. Thus, there are many standards a health record should follow to protect the healthcare organization.

For a health record to be used as evidence in a court case, it needs to

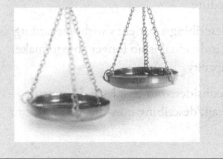

follow four basic principles. The record must be:

- documented following normal routines.
- kept in the regular course of healthcare business.
- recorded during or close to the time the event happened.
- recorded by a person with knowledge of the events.

Healthcare facilities must routinely assess policies and procedures regarding record keeping to ensure their records are legally sound.

Financial Data

Financial data consists of insurance and employer information. A copy of the patient's insurance coverage, when available, may also be included. There may be times when a patient pays for healthcare services with a payment plan or another type of financial arrangement. The financial data section of the health record would note this agreement. Figure 2.6 shows a financial data form that a patient may be asked to complete at the time of the visit. Financial data is often combined with administrative data, meaning that both types of data are collected on the same form.

Figure 2.6   Financial Data Form

Patient Insurance Information

Primary Policyholder Information

Insurance Plan: _____

Policyholder's Name: _____

Address: _____

_____

Home Phone: _____ Work Phone: _____ Cell Phone: _____

Birth Date: _____

Relationship to Patient: _____

Employer Name: _____

Employer Address: _____

Consider This

The EHR must meet the same requirements of a paper health record to be considered a legal document. Healthcare providers must accurately document vital signs, chief complaints, history, orders, plans, and prescriptions. The procedures and tools must also comply with the state's and organization's requirements. Documentation must be original, corrected, clarified, and amended. The EHR must maintain clinical messages, reports, and auditing tools. In addition, healthcare organizations must implement policies to include how unique health records are created and maintained; how content is chosen to be required; how they are authenticated and accessed; how privacy, confidentiality, and security are maintained; and how amendments and corrections are made. Healthcare organizations must create policies for record retention, archiving, destruction, abstracting, and reporting. Healthcare organizations should work with vendors to ensure that their EHR software adheres to the regulations to maintain a legal health record. What else can healthcare organizations do to maintain the legal health record in an EHR system? What might EHR vendors do to help healthcare organizations maintain a legal health record?

National Committee on Vital and Health Statistics Core Data Elements

In 1996, the **National Committee on Vital and Health Statistics (NCVHS)** completed a review of core health data elements and developed a list and definitions of the 42 core elements that can be used in a variety of healthcare settings. The patient provides the patient/enrollment data at the initial visit with the healthcare provider or facility, not at subsequent visits. Table 2.1 lists these core data elements and their definitions.

In addition to the core data elements proposed by NCVHS, other data sets have been proposed as national guidelines to encourage the exchange of information across healthcare providers and settings. The American Health Information Management Association (AHIMA) developed a core data set for the physician practice EHR, with its core elements divided into demographic and administrative information, vital signs, reason for the visit, present illness, medical history, physical examination, problem and medication list, screenings, immunizations, summary, referrals, and authentication.

Table 2.1 National Committee on Vital and Health Statistics Core Data Elements

Core Data Element	Definition
Patient/Enrollment Data	
Personal/Unique Identifier	Two options: A. Name—Last, first, middle, suffix B. Numeric identifier Without a universal unique identifier or a set of data items to form a unique identifier, it is challenging to link data across healthcare facilities and providers.
Date of Birth	MM/DD/YYYY
Gender	M/F/Unknown/Not stated

Race and Ethnicity	Recommendation to be self-reported
	Race
	  1. American Indian/Eskimo/Aleut
	  2. Asian or Pacific Islander
	  3. Black
	  4. White
	  5. Other (specify)
	  6. Unknown/Not stated
	Ethnicity
	  1. Hispanic origin (specify)
	  2. Other (specify)
	  3. Unknown

Residence	Full address and ZIP code

Marital Status	1. Married—currently married (classify common-law marriage as married)
	  a. Living together
	  b. Not living together
	2. Never married—never married or annulled
	3. Widowed—person widowed and not remarried
	4. Divorced—person divorced and not remarried
	5. Separated—person legally separated
	6. Partner—civil unions (some forms now include this option)
	7. Unknown/Not stated

Living/Residential Arrangement	Living Arrangement
	  1. Alone
	  2. With spouse (alternate: with spouse or unrelated partner)
	  3. With children
	  4. With parent or guardian
	  5. With relatives other than spouse, children, or parents
	  6. With nonrelatives
	  7. Unknown/Not stated
	Residential Arrangement
	  1. Private residence/household
	  2. Homeless shelter
	  3. Housing with services or supervision
	  4. Jail/correctional facility
	  5. Healthcare institutional setting
	  6. Homeless
	  7. Other residential setting

Continues

Table 2.1 *Continued*

Core Data Element	Definition
Self-Reported Health Status	There is no consensus on how to define health status, but a common measure is the following: Excellent Very good Good Fair Poor
Functional Status	The functional status of a person is an increasingly important health measure shown to be strongly related to medical care utilization rates. Many scales have been developed that include both (a) self-report measures such as limitations of activities of daily living and instrumental activities of daily living, and National Health Interview Survey age-specific summary, and (b) clinical assessments such as the International Classification of Impairments, Disabilities, and Handicaps, and the Resident Assessment Instrument. Self-report measures and clinical assessments are both valuable and informative.
Years of Schooling	Years of schooling completed by the enrollee/patient as a proxy for socioeconomic status. This core data element is highly predictive of health status and healthcare use.
Patient's Relationship to Subscriber/Person Eligible for Entitlement	1. Self 2. Spouse 3. Child 4. Other
Current or Most Recent Occupation/Industry	Used to track occupational diseases
Encounter Data	
Type of Encounter	1. Inpatient 2. Outpatient 3. Emergency department 4. Observation 5. Ambulatory 6. Other
Admission Date (inpatient)	Format MM/DD/YYYY
Discharge Date (inpatient)	Format MM/DD/YYYY
Date of Encounter (ambulatory and physician services)	Format MM/DD/YYYY
Facility Identification	Identifier for hospitals, ambulatory surgery centers, nursing homes, and hospices, among others
Type of Facility/Place of Encounter	Identifier for type or place of encounter; part of the National Provider Identifier (NPI)
Healthcare Provider Identification (outpatient)	The NPI enables each provider to have a universal unique number across the system
Provider Location or Address of Encounter (outpatient)	Full address and ZIP code for the location of the provider
Attending Physician Identification (inpatient)	The unique national identification assigned to the clinician of record at discharge

Table 2.1 *Continued*

Core Data Element	Definition
Operating Physician Identification (inpatient)	The unique national identification assigned to the clinician who performed the principal procedure
Provider Specialty	Part of the NPI system that identifies the provider's specialty
Principal Diagnosis (inpatient)	The condition determined to be chiefly responsible for patient admission
Primary Diagnosis (inpatient)	The diagnosis responsible for the majority of the care given to the patient
Other Diagnoses (inpatient)	Conditions should be coded that affect patient care in terms of requiring the following: 1. Clinical evaluation 2. Therapeutic treatment 3. Diagnostic procedures 4. Extended length of hospital stay 5. Increased nursing care/monitoring
Qualifier for Other Diagnoses (inpatient)	The following should be applied to each diagnosis coded under *other diagnoses*: 1. Onset prior to admission 2. Onset not prior to admission 3. Onset uncertain
Patient's Stated Reason for Visit or Chief Complaint (ambulatory)	Reason at the time of the encounter for seeking attention or care
Diagnosis Chiefly Responsible for Services Provided (ambulatory)	Contains the code(s) for the diagnosis, condition, problem, or the reason for encounter/visit chiefly responsible for the services provided
Other Diagnoses (ambulatory)	Additional code(s) that describe any conditions coexisting at the time of the encounter/visit that require management
External Cause of Injury	Code for the external cause of an injury, poisoning, or adverse event; completed whenever there is a diagnosis of an injury, poisoning, or adverse event
Birth Weight of Newborn (inpatient)	Specific birth weight of the newborn recorded in grams or in pounds and ounces
Principal Procedure (inpatient)	The principal procedure is one that was performed for definitive treatment, rather than one performed for diagnostic or exploratory purposes, or necessary to take care of a complication. If there appear to be two procedures that are principal, then the one most related to the principal diagnosis should be selected as the principal procedure. 1. Is surgical in nature 2. Carries a procedural risk 3. Carries an anesthetic risk 4. Requires specialized training
Other Procedures (inpatient)	All other procedures that are considered significant. A significant procedure is one of the following: 1. Is surgical in nature 2. Carries a procedural risk 3. Carries an anesthetic risk 4. Requires specialized training
Dates of Procedures (inpatient)	MM/DD/YYYY
Services (ambulatory)	Describe all diagnostic services of any type, including history and physical examinations, laboratory studies, x-rays, and others performed and pertinent to the patient's reasons for the encounter; all therapeutic series; all preventive services and procedures at time of encounter.
Medications Prescribed	All medications prescribed by the healthcare provider at the time of the encounter. Include dosage, strength, and amount prescribed.

Continues

Table 2.1 *Continued*

Core Data Element	Definition

Disposition of Patient (inpatient)	1. Discharge status
	  a. Discharged alive
	  b. Discharged dead
	  c. Status not stated
	2. Discharge setting
	  a. Discharged to home or self-care
	  b. Discharged to acute care hospital
	  c. Discharged to a nursing facility
	  d. Discharged to other healthcare facility
	  e. Discharged home to be under care of a home health services agency
	  f. Left against medical advice

Disposition (ambulatory)	Provider's statement of the next steps in care of patient. The following are the suggested classifications:
	  1. No follow-up planned
	  2. Follow-up planned or scheduled
	  3. Referred elsewhere

Patient's Expected Sources of Payment	Name of each source of payment including primary and secondary sources
Injury Related to Employment	Yes or No
Total Billed Charges	Copayment or update payment data when available

CHECKP⊕INT 2.1

1. Define *data*, *information*, and *record*.

_____

_____

_____

_____

_____

2. Describe several types of information that may be found within a health record.

_____

_____

_____

_____

_____

2.4 Health Record Format

The **format** of the paper health record refers to the organizing principle for health documents from all departments in a healthcare facility. There are no specific requirements on how paper health records are formatted, as long as an organization uses the same format throughout its facility. There are three organizational formats used in paper health records: source-oriented record, integrated health record, and problem-oriented record.

Source-Oriented Record

The **source-oriented record (SOR)** is the most common format used by healthcare facilities. This format organizes the health documents into sections that contain information collected from a specific department or type of service; for example, all progress notes, laboratory reports, and radiology reports are assembled together in their respective sections. Within each section, the health record content is organized in chronologic order. (Most healthcare facilities using the source-oriented format keep the health content in chronologic rather than reverse chronologic order.) SORs permit rapid retrieval of health content, although the format can make it challenging to view the complete health status of the patient.

Integrated Health Record

The second format type is the **integrated health record**, which is organized either in chronologic or reverse chronologic order. The health content is not separated by department or type of service; therefore, health documentation is viewed by date. Healthcare facilities may use the integrated health record format in several ways. The paper health record may place all forms together or be organized by healthcare setting (e.g., dental forms in one section, primary care documents in another). The integrated health record provides a complete view of the health status of the patient, although this format makes it difficult to compare findings from the same type of service, such as comparing two radiology reports completed at the beginning and at the end of a patient's stay.

Problem-Oriented Record

The third format type is the **problem-oriented record (POR)**. As discussed previously, Dr. Lawrence L. Weed and Jan Schultz developed the POMR because the SOR did not provide a complete view of the patient's health status. The POR focuses on assessment of the clinical documentation by healthcare providers and the creation of a plan that addresses the patient's health concerns. This type of format promotes a collaborative approach to documentation through the use of the SOAP progress note format that comprises the following documentation:

- S (Subjective): the reason the patient is at the healthcare facility for care, as well as comments from the patient or patient's family about the existing condition

- O (Objective): specific notes such as results from a laboratory test completed during the patient's visit

- A (Assessment): the healthcare provider's opinion on the condition or diagnosis

- P (Plan): the healthcare provider's plan to diagnose or treat the patient

The SOAP progress note format is used in both paper and electronic records.

CHECKPOINT 2.2

1. Describe the source-oriented health record format.

_____

_____

_____

_____

2. What are the four components of the SOAP progress note format?

a. _____

b. _____

c. _____

d. _____

2.5 Health Record Content

The content of a health record will vary depending on the type of healthcare facility. Chapter 4 will go into greater detail on the types of healthcare facilities. In this chapter, the health record content of patients in acute and ambulatory settings will be discussed. Note the variances in the patient records of these two types of facilities.

Acute Care Setting

Facilities that provide acute care include acute care hospitals and long-term care hospitals (LTCHs). Patients who are admitted to these facilities are called *inpatients*. An **inpatient** occupies a hospital bed for at least one night in the course of treatment, examination, or observation.

Record Content

For an inpatient admitted to an acute care setting, a health record usually contains the following content:

- Admission record: state of the patient when they are admitted to an acute care facility
- History and physical: information regarding the patient's past and current health condition, assessment, and treatment or diagnostic work-up plan
- Progress notes: entries of the patient's care and progress reported by the healthcare providers

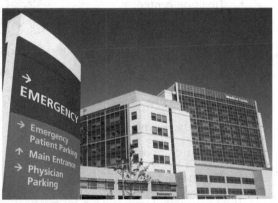
A hospital is an acute care facility.

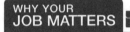

WHY YOUR JOB MATTERS

The accuracy of the health record is more important than ever because it is no longer just historical health information that is filed away. The EHR of today is digitized, real-time health information that is more accessible to patients and providers, resulting in improved patient outcomes.

- Laboratory tests: test and laboratory results ordered by healthcare providers

- Diagnostic tests: medical tests that assist in the diagnosis of the patient's health issue

- Operative notes: notes immediately written after surgery that document the procedure and results

- Pathology reports: detailed information on the review of specimens from tissue or cell biopsy

- Physician orders: orders given by the physician for medications, fluids, patient testing, etc.

- Consents: authorizations for treatment

- Consultations: reports provided by other healthcare providers that review the patient's health issues

- Emergency department encounters: documentation of visits or encounters in the emergency department

- Discharge summary: summary of the patient's course of care signed by the attending physician

The content in each record may be supplied in different formats but typically contains similar data.

Ambulatory Care Setting

Ambulatory care is an increasingly popular mode of healthcare delivery. Some ambulatory care settings include:

- Physician's offices

- Clinics

- Surgery centers

- Dental offices

- Imaging centers

- Occupational health centers

- Oral and maxillofacial care offices

- Podiatrist offices

- Pain management centers

- Community or college health centers

- Urgent care centers

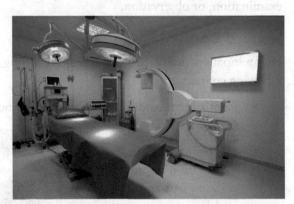
A surgery center is an example of an ambulatory care facility.

The term *ambulatory* is used for medical care, including diagnosis, observation, treatment, and rehabilitation services. Patients receiving treatment in an ambulatory setting are called *outpatients*. An **outpatient** is a patient who does not spend more than 24 hours in a healthcare facility and/or is not admitted to the hospital.

Record Content

Each facility, unless part of an organization, creates and maintains its own health record for a patient. The ambulatory care record typically contains the following content:

- Demographic information: patient's name, address, date of birth, and other information not medical in nature

- Contact information: various telephone numbers and email addresses, as well as emergency contacts

- History and physical: health history, a review of vital signs, and a complete organ-specific physical examination

- Immunization records: comprehensive list of dates and types of vaccines received as a child, as well as additional vaccines such as flu, tetanus, and hepatitis

- Problem lists: list of the patient's current health issues

- Allergy lists: list of medications, food, and other items to which a patient is allergic

- Prescription lists: list of current medications, including dosages

- Progress notes: updates to the patient's healthcare issues; may be in SOAP format

- Assessment: summary of the likely causes of the patient's current health issues; provides a course of action to address health issues

- Consultations: documentation of a patient's visit to another healthcare provider and what that healthcare provider recommends or concludes

- Referrals: permission or suggestions for the patient to be seen by another healthcare provider

- Treatment plans: plan for treatment of the patient's health issues

- Patient instructions: directions and orders to be followed by the patient to help with their health issues

- Laboratory tests and results: test and laboratory results ordered by the healthcare provider

- Consents: authorizations for treatment

- Communication: letters, emails, messages taken by phone, or any other documented communication

- External correspondence: communication between the healthcare provider and any other provider or carrier that provides information about the patient

- Financial information: payment arrangements and insurance information

Each specialty practice may provide the health information in a slightly different way, but the concept and purpose of each category are the same.

EXPAND YOUR LEARNING

The current patient record in an EHR contains a large amount of information, but it is often difficult to find the exact data needed to develop an appropriate treatment plan. Is it time for a new type of EHR? Read about how technology can be used to create a new kind of EHR at https://EHR3.ParadigmEducation.com/NewEHR.

CHECKPOINT 2.3

1. Name five content areas found in an acute care health record.

   a. _____

   b. _____

   c. _____

   d. _____

   e. _____

2. Name five content areas found in an ambulatory care health record.

   a. _____

   b. _____

   c. _____

   d. _____

   e. _____

2.6 Documentation in the Health Record

Each healthcare facility is responsible for the quality of care provided to its patients. Direct documentation of this care must be provided in a paper record or EHR system and is the responsibility of the healthcare provider. This documentation must be accurate, timely, and complete, reflecting all procedures, treatments, medications, tests, assessments, observations, and communications involved with patient care. Remember the saying, "If it's not documented, it didn't happen."

The maintenance and accuracy of the health record are important responsibilities of health information staff, whose duty is to ensure that healthcare records are readily available when patients arrive for care. The staff must also ensure that all forms are in each patient's record, verify that the healthcare provider has documented care, validate the accuracy of the coding of service, and adhere to established healthcare data standards.

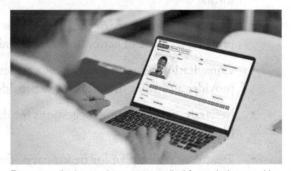

Paper medical records must be pulled from shelves and be readily available when patients arrive at a healthcare facility, but an EHR can be pulled up on an electronic device within seconds.

Documentation Guidelines

Every healthcare organization should establish policies and procedures specifying health record documentation guidelines, for both paper and electronic health records, to ensure that health record documentation is accurate, timely, and supportive of assessment, diagnosis, and treatment. Documentation guidelines are established based on the laws, rules, and standards of licensing agencies, accrediting bodies, and payers of healthcare treatment and services. Some of the typical documentation guidelines for paper and electronic records are compared and listed in Table 2.2.

When working with health records, healthcare personnel need to be aware of three areas of concern that affect patient safety: the legibility of the entries, the use of only

ON THE JOB

A medical scribe is a profession that has come about because of EHRs. A medical scribe maintains data in the EHR, gathers information for the patient's visit, and assists physicians in locating information from the health record.

Table 2.2   Documentation Guidelines for Paper and Electronic Health Records

Paper Health Records	Electronic Health Records
A separate, physical paper record is established for each patient.	A separate, electronic record is established for each patient.
Paper documents are assembled in an established chart order, including chronologic or reverse chronologic order.	Electronic documents are organized in an organized fashion that promotes fast, easy retrieval of information.
Proper authentication (all documents signed/initialed with pen)	Proper authentication (electronic signatures on all documents)
All documentation dated and timed, including signatures authenticating verbal and telephone orders	All documentation dated and timed, including signatures authenticating verbal and telephone orders
Timely documentation handwritten or dictated/transcribed (e.g., history and physical documented within 24 hours of admission, progress notes documented at the time of the visit/treatment)	Timely documentation typed or dictated/transcribed (e.g., history and physical documented within 24 hours of admission, progress notes documented at the time of the visit/treatment)
Legible handwriting	N/A
Complete documentation to support diagnoses and procedures	Complete documentation to support diagnoses and procedures
Patient identifiers on each piece of paper (patient name, medical record number, patient account number, date of birth, etc.)	Patient identifiers on each electronic document (patient name, medical record number, patient account number, date of birth, etc.)
Results of all tests and procedures are filed in the paper medical record in a timely fashion.	Results of all tests and procedures are electronically filed in the EHR in a timely fashion.
Correction of errors: single ink line through the documentation with date and initials of author. Documentation is *never* obliterated or destroyed from a paper record.	Correction of errors: strike through documentation in error and include the date and author initials or documentation moved to a separate, retrievable electronic file. Information/documentation is *never* completely deleted from the EHR.

approved abbreviations and acronyms in the documentation, and the protocol for changing or correcting documented entries. Specifics of these safety concerns are outlined next.

Legibility of Entries

When working with paper record entries, interpreting the handwriting of healthcare providers may be difficult (see Figure 2.7). Consequently, healthcare personnel must query the appropriate staff members about any unclear entries. This verification protects both the safety of the patient and the liability of the healthcare worker and the facility.

Using Abbreviations and Acronyms

Abbreviations and acronyms are often used in the health record. Therefore, to ensure clear communication, there are standards for abbreviations and symbols that should be followed when documenting information. Some examples of approved abbreviations are provided in Table 2.3. Healthcare facilities can place additional rules in their bylaws that indicate other acceptable abbreviations per facility preference.

The Joint Commission developed an official "Do Not Use" List of abbreviations as part of its information management standards that healthcare organizations must follow. In addition, the commission has proposed a list for possible future inclusion in the official "Do Not Use" List. The "Do Not Use" List is found in Figure 2.8.

Changing or Correcting Documented Entries

Healthcare personnel need to follow established procedures when changing or correcting documented entries in a paper health record. Information must not be erased.

When correcting information in an EHR, authors strike through the error and include the date and author initials or they move the documentation to a separate, retrievable electronic file. Information/documentation is never completely deleted from the EHR. Healthcare personnel may also document an addendum to clarify documentation. The health record should be flagged along with an explanation of the error and how the error was corrected.

Figure 2.7 Handwritten Physician Order

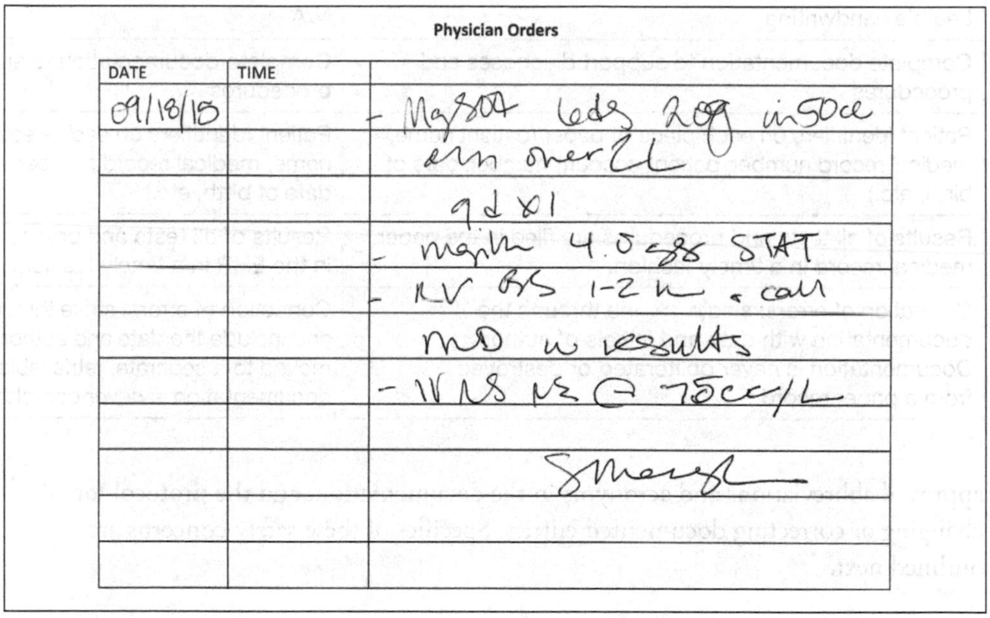

Table 2.3 Health Record Abbreviations and Acronyms

Abbreviation	Meaning	Abbreviation	Meaning
ABN	Advanced beneficiary notice	MD	Medical doctor
BMI	Body mass index	MMR	Measles, mumps, and rubella
BP	Blood pressure	MS	Multiple sclerosis
CV	Cardiovascular	Neuro	Neurologic
DOB	Date of birth	NPP	Notice of privacy practices
DPT	Diphtheria, pertussis, and tetanus	O2, O_2	Oxygen
ENMT	Ears, nose, mouth, and throat	OR	Operating room
ETOH	Alcohol	p.o.	By mouth
GI	Gastrointestinal	PCP	Primary care provider
GYN	Gynecologic	PRN	As needed
HPI	History of present illness	ROS	Review of systems
IM	Intramuscularly	Temp	Temperature
LMP	Last menstrual period	VIS	Vaccine information sheet

Figure 2.8   The Joint Commission's Official "Do Not Use" List of Abbreviations

The Joint Commission.

Official "Do Not Use" List

The Joint Commission
FACT
SHEET

- This list is part of the Information Management standards
- Does not apply to preprogrammed health information technology systems (i.e. electronic medical records or CPOE systems), but remains under consideration for the future

Organizations contemplating introduction or upgrade of such systems should strive to eliminate the use of dangerous abbreviations, acronyms, symbols and dose designations from the software.

For more information

- Complete the Standards Online Question Submission Form.
- Contact the Standards Interpretation Group at 630-792-5900.

Official "Do Not Use" List[1]

Do Not Use	Potential Problem	Use Instead
U, u (unit)	Mistaken for "o" (zero), the number "4" (four) or "cc"	Write "unit"
IU (International Unit)	Mistaken for IV (intravenous) or the number 10 (ten)	Write "International Unit"
Q.D., QD, q.d., qd (daily)	Mistaken for each other	Write "daily"
Q.O.D., QOD, q.o.d, qod (every other day)	Period after the Q mistaken for "I" and the "O" mistaken for "I	Write "every other day"
Trailing zero (X.0 mg)* Lack of leading zero (.X mg)	Decimal point is missed	Write X mg Write 0.X mg
MS	Can mean morphine sulfate or magnesium sulfate	Write "morphine sulfate" Write "magnesium sulfate"
MSO_4 and $MgSO_4$	Confused for one another	

[1]Applies to all orders and all medication-related documentation that is handwritten (including free-text computer entry) or on pre-printed forms.

*Exception: A "trailing zero" may be used only where required to demonstrate the level of precision of the value being reported, such as for laboratory results, imaging studies that report size of lesions, or catheter/tube sizes. It may not be used in medication orders or other medication-related documentation.

Development of the "Do Not Use" List
In 2001, The Joint Commission issued a *Sentinel Event Alert* on the subject of medical abbreviations. A year later, its Board of Commissioners approved a National Patient Safety Goal requiring accredited organizations to develop and implement a list of abbreviations not to use. In 2004, The Joint Commission created its "Do Not Use" List to meet that goal. In 2010, NPSG.02.02.01 was integrated into the Information Management standards as elements of performance 2 and 3 under IM.02.02.01.

8/20

2.7 Health Record Standards

Several accreditation, professional, and federal organizations provide guidelines and support on maintaining the integrity of patient health records. By affiliation with these organizations and meeting their professional standards and goals, healthcare facilities can distinguish their services from others as well as reduce the number of state and federal reviews. A focus of all of these organizations is to improve the quality of patient care and health record documentation.

Accreditation Organizations

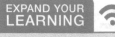

EXPAND YOUR LEARNING

Search for these organizations on the internet to learn more about how they promote high standards in documenting health information.

The **Commission for Accreditation of Rehabilitation Facilities (CARF)** is an independent, nonprofit organization that focuses on aging services, behavioral health, child and youth services, employment and community services, medical rehabilitation, and opioid treatment programs. **The Joint Commission**, formerly known as the Joint Commission on Accreditation of Healthcare Organizations (JCAHO), is an independent, not-for-profit organization that accredits and certifies a variety of healthcare organizations, ranging from dental to behavioral health to acute care facilities. Health record content standards are addressed in each field of health care.

The **National Committee for Quality Assurance (NCQA)** is an independent, nonprofit organization that focuses on healthcare quality. Healthcare organizations such as individual or group healthcare providers and health plans that seek NCQA accreditation do so voluntarily.

The **Community Health Accreditation Program (CHAP)** and the **Accreditation Association for Ambulatory Health Care (AAAHC)** are two examples of specialty accrediting organizations.

Professional Organizations

The following three professional organizations support healthcare information personnel in maintaining quality assurance of health records.

The **Association for Healthcare Documentation Integrity (AHDI)** has vowed "to set and uphold standards for education and practice in the field of clinical documentation that ensure the highest level of accuracy, privacy, and security for the US healthcare systems in order to protect public health, increase patient safety, and improve quality of care for healthcare consumers."

The American Health Information Management Association (AHIMA) is a professional organization that provides resources, education, and networking with other professionals. AHIMA focuses on the quality of health information used in the delivery of health care. Initially, the organization focused on hospital records, but it now supports ambulatory, community health, and many other healthcare delivery (HCD) organizations.

The Healthcare Information and Management Systems Society (HIMSS) focuses on using information technology and management systems to improve the quality and delivery of health care.

Federal Organizations

Lastly, the following federal organizations are actively involved in setting standards for health records.

The **Agency for Healthcare Research and Quality (AHRQ)** focuses on improving the safety and quality of health care. Their core competencies are focused on data, analytics, health system research, and practice improvement.

The Centers for Medicare & Medicaid Services (CMS) is a federal government agency that oversees federal healthcare programs, including Medicare Conditions of Participation (CoPs). In 2009, CMS expanded its role to include the implementation of EHR incentive programs, meaningful use of certified EHR systems, drafting standards for certified EHR technology, and updating privacy and security regulations under HIPAA. The **Health Resources and Services Administration (HRSA)** is an agency of the US Department of Health and Human Services. This agency focuses on improving health and health equity through innovative programs and a skilled health workforce and providing access to services to those who are economically or medically vulnerable.

A **Quality Improvement Organization (QIO)** is a group of health experts, providers, and consumers who are dedicated to improving the quality of care for people with Medicare.

2.8 Ownership and Stewardship of Health Records and Health Information

Health record and health information ownership and stewardship are controversial topics that have grown increasingly complex as healthcare facilities transitioned from paper health records to EHRs.

Ownership of Health Records

Historically, state laws and healthcare professional associations have accepted that the healthcare facility that created the health record owns the physical health record. For example, a sole practitioner (a single, independent healthcare practice) owns the record created in their practice just as a hospital or other inpatient facility owns records for all patients admitted or treated at the facility.

Ownership of Health Information

Historically, there have also been discussions and attempts to separate the ownership of the physical health record from the ownership of the health data contained in the record. Is the patient the owner because they are the subject of the record? Or is the healthcare facility the owner because it generated the information and physically has possession of the record? Many leaders in health information management anticipate that future legislation will address the subject of the ownership of health information, ultimately creating a uniform definition of *ownership*.

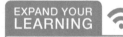

EXPAND YOUR LEARNING

To see how your state handles the ownership of health information, visit https://EHR3 .ParadigmEducation .com/MedRecordOwner.

Ownership versus Stewardship

While clarification of the ownership of health records and health information is needed, the concept of stewardship is a way to address the responsibilities of retention, privacy, and maintenance of health records and health data without having to solve the issue of ownership. Since stewardship implies careful and responsible management, as stewards, all healthcare providers and staff involved in the creation, use, maintenance, and retention of health records and data are responsible for ensuring that health data is generated, used, and stored in a manner that complies with all required laws, rules, standards, and guidelines.

Obtaining a Health Record

Patients have the right to access and/or obtain a copy of their health records, whether paper or electronic, depending on federal and state laws. To request a copy of the health record from the healthcare provider, typically a patient provides a written request, signs a HIPAA-compliant release of records form, and then pays the necessary fees. The cost of a copy, paper or electronic, of the health record varies depending on the provider and facility. See Figure 2.9 for an example of a release of information authorization form for a patient's health record. As EHRs have developed, new ways to authorize the release of medical records have evolved, including digital download and electronic sharing and access.

Figure 2.9 Release of Information

Northstar Medical Center MRN/Chart #________

PATIENT INFORMATION

Name Address City State ZIP

Date of Birth Daytime Phone Previous Name (if applicable)

AUTHORIZES

Name of Healthcare Provider/Plan

Address

TO DISCLOSE TO

❑ Self

Delivery Options: ❑ Pick Up ❑ View on Site ❑ Mail to Address Above

❑ To Be Picked Up By Another Person

I hereby authorize ______________ to pick up my records.

Send to: ❑ ________

Name of Healthcare Provider/Plan

Address Fax Number

DATE(S) OF INFORMATION TO BE DISCLOSED: From ________ to ________. If left blank, only information from the past two (2) years will be disclosed.

INFORMATION TO BE DISCLOSED:

❑ All medical records related to (specify condition, treatment, etc.): ________

❑ All billing records related to (specify condition, treatment, etc.): ________

❑ Radiology films/images (specify test): ________

❑ Other records: ________

DO NOT DISCLOSE THE FOLLOWING INFORMATION:

❑ Alcohol/drug use ❑ HIV test results ❑ Mental health status ❑ Developmental disabilities

PURPOSE (check all that apply):

❑ Further Medical Care ❑ Legal ❑ Insurance ❑ Personal ❑ Other:________

YOUR RIGHTS WITH RESPECT TO THIS AUTHORIZATION

I am aware that I have the right to inspect and receive a copy of the health information I have authorized to be used and/or disclosed by this authorization. I understand that I may be charged a fee for record copies. In addition, I understand that I do not need to sign this authorization in order to receive treatment. I understand that I may revoke this authorization by notifying the disclosing medical records/health information department in writing. However, I understand that my revocation will not be effective as to uses and/or disclosures: (1) already made in reliance upon this Authorization; or (2) needed for an insurer to contest a claim/policy as authorized by law if signing the Authorization was a condition to obtaining insurance coverage. I realize that the information used and/or disclosed pursuant to this Authorization may be subject to redisclosure and no longer protected by federal privacy law.

SIGNATURE OF PATIENT/LEGAL REPRESENTATION

________ DATE: ________

Now that health records are housed in an EHR system, patients often request an electronic copy of their records. The ability to receive electronic records is discussed in more detail in Chapter 6.

2.9 Importance of EHR Transition

Unfortunately, it took a natural disaster to underscore the importance of transitioning from paper health records to EHRs. In 2005, Hurricane Katrina made landfall in southeastern Louisiana. The resulting breach of the levee system in New Orleans caused many parts of the city to flood, washing away thousands of paper records and causing many residents to lose all of their medical information. In addition, many healthcare providers fled New Orleans, leaving many patients with no record of their health history, current health status, or medication information and no way to contact their healthcare providers. In response, the federal government, along with public and private organizations, created the KatrinaHealth.org website to help healthcare providers and pharmacies obtain access to patients' prescription information. Although this service helped many New Orleans residents, one segment of the city's population had maintained access to their medical records. The Veterans Health Administration's VistA system enabled displaced veterans to access their records no matter where they chose to relocate.

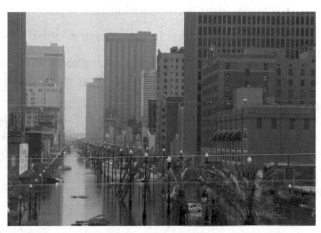

Many paper health records were destroyed in Hurricane Katrina.

Hurricane Katrina highlighted the necessity for health information to withstand natural disasters, an important lesson that supports the initiative for the development of EHRs.

Conversion from Paper Health Records to EHRs

As most healthcare organizations have transitioned from paper health records to EHRs for current healthcare record keeping, many organizations still have paper records in storage that are being digitally scanned to be included in their EHR system. This is a slow process but one that is necessary to ensure that all of a patient's health data is electronically available to healthcare staff.

Consider This

In 2018, over 200 hospitals, nursing homes, and medical facilities in North and South Carolina were in the path of Hurricane Florence. Some hospitals used health information exchanges that allowed their staff to access patient data from other healthcare systems when they could not access their own EHR systems.

Limitations of Paper Records

Paper health records have served an important role in patient health care for many decades. However, they also present many challenges to healthcare providers, including the following:

- Increasing complexity of healthcare delivery

- Single location of records

- Restricted access, allowing only one user to view records at a time

- Inconsistent documentation

- Unsecured storage in the event of a natural disaster or human error

In addition, managing the paper health record can be time consuming and labor intensive. Figure 2.10 shows a typical workflow for a paper health record in an ambulatory care setting.

Due to the challenges presented by this time-consuming workflow, and the increasing amount of patient and provider information required to be documented, the concept of using an EHR system became increasingly embraced by healthcare practitioners.

Figure 2.10 Paper Health Record Workflow

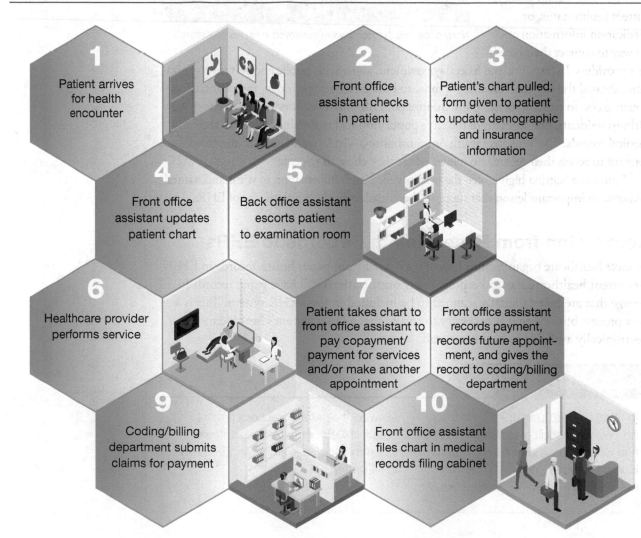

Advantages of EHRs

As discussed in Chapter 1, an EHR is not just an electronic version of a paper record, although the two have common data elements. Rather, an EHR begins with a database populated with health content from the patient's healthcare encounters. It includes demographic information, progress notes, assessments, results, consultations, and many of the other documents found in a paper health record. The database of the patient's healthcare encounters is updated each time the patient seeks medical care. Figure 2.11 demonstrates how data flows and is accessed in an EHR.

Healthcare providers can enter information in an EHR using laptops, desktop computers located in patient examination rooms, or wireless devices used during patient encounters. This easy accessibility to a patient's health record is a key advantage over a paper record that must be accessed from one location. The provider can log in to the EHR using a unique username and a secure password. Once the record is accessed by the provider, their activities within the record are tracked by the system.

The record itself offers a standardized format containing drop-down menus, lists, icons, and free-text areas for practitioners to enter health information into the database. Because of this standardization, EHRs can be easily searched for specific patient information and programmed to automatically prompt clinicians to send reminders and follow up with patients. The electronic data format provides users with a complete picture of a patient's overall health status.

Figure 2.11   EHR Data Flowchart

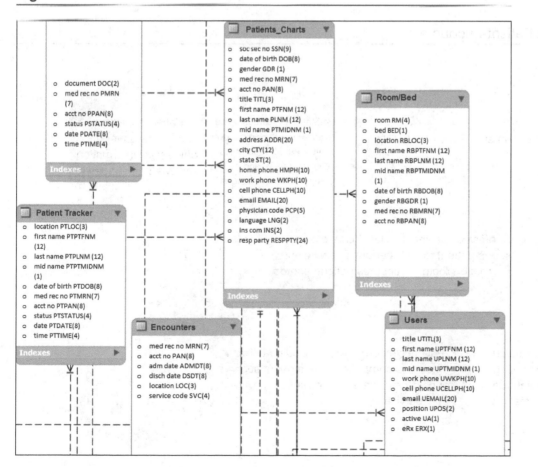

The workflow of an EHR differs from the pathway of a paper health record. As shown in Figure 2.12, the process is more streamlined for healthcare personnel.

Challenges of EHR Transition

Implementing an EHR system also presents some challenges. Converting the paper records into an electronic format is both time consuming and costly. As HCD systems convert from paper to an electronic format, portions of patient records will be stored electronically and on paper, resulting in a **hybrid health record**. Healthcare providers with small patient populations are likely to be able to convert to EHRs in a shorter time frame than healthcare providers with large patient populations, such as major hospitals. For these larger facilities, the conversion may take several years and, consequently, hybrid health records will need to be implemented.

There may be additional challenges in converting from paper health records to EHRs, such as dealing with duplicate records, establishing the identities of patients/unique patient identifiers, detecting insurance fraud, and identifying questionable identities of patients in various components in the EHR system.

Once all the records have been converted, healthcare workers must review records to ensure accuracy. Even with EHRs, there is room for error during the data entry or data conversion process. Removing erroneous information from an EHR is not allowed, and doing so may be seen as fraud if it is attempted.

Figure 2.12 EHR Patient Encounter

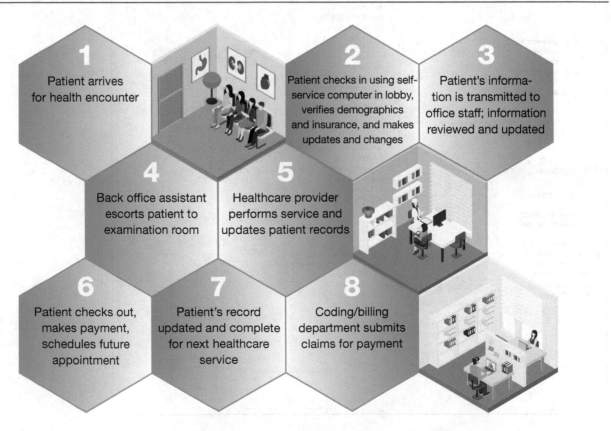

1 Patient arrives for health encounter

2 Patient checks in using self-service computer in lobby, verifies demographics and insurance, and makes updates and changes

3 Patient's information is transmitted to office staff; information reviewed and updated

4 Back office assistant escorts patient to examination room

5 Healthcare provider performs service and updates patient records

6 Patient checks out, makes payment, schedules future appointment

7 Patient's record updated and complete for next healthcare service

8 Coding/billing department submits claims for payment

Training all users of the EHR system to use EHR content can be difficult. Employees may lack the necessary technologic skills, and some users may be reluctant to learn a new system.

The goal of an EHR system is to improve patient health care by allowing access to multiple providers across all aspects of health care and involving the patient more directly, so that all players have current information on the patient's past and present health status. Having accurate and accessible EHRs will result in improved patient care and outcomes.

Chapter Summary

Some of the earliest US hospitals began keeping patient records in the early 1800s, although the first known health record was kept by Chunyu Yi, a famous Chinese physician. In 1917, the American College of Surgeons developed a hospital standardization program that established the minimum standards for elements that should be included in health records to report care and treatment. These standards are in use today. Paper health records continued to be used for many years, with the first EHR implementation occurring in the 1990s by the US Department of Veterans Affairs. EHR implementations have occurred and continue to occur in most healthcare facilities nationwide.

A health record is an accumulation of information about a patient's past and present health. The primary purpose of the health record, whether recorded electronically or on paper, is to document the health history of the patient. The health record is composed of data that includes the descriptive or numeric attributes of one or more variables. Data collected and analyzed becomes information. A record is a collection, usually in writing, of an account or an occurrence.

There are five primary uses of an EHR system, including the delivery of patient care, the management of patient care, financial processes, administrative processes, and patient self-management.

There are four secondary uses of an EHR system, including education, regulation, research, and public health.

There are four major categories of data in the health record, including administrative, clinical, legal, and financial data. The data in the health record is based on elements developed by the National Committee on Vital and Health Statistics. The information in the paper health record follows one of three formats: the source-oriented record, the integrated health record, or the problem-oriented record. Different formats of the health record are used depending on the healthcare setting.

Every healthcare organization should establish policies and procedures specifying health record documentation guidelines, for both paper and electronic health records, to ensure that health record documentation is accurate, timely, and supportive of assessment, diagnosis, and treatment. Documentation guidelines for data entries must be followed by healthcare personnel.

There are several organizations that provide standards for health records, including The Joint Commission, the National Committee for Quality Assurance, the Community Health Accreditation Program, the Accreditation Association for

Ambulatory Health Care, the American Health Information Management Association, and the Association for Healthcare Documentation Integrity.

Health record and health information ownership is a controversial topic that has grown increasingly complex as healthcare facilities transitioned from paper health records to EHRs. Historically, state laws and healthcare professional associations have accepted that the healthcare facility that created the health record owns the physical health record. The concept of stewardship is a way to address the responsibilities of retention, privacy, and maintenance of health records and health data without having to solve the issue of ownership. As stewards, all healthcare providers and staff involved in the creation, use, maintenance, and retention of health records and data are responsible for ensuring that health data is generated, used, and stored in a manner that complies with all required laws, rules, standards, and guidelines.

Review and Assessment

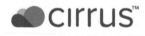

The following Review and Assessment activities are also available online in the Cirrus online course. Your instructor may ask you to complete these activities online. Cirrus also provides access to flash cards, a crossword puzzle, and practice quizzes to help strengthen your understanding of the chapter content.

Acronyms/Initialisms

Study the following acronyms discussed in this chapter. Go to the online course for flash cards of the acronyms and other chapter key terms.

AAAHC: Accreditation Association for Ambulatory Health Care

ACS: American College of Surgeons

AHDI: Association for Healthcare Documentation Integrity

AHIMA: American Health Information Management Association

ARRA: American Recovery and Reinvestment Act of 2009

CHAP: Community Health Accreditation Program

CMS: Centers for Medicare & Medicaid Services

CoPs: Medicare Conditions of Participation

CPRS: Veterans Health Administration's Computerized Patient Record System

HCD: healthcare delivery

HIMSS: Healthcare Information and Management Systems Society

HIPAA: Health Insurance Portability and Accountability Act of 1996

HMD: Health and Medicine Division

NCQA: National Committee for Quality Assurance

NCVHS: National Committee on Vital and Health Statistics

NPI: National Provider Identifier

POMR: problem-oriented medical record

POR: problem-oriented record

PROMIS: Problem-Oriented Medical Information System

SOAP format: subjective, objective, assessment, plan

SOR: source-oriented record

Check Your Understanding

To check your understanding of this chapter's key concepts, answer the following questions.

1. An ambulatory healthcare facility may be all of the following *except* a(n)

    a. surgery center.

    b. intensive care unit.

    c. dental office.

    d. psychologist office.

2. The four major categories of information in the health record include administrative, clinical, financial, and

    a. demographic.

    b. diagnostic.

    c. procedural.

    d. legal.

3. What type of information would be found in an acute health record, but *not* in an ambulatory health record?

    a. laboratory tests and referrals

    b. progress notes and consults

    c. admission record and discharge summary

    d. history and physical exam and problem lists

4. The treatment plan is a(n)

    a. itemized list of the patient's health problem(s).

    b. organized collection of the patient's health problem(s).

    c. list of reasons why the patient is at the healthcare facility.

    d. plan for treatment of the patient's health problem(s).

5. Information standards include an official "Do Not Use" List of abbreviations. Which organization developed this list?

    a. American College of Surgeons

    b. The Joint Commission

    c. National Committee for Quality Assurance

    d. Association for Healthcare Documentation Integrity

6. True/False: The health record is limited to a patient's acute care health information.

7. True/False: An advantage of an electronic health record (EHR) is accessibility by multiple healthcare providers.

8. True/False: The second step in the workflow of an EHR is that the patient checks in using a self-service computer, verifies demographics and insurance information, and makes updates and changes to their record.

9. True/False: Abbreviations and acronyms are often used in the medical record. The abbreviation for "by mouth" is *p.o.*

10. True/False: An ambulatory care setting is where the patient stays longer than 24 hours.

Go on the Record

To build on your understanding of the topics in this chapter, complete the following short-answer activities.

1. Discuss the importance of the workflow of paper health records and EHRs. Include in your discussion what would happen if a paper or electronic record missed a step in the workflow process.

2. Explain the purpose of the health record.

3. Compare and contrast the various accreditation, professional, and regulatory organizations involved in paper health records and EHRs.

4. Identify the four types of data found in the health record. Provide an example of each type of data.

5. Explain the concept of health record ownership.

6. How do EHRs change the day-to-day responsibilities if you are part of the health administrative staff?

7. How might your role evolve as more of your duties are electronically performed?

Navigate the Field

To gain practice in handling challenging situations in the workplace, consider the following real-world scenarios and identify how you would respond to each.

1. You are in charge of the medical records department. Your healthcare facility is preparing for a state department of health review, and you want to ensure that your facility's health records follow the suggested standards. There are several organizations that provide accreditation standards as well as guidance on the content and format of the health record. Select two of the following organizations and prepare a report on the importance of the organization: The Joint Commission, the National Committee for Quality Assurance, the Community Health Accreditation Program, the Accreditation Association for Ambulatory Health Care, the American Health Information Management Association, and the Association for Healthcare Documentation Integrity. After researching the two organizations, develop a checklist for reviewing your department's medical records based on the guidelines suggested by the two organizations.

2. As director of health information, you are in charge of training the new physicians and nurses on the official "Do Not Use" List of abbreviations developed by The Joint Commission. Prepare a summary document that the providers can use after the training session.

Think Critically

Continue to think critically about challenging concepts and complete the following activities.

1. Match the following description of the problem-oriented medical record with the SOAP format.

   a. Subjective

   b. Objective

   c. Assessment

   d. Plan

   _____ A. X-rays of the right hand will be ordered. If a fracture is seen, the patient will be referred to the orthopedic surgeon. The patient will be given a tetanus booster because he has not had one in the past 10 years. His wounds will be cleaned today, and antibiotic ointment and light bandages will be applied. He will be restricted from using his right hand at work for the next three days with no gripping. He will keep his wounds clean and watch for infection. He will follow up in the clinic in four days to reassess his injury and hopefully return back to full duty.

   _____ B. Mr. Smith is a 35-year-old man who was operating a cherry picker forklift today at work when he backed up and smashed his right hand in between the handle of his lift and a wooden pallet. He complains of pain in his second, third, and fourth fingers. He notes that his fingers are swollen and that they hurt when he tries to bend them. He has not noted any numbness in the fingers but says they are throbbing in pain. He also states that there are several cuts on his hand. He was seen by the company nurse who cleaned his wounds and put bandages on them. He was sent here by his company for evaluation.

   _____ C. VS BP 120/72 P74 Temp 98.7° F

   Right hand: The second, third, and fourth fingers are swollen from the PIP joints to the MCP joints. Bruising is present. ROM of the PIP joints is limited. There is normal ROM of the DIP and MCP joints. Extensor and flexor tendon strength is intact. Distal sensation is intact. Capillary refill is brisk. There are several abrasions noted on each finger. The remainder of the hand and wrist is free of injury.

   _____ D. 1. Right hand contusion

   2. Abrasions right hand

2. A 56-year-old woman with sudden onset upper back pain presents to the emergency department. This is the patient's first visit to Northstar Medical Center. Use the sample medical record located in Appendix B to identify the components of the medical record.

   A. Demographic information—including the patient's name, address, and date of birth

    B. Contact information—home, work, and cell phone numbers and email address

    C. History and physical—health history, review of vital signs, and complete organ-specific physical examination

    D. Problem list—list of current health issues

    E. Allergy list—list of medications, food, and other items, if any, to which a patient is allergic

    F. Prescription list—list of current medications, including dosages

Make Your Case

Consider the scenario and then complete the following project.

This chapter illustrated how Hurricane Katrina affected medical records. Dig deeper into this topic by locating five reputable websites that discuss the impact of the hurricane on the medical records of local citizens. Read and consider the information carefully. Then create a preparedness plan that would prevent a loss of medical information in a future catastrophe.

Explore the Technology

To expand your mastery of EHRs, explore the technology by completing the following online activities.

1. Conduct an internet search for patient registration/admission forms at two acute and two ambulatory care facilities. Identify and explain the registration/admission process at each type of facility. Is the patient required to complete the forms before the admission/visit? If so, are there forms the patient downloads and completes? Does the patient register online? If so, how does the patient do this? Is there a patient portal that requires the patient to create an account? If so, are the instructions clear? What are the advantages and disadvantages of the system the care facility is using?

2. Research the three different formats of the health record. Explain the advantages and disadvantages of each type of format.

3. Locate three websites that provide information and resources on proper health record documentation. Do the three sources provide different guidelines for proper health record documentation? How are they similar and different?

4. Research why the NCVHS list of 42 core elements is important. How will the core elements affect the EHR?

Chapter **3** Introduction to Electronic Health Record Software

Field Notes

"Electronic prescribing has had a positive effect on the practice of pharmacy and the quality of care of patients. It allows healthcare providers to send prescriptions to the pharmacy more quickly, meaning medications are ready for the patients when they arrive at the pharmacy, reducing their wait time. Electronic prescribing also reduces medication errors, since handwriting is not a factor. Overall, electronic prescribing is improving patients' quality of care as well as their safety."

– Michelle Watters, PharmD, Pharmacist

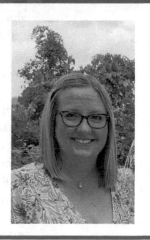

Learning Objectives

3.1 Understand the terms *input*, *output*, *processing*, *storage*, and *local area network*.

3.2 Explain the importance of backing up the EHR system.

3.3 Examine mobile features in an EHR system.

3.4 Describe the password and security measures of an EHR system.

3.5 Demonstrate how to navigate an EHR system.

3.6 Identify menu options in the EHR Navigator.

3.7 Examine charting features in the EHR Navigator.

3.8 Review the various scheduling features of the EHR Navigator.

3.9 Examine secure messaging, document management, laboratory integration, and e-prescribing features of the EHR Navigator.

An electronic health record (EHR) system manages all aspects of a patient visit, from the time a patient contacts the healthcare facility to the time the insurance and billing are both processed. This system can be accessed by healthcare personnel who work in an acute care setting as well as those individuals who work in an ambulatory care facility. As defined in Chapter 2, an acute care facility treats patients who have acute health issues that require inpatient care. An ambulatory care setting services outpatients, or patients who do not require admission to an acute care facility. There are many types of ambulatory care facilities, such as a physician's office, a hospital emergency department, a dental office, a surgery center, or a health clinic. An EHR system provides interoperability among various healthcare facilities, which allows the facilities to communicate with each other and view the patient's health record. To help you understand how an EHR system operates, you must become familiar with the system's features and have plenty of opportunities for practice. The EHR Navigator will help you do just that.

The EHR Navigator is a comprehensive EHR and practice management system that provides hands-on experience within a realistic EHR system. This practice software, accessed through your online course, provides you with the necessary skills to work in any EHR system you might encounter in either an acute care or ambulatory care setting. You will become

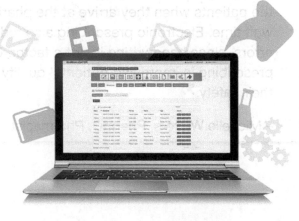

familiar with patient management, scheduling, medical charting, laboratory integrations, medical documents, e-prescribing, clinical collaboration, reporting, coding, and billing. You will also practice patient portal activities.

In addition to an overview of the user interface of the EHR system, this chapter examines security settings and requirements of a typical EHR system, discusses the importance of having a backup system, and discusses the hardware used in conjunction with EHR systems. As you progress through the chapter, you will have opportunities to explore the EHR Navigator and see how these concepts are applied in the software.

3.1 Information Processing Cycle

The **information processing cycle** provides the building blocks for the EHR system and includes four components: input, processing, output, and storage (see Figure 3.1). The information processing cycle converts data entered into the computer into valuable information for healthcare personnel.

The **input** component is the data entered by the user of an EHR system (e.g., the patient's first name, last name, identification number, and test results).

The **processing** component permits data to be usable by analyzing that data or comparing it against the same values of another data set, such as the patient's previous health data or a relevant patient population. For example, in an EHR, the processing component can determine whether entered test results are values within a critical or normal range.

The **output** component is the processed and organized data that provides meaningful information for the user. A report on a patient's laboratory test results is an example of an output in an EHR system. A healthcare provider may use the report to guide treatment decisions.

Storage is the fourth component of the information processing cycle. Patient information is stored so that it can be retrieved, added to, or modified for later use. There are various types of **storage devices** that an EHR system uses. EHR systems may be stored on a dedicated server at the healthcare facility or on a server provided by a vendor. If an EHR

Figure 3.1   Information Processing Cycle

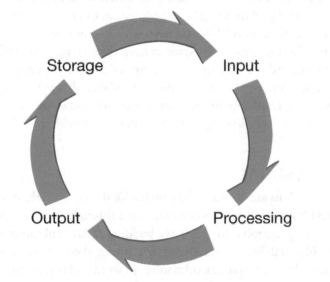

system is networked, then the storage may exist on the healthcare system's server. **Cloud storage** refers to virtual servers where data and the EHR system are backed up.

As technology continues to develop, EHR systems become easier to use. Internet and intranet technologies will allow you to access and share an EHR system in one building as well as in remote locations. This accessibility can be a liability, which is why an EHR system must be secure and accessed based on necessary functions to perform a specific job. As an additional security measure, the data entered into and extracted from the EHR system is encrypted to maintain security and protect patient privacy.

Hardware Support

An EHR system is most commonly accessed through a computer workstation. A typical **workstation** includes a computer and input and output devices. Healthcare

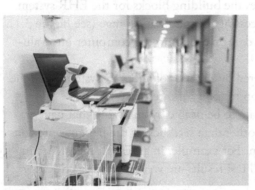

EHR systems are commonly accessed through a computer workstation.

providers may also be supplied with digital mobile devices not wired to a workstation. Both computer workstations and digital devices can be found in healthcare facilities today. An **input device**—such as a keyboard, mouse, scanner, microphone, camera, stylus, or touch screen—is used to enter data into an EHR system. An **output device**—such as a computer monitor, digital device screen, or printer—displays the results from EHRs. Because the printing functionality of an EHR is a security issue, healthcare staff members must adhere to their facilities' policy and procedure manuals for the permissible circumstances for printing a patient's health record.

EHR Accessibility

The expense of having a computer workstation in every service room may prevent providers from expanding an EHR system as widely as necessary for maximum efficiency. However, not having access to a workstation may cause a delay in updating and adding information to an EHR for other healthcare providers to view. One solution for this accessibility issue is the use of mobile and digital devices at an increased rate by all hospital workers. Mobile and digital devices will be explored later in this chapter.

Data may be entered into EHRs via keyboard, microphone, touch screen, or alternative input device. Some EHR systems have voice recognition software that will adapt to your voice and speech patterns and input data into the system. Electronic handwriting or touch screen input may also be available, depending on the EHR system design. Some EHR systems have templates that allow you to select text options from a drop-down menu, allowing standard data to be quickly added to the patient's record.

Network Systems

Computer workstations are networked through a local area network. A **local area network (LAN)** is a group of computers connected through a network confined to a single area or small geographic area such as a building or hospital campus. The network is secure and reliable, enabling safe transfer of data among the workstations. The networked computer system allows computer workstations to work and communicate together.

Figure 3.2 Network System

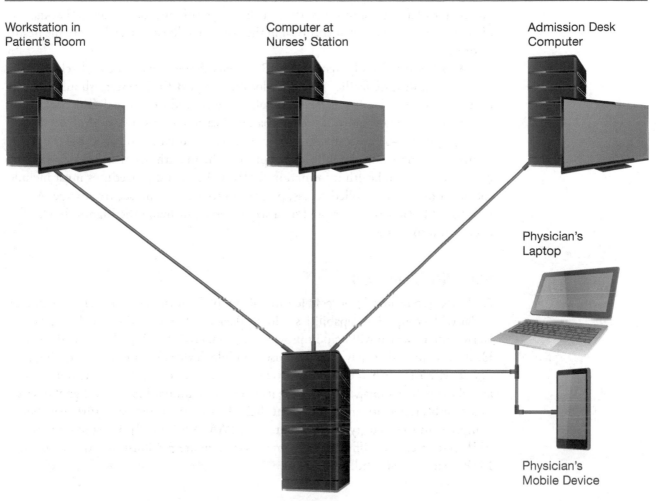

Workstation in
Patient's Room

Computer at
Nurses' Station

Admission Desk
Computer

Physician's
Laptop

Physician's
Mobile Device

Hospital Server

The network should provide a great deal of flexibility and should be adaptable to new technologies, such as fiber-optic cables, new software, and wireless communication. The LAN utilizes a dedicated server for the workstations. The network is connected through either wired or wireless connections. The advantage of a wireless connection is that the healthcare provider may be anywhere and still have access to an EHR system. Figure 3.2 shows a visual representation of a network system.

A **wide area network (WAN)** is a network that covers a broader area than a LAN. It is a computer network that spans regions, countries, or the world. As health care becomes more global and interoperable, more WANs will be used to connect the LANs of separate healthcare facilities.

3.2 Backing Up and Accessing EHR Systems

EHR systems can be web based or locally installed. Regardless, the EHR system data belongs to the healthcare facility. If the healthcare facility decides to switch from a web-based to a locally installed EHR system, the data may be exported from a cloud-based server into the local EHR system.

Backup System

No matter what type of server is used, the EHR system must have a secure backup plan. This contingency plan is critical in the event of a disaster that destroys the health records.

Web-based or locally installed EHR systems should have a secure backup system. A healthcare facility that has a locally installed EHR system should have its backup plan recorded in the facility's policy and procedure manual. The backup system must provide an exact copy of patient health records. Depending on the backup system—be it on site, magnetic storage, cloud based, or off site—the same security measures must be followed to prevent the unauthorized access or release of patient's protected health information (PHI). Policies and procedures must include specifications for controlled access, password protection, and secure storage. A web-based EHR system is stored on a secure server, utilizing the highest levels of encryption software.

Mobile Devices

An EHR system may be accessible through a mobile device such as a smartphone or tablet with computing capabilities. Mobile devices allow you to remotely access the EHR system, which will help improve your productivity and quality of patient care. Healthcare providers may choose to use a mobile device because they can bring the device with them when caring for patients. These easy-to-use devices help inform and show patients images such as the location of an injury. However, digital devices in a healthcare facility are not without their challenges; you must ensure that they comply with the security requirements of HIPAA. Additionally, integration with the EHR system can be difficult with some devices. Figure 3.3 illustrates the use of an EHR system on an iPad.

Figure 3.3 Patient Tracker on iPad
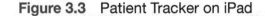

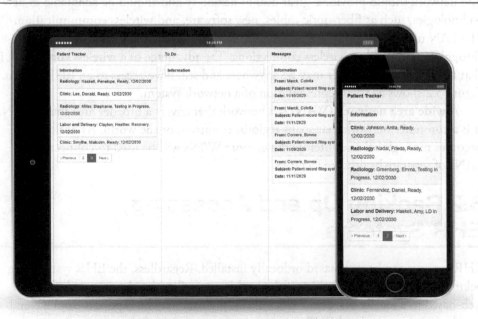

Consider This

Mobile health (mHealth) technology played a role in treating patients impacted by the coronavirus pandemic. mHealth technologies include wearable sensors, digital contact tracing, and electronic patient outcomes screening systems. This technology can be used to monitor patient's symptoms, including temperature, heart rate, and oxygen saturation. Using mHealth can allow healthcare providers to intervene at the appropriate time and monitor patients after discharge. mHealth also helped healthcare providers track and monitor patient conditions to prevent the healthcare organization from becoming overwhelmed. Review the study on using mHealth technology to mitigate the effects of the coronavirus pandemic at https://EHR3.ParadigmEducation.com/mHealthStudy and the study by Fitbit that found that wearable devices could detect nearly 50% of those infected by COVID one day before the onset of symptoms at https://EHR3.ParadigmEducation.com/FitbitStudy.

CHECKPOINT 3.1

1. Name the four components of the information processing cycle.

   a. _____

   b. _____

   c. _____

   d. _____

2. Explain how a LAN affects the use of an EHR system.

   _____

   _____

   _____

   _____

3.3 Privacy and Security in the EHR System

The privacy and security settings of an EHR system must conform to Health Insurance Portability and Accountability Act of 1996 (HIPAA) regulations. (For more information on HIPAA regulations, refer to Chapter 6.) These settings include the use of passwords and user permissions.

Password Protection

An EHR system must allow acute and ambulatory care facilities to create, change, and safeguard passwords. Facilities must have policies and procedures in place for managing these passwords. Typically, passwords are six to eight characters long, with a combination of alphanumeric characters, and typically contain at least one uppercase letter. When you enter your password, characters appear as dots, asterisks, or other symbols, thus preventing other users from seeing the password. Generally, you must change your password every 90–120 days. In addition to using a password to enter the system, specific areas of an EHR system may also be password protected to maintain

ON THE JOB

A six-character password takes a hacker about 10 minutes to crack, and the most common passwords are *123456* or *password*. To ensure security, passwords in an EHR system should include an uppercase letter, two numerical digits, and one special character.

the privacy and security of patient health records. The password is encrypted in the transmittal process between your workstation and an EHR system. An audit manager or administrator records the user log-ins and log-outs to monitor use of the EHR system. EHR systems allow for backend auditing so there is an objective record available that indicates all users who have accessed a patient's chart. Audit records can be reproduced to address access issues or HIPAA noncompliance.

When you first log in to an EHR system, you key in a default password, then follow the prompts to change your password. Typically, you can attempt to log in three times before being locked out and required to reset the password with the help of the administrator or information technology (IT) manager at the facility.

User Permissions

An EHR contains a patient's protected health information (PHI). *PHI* is any personal health information that may identify an individual, that was created, used, or disclosed during a healthcare visit that may include diagnoses, healthcare services provided, treatments, and/or payments for services. HIPAA rules mandate PHI protections, therefore, if you are an employee of an acute care or ambulatory care facility, you must have a unique username that registers your identity and tracks your activity in an EHR system. Each user's access to information is based on the type of information they will need to view or modify. Therefore, users are assigned access according to their job functions (e.g., healthcare provider, nurse, health information professional, or registrar). For example, a registration or an admission clerk may not have access to a patient's x-rays but would have access to the patient's insurance information. This assigned access ensures the security and confidentiality of patient records. Figure 3.4 illustrates how an administrator can assign you permission to access various areas of an EHR system based on your job position.

Figure 3.4   Assign User Permissions

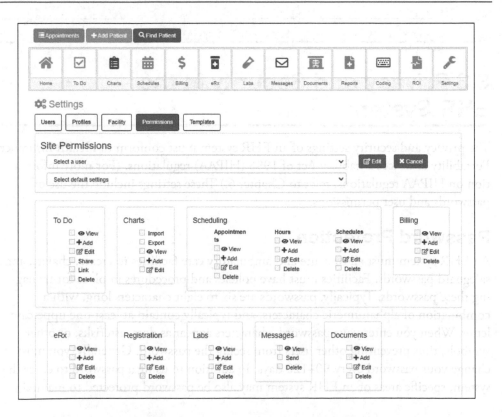

These permissions define the areas of the software in which a user may view, add, edit, or delete information. For example, a front desk clerk at an outpatient facility may see a screen similar to the one shown in Figure 3.5 when accessing the EHR Navigator. When admitting a patient, an admission clerk would view a screen similar to the one shown in Figure 3.6.

Figure 3.5   Home Screen—Outpatient

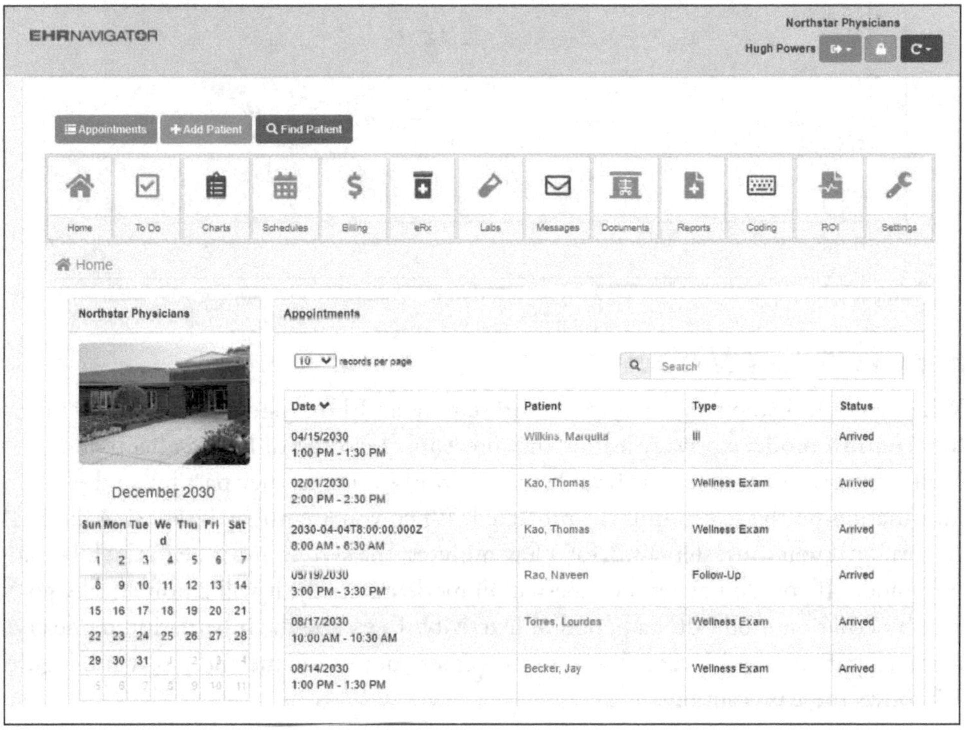

Figure 3.6   Patient Admission—Inpatient

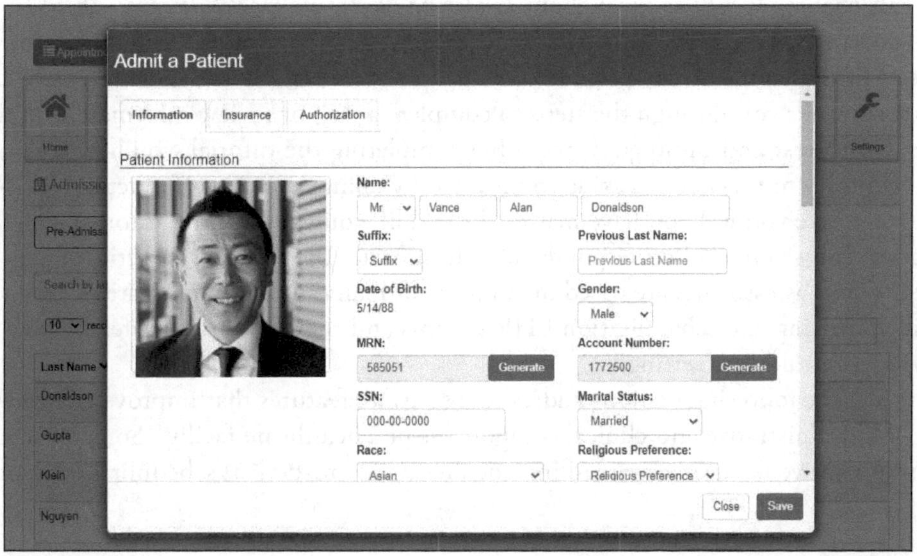

Figure 3.7 Log-in Prompt and Hibernation Mode

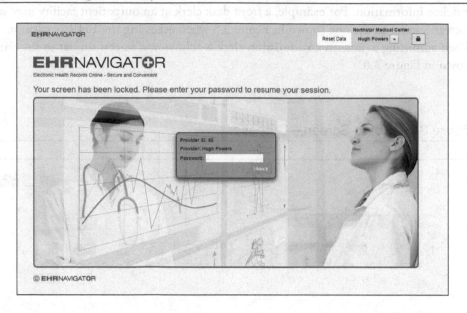

Hibernation Mode

When you must step away from your workstation, an EHR system should be set to **hibernation mode**, a privacy feature that prevents disclosure of PHI. Patients and healthcare providers alike may be able to see a workstation as they pass by, so the information on the screen must be protected. When you are not actively using the EHR system, or if you must step away for a few minutes, the system must be in the hibernation mode. If you do not set the hibernation mode manually, it will automatically go into hibernation mode after a period of inactivity. To escape the hibernation mode and reopen a patient's health record, you must reenter your username and password. Figure 3.7 shows these precautions.

3.4 Accessing and Using the EHR Navigator

In this chapter as well as throughout *Exploring Electronic Health Records*, Third Edition, hands-on tutorials, practice assessments, and assessments using the web-based EHR Navigator will provide you with practical experience. Each interactive tutorial walks you through the steps to complete a task or review information in the EHR with text and audio guidance. After completing the tutorial, you have the opportunity to practice the skills you learned by taking a variety of practice assessments. Once you feel you have mastered the skill, you can take the automatically graded assessment that corresponds to each tutorial. The tutorials, practice assessments, and assessments are based on a review of many inpatient, outpatient, and skilled nursing and rehabilitation EHR systems and therefore are transferable to a variety of healthcare settings.

The following sections address the software features that improve efficiency in the administrative and clinical components of a healthcare facility. Some of the administrative features examined include messaging, to-do list, scheduling, patient management, billing, and coding. Several features that are used in a clinical setting are also discussed, including medical charting, clinical collaboration, results reporting, clinical decision support, and patient portals.

Capabilities of EHR Systems

The Office of the National Coordinator for Health Information Technology (ONC) has defined the capabilities that are necessary for the meaningful use of EHR technology. These capabilities were originally defined by the Certification Commission for Health Information Technology (CCHIT), the organization that was previously responsible for certifying EHR systems. These capabilities include functionality, interoperability, and security. **Functionality** is the ability to create and manage EHRs for all patients in a healthcare facility and includes the ability to automate workflow in a healthcare facility. **Interoperability** is the ability of an EHR system to exchange data with other sources of health information, including pharmacies, laboratories, and other healthcare providers. Interoperability is achieved through standards such as Health Level Seven International (HL7), which aims to facilitate sharing and transferring clinical information from one system to another. **Security** is the standard that prevents data loss and ensures that patient health information is private.

The EHR Navigator encompasses inpatient, outpatient, and skilled nursing and rehabilitation EHR systems. Within each menu are submenu options. Figure 3.8 illustrates the inpatient system, Northstar Medical Center. The outpatient system, Northstar Physicians, is shown in Figure 3.9, and the Northstar Skilled Nursing and Rehab system is shown in Figure 3.10.

Figure 3.8   EHR Overview—Inpatient

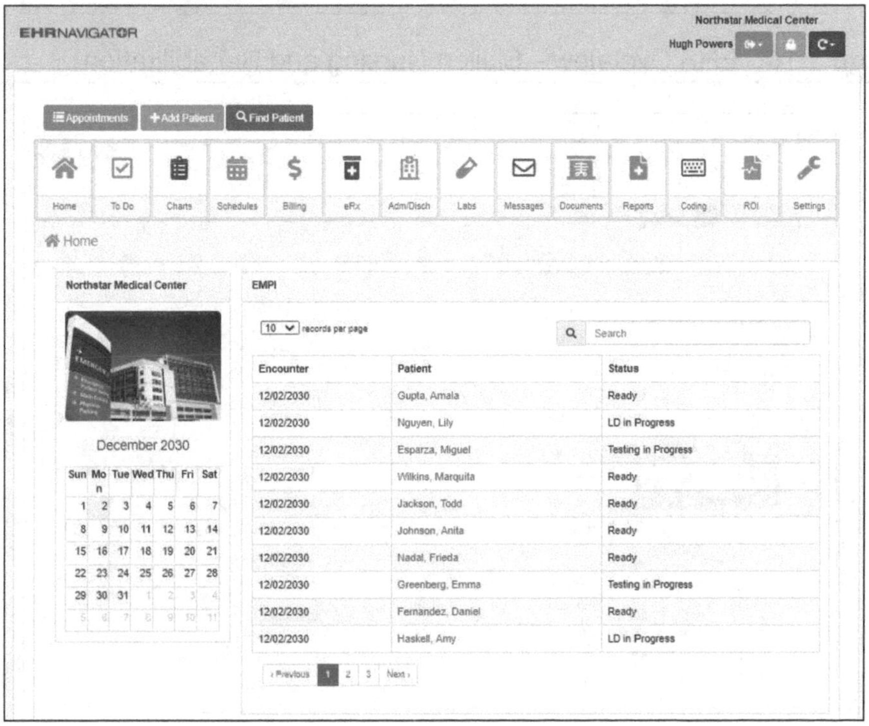

Figure 3.9   EHR Overview—Outpatient

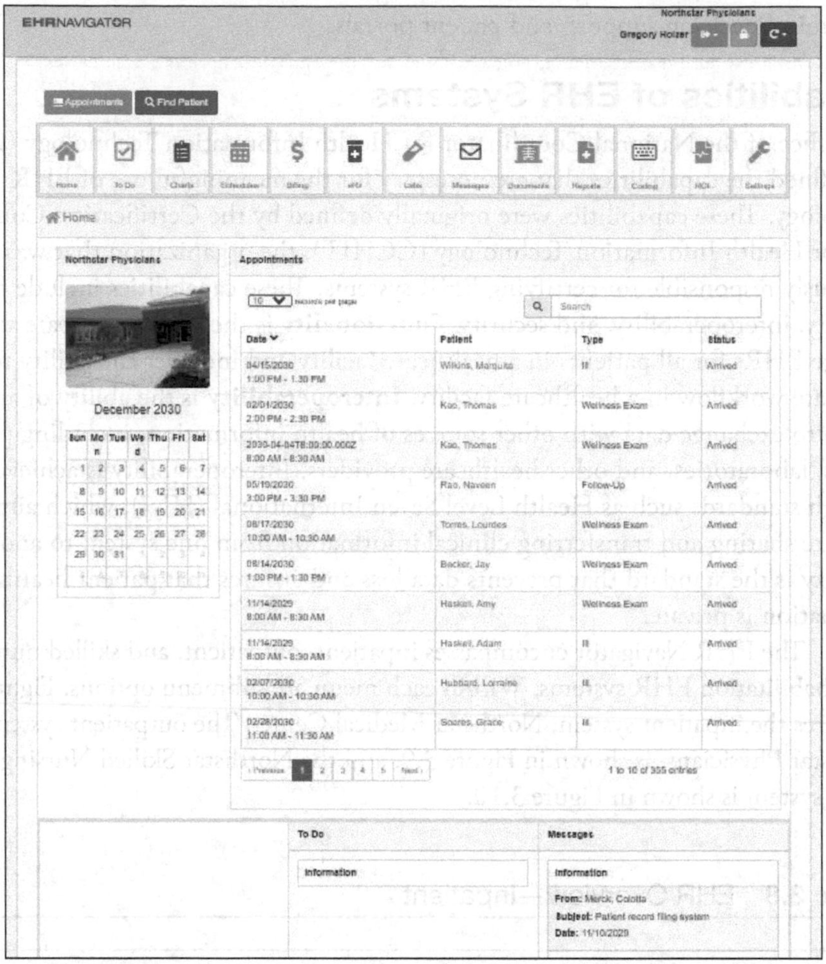

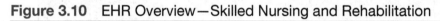

Figure 3.10   EHR Overview—Skilled Nursing and Rehabilitation

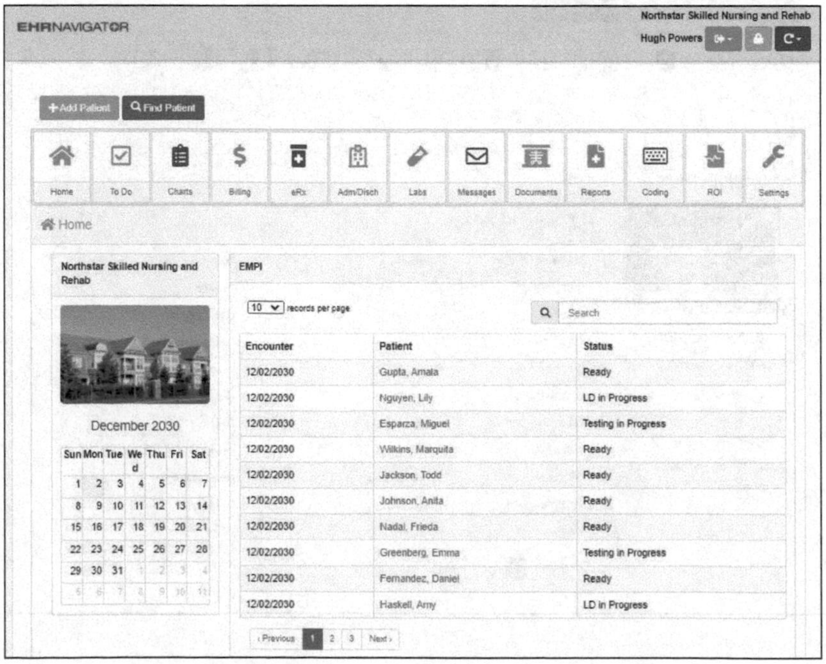

Figure 3.11   Menu—Inpatient

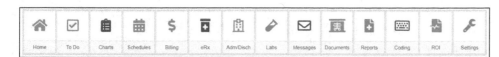

Figure 3.12   Menu—Outpatient

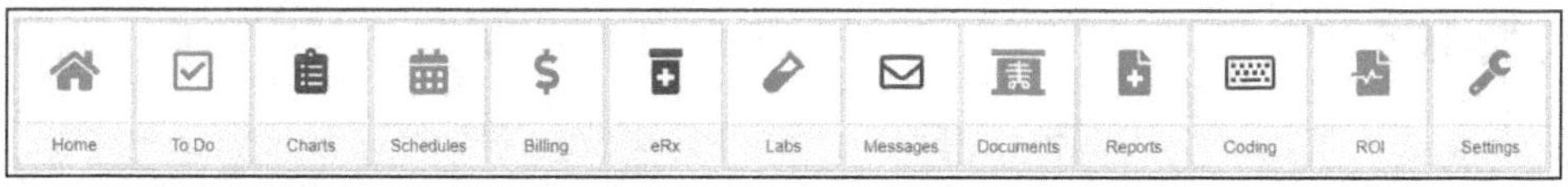

Figure 3.13   Menu—Skilled Nursing and Rehabilitation

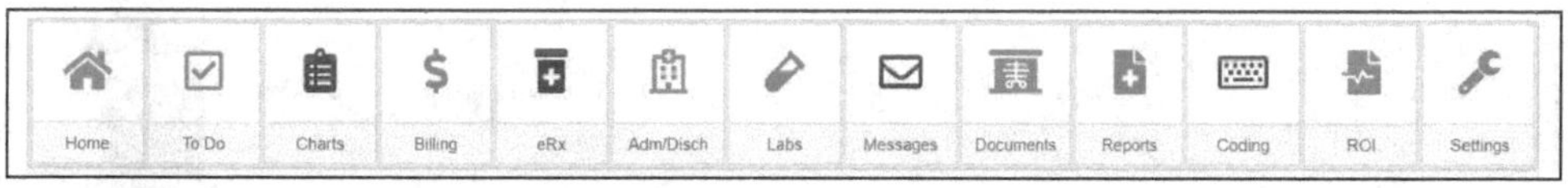

Menus

The menu bar is at the top of the screen. The options on the Northstar Medical Center menu bar are *Home, To Do, Charts, Schedules, Billing, eRx, Admission/Discharge, Labs, Messages, Documents, Reports, Coding, ROI* (release of information), and *Settings* (see Figure 3.11).

The options on the Northstar Physicians menu bar are *Home, To Do, Charts, Schedules, Billing, eRx, Labs, Messages, Documents, Reports, Coding, ROI,* and *Settings* (see Figure 3.12).

The options on the Northstar Skilled Nursing and Rehab menu bar are *Home, To Do, Charts, Billing, eRx, Admission/Discharge, Labs, Messages, Documents, Reports, Coding, ROI,* and *Settings* (see Figure 3.13). When you click each of the menu options, a list of functions appears below the menu option.

⚙ Settings

The EHR Navigator has a *Settings* feature that allows the healthcare facility to add users, edit facility information, grant user permissions, and customize features to meet the needs of the healthcare facility. Figure 3.14 illustrates the *Settings* feature for both inpatient and outpatient facilities.

Figure 3.14   Settings

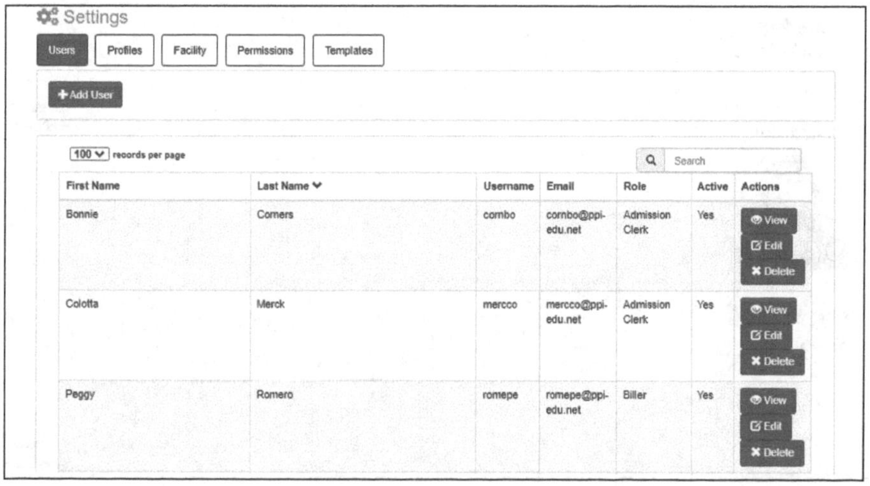

⚙ Settings

| Users | Profiles | Facility | Permissions | Templates |

+ Add User

100 ⌄ records per page   🔍 Search

First Name	Last Name ⌄	Username	Email	Role	Active	Actions
Bonnie	Corners	cornbo	cornbo@ppi-edu.net	Admission Clerk	Yes	👁 View / ✏ Edit / ✖ Delete
Colotta	Merck	mercco	mercco@ppi-edu.net	Admission Clerk	Yes	👁 View / ✏ Edit / ✖ Delete
Peggy	Romero	romepe	romepe@ppi-edu.net	Biller	Yes	👁 View / ✏ Edit / ✖ Delete

Figure 3.15   Users Submenu

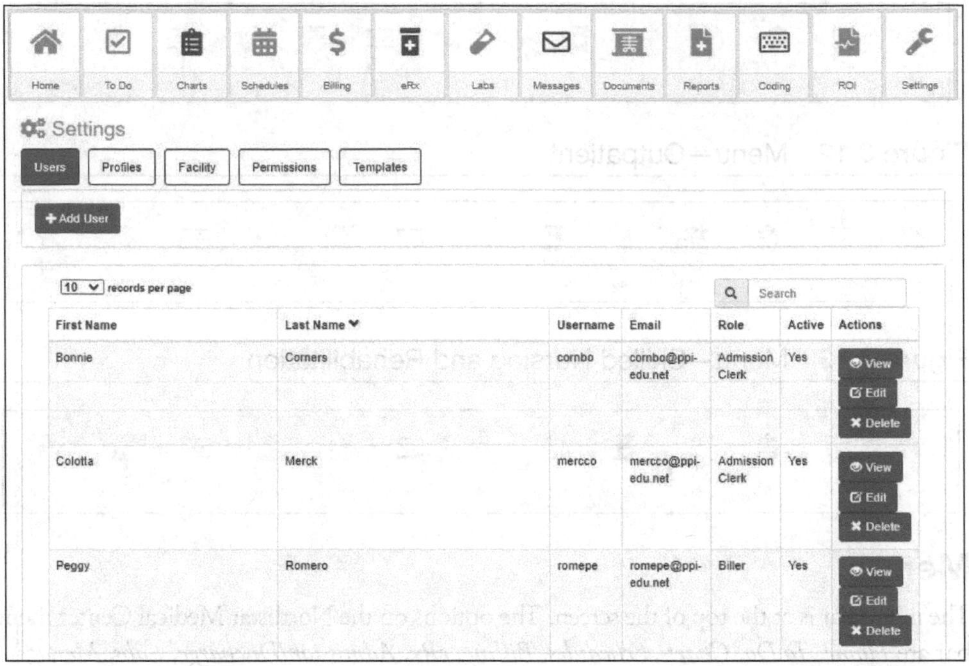

Users

In the *Users* submenu option, all users are listed along with their respective roles (e.g., physician, HIM professional, unit clerk, or pharmacist). This submenu is also where the EHR administrator or office manager can add or edit users (see Figure 3.15).

Profiles

By selecting *Profiles*, you may update your basic information (see Figure 3.16).

Figure 3.16   Profiles Submenu

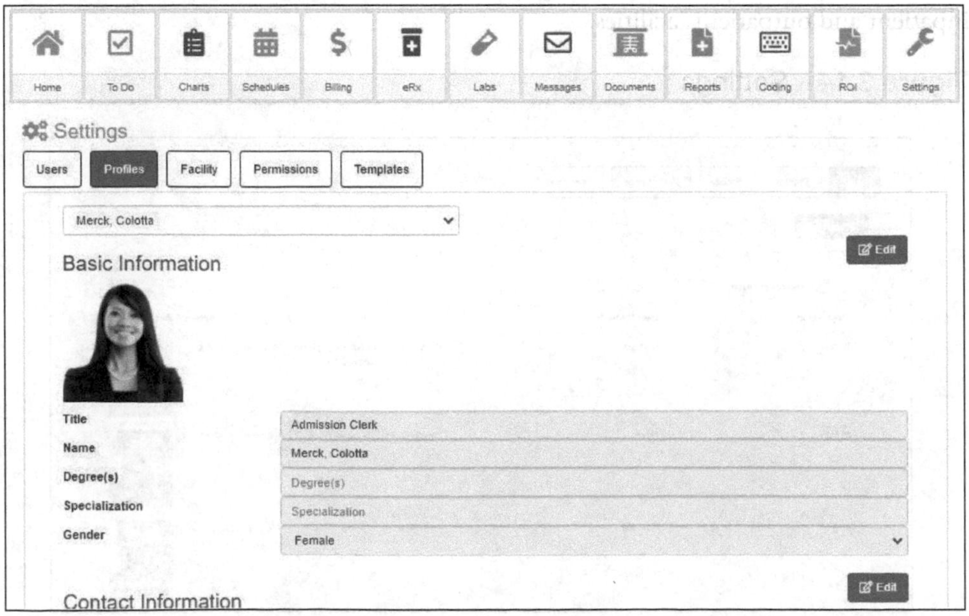

Facility

The *Facility* submenu of the EHR Navigator (see Figures 3.17 and 3.18) allows you to view basic information about the facility, including the following:

- Identifiers such as a National Provider Identifier (NPI); Employer Identification Number (EIN); and Medicare, Medicaid, and the TRICARE provider numbers

- Healthcare organizations list (details a list of related healthcare organizations)

- Payer list (details a list of payers)

Figure 3.17 Facility Submenu

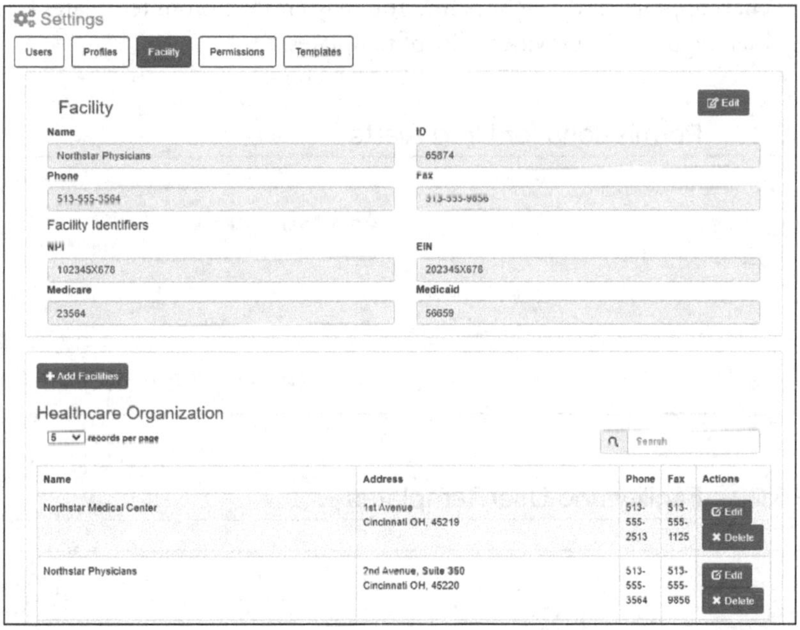

Figure 3.18 Facility Submenu (continued)

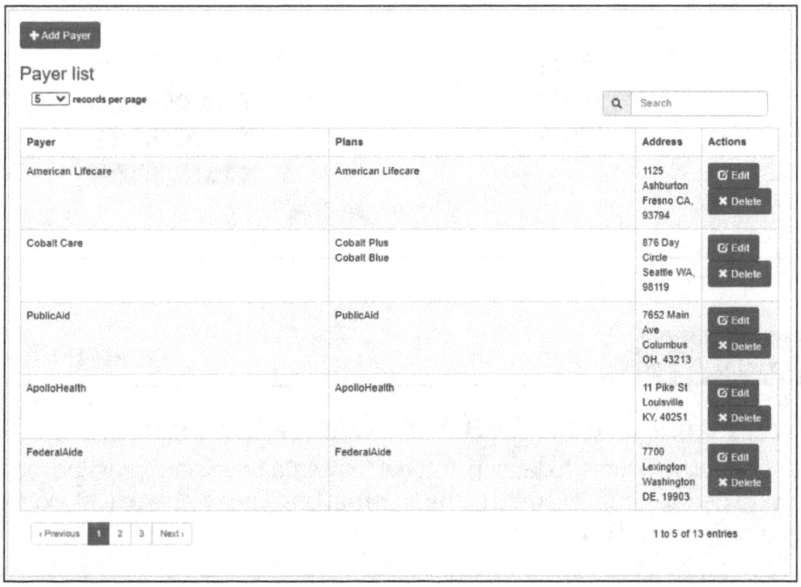

Permissions

The *Permissions* submenu in the EHR Navigator is where employee access to EHR functions is managed. Options to view, add, edit, and delete permissions are selected for each user. For example, all users are granted access to the *To Do* option on the *Users* menu, but only certain healthcare personnel that can order medications (e.g., physicians, physician assistants, nurse practitioners, and pharmacists) can override drug allergies. Figure 3.19 provides an example of how adjustments for permissions may be made to drug-drug and drug-allergy alerts.

Templates

The *Settings* menu allows you to manage charting templates. When you select *Templates*, facility templates appear on the left panel, and a list of templates you may like to use in a patient's chart appears on the right panel. You may create custom templates by selecting *Add Templates*. Figure 3.20 provides a list of templates.

Figure 3.19   Permissions for Drug Alerts

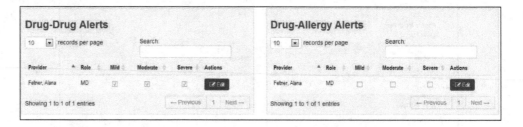

Figure 3.20   Facility and User Templates

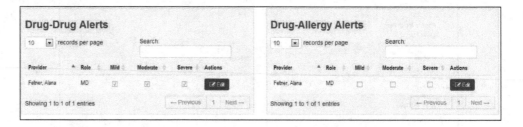

Tutorial 3.1   **EHR**NAVIGAT⊕R

Viewing Features in the EHR and Adding a Template

Go to your online course to launch Tutorial 3.1. As a physician, practice logging in, viewing permissions, examining the hibernation feature, and unlocking the system using the EHR Navigator.

Tutorial 3.2   **EHR**NAVIGAT⊕R

Adding a New Employee and Assigning Rights to the EHR
Go to your online course to launch Tutorial 3.2. As an IT administrator, practice adding a new employee and assigning rights using the EHR Navigator.

3.5 Administrative Features

The administrative features in the EHR Navigator include reports, messages, scheduling, billing, some charting information, and documents.

🏠 Home

On the *Home* menu, there are six areas: *Calendar*, *To Do*, *Appointments*, *Patient Tracker*, and *Messages* (see Figure 3.21). The *Calendar* provides quick access to specific dates, and the *To Do* section allows you to create reminders, prioritize activities, and organize lists to be more efficient and effective on the job. *Appointments* displays appointments for the current week, and *Patient Tracker* identifies a patient's physical location while they are in the facility. *Messages* is an internal communication tool for all users of the EHR Navigator.

Figure 3.21   Home Menu

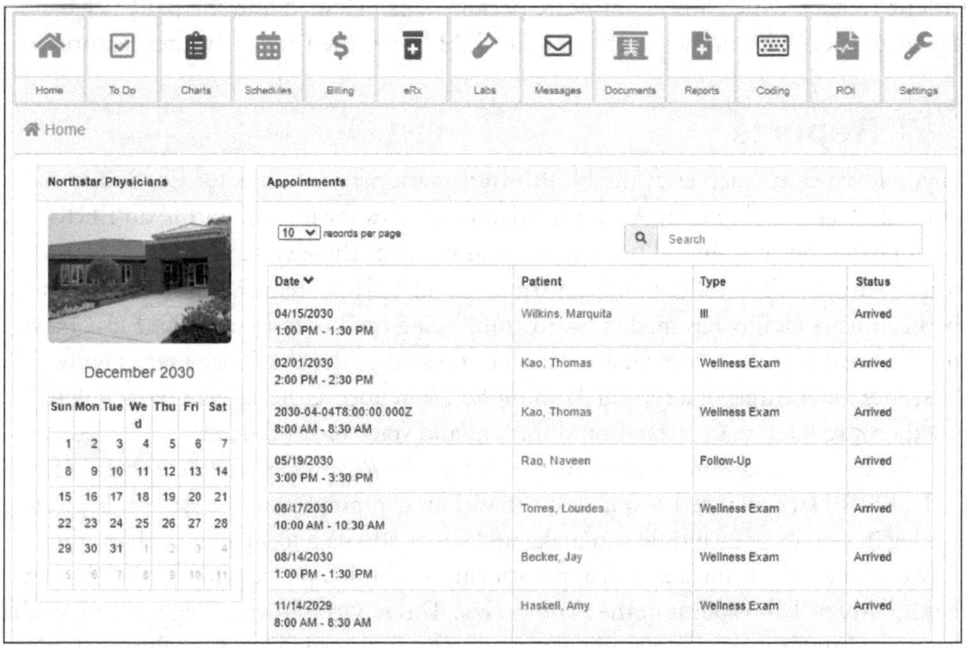

Figure 3.22   Patient Tracker Status

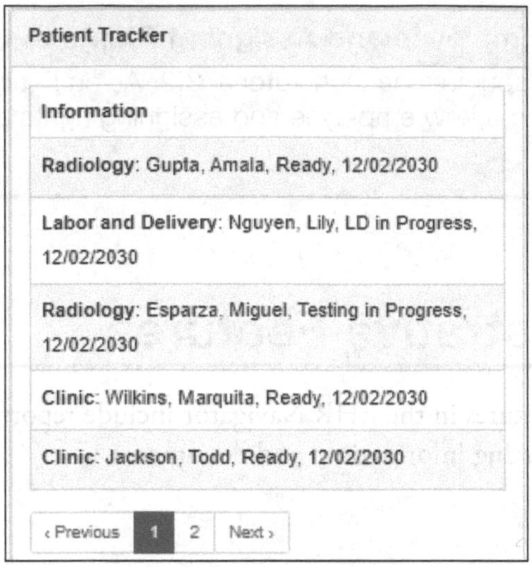

Patient Tracker

Information
Radiology: Gupta, Amala, Ready, 12/02/2030
Labor and Delivery: Nguyen, Lily, LD in Progress, 12/02/2030
Radiology: Esparza, Miguel, Testing in Progress, 12/02/2030
Clinic: Wilkins, Marquita, Ready, 12/02/2030
Clinic: Jackson, Todd, Ready, 12/02/2030

‹ Previous   1   2   Next ›

Patient Tracker

In the *Home* menu, *Appointments* area, a *Status* feature allows you to view the status of the patient. For instance, the patient status may change from *Scheduled* to *Arrived*, *No Show*, or *Canceled*. This allows the administrative staff to easily track patients.

Once a patient's status is changed to *Arrived*, the patient is displayed in the *Patient Tracker*. As the visit progresses and the patient is moved from room to room, the administrative staff or healthcare worker accompanying the patient updates the tracker to reflect the location and status. When the information is updated, it is reflected in the Patient Tracker, which other healthcare personnel can view to find the patient when it is time to meet with or move them. Figure 3.22 shows the Patient Tracker feature.

📁 Reports

As you learned in Chapter 1, the Health Information Technology for Economic and Clinical Health (HITECH) ACT provided incentives for implementing an EHR system based on meaningful use criteria, and many of these systems have a dashboard to track this use. Typically, an administrator of an EHR system monitors the progress the healthcare facility has made toward completing each criterion. In the EHR Navigator, the meaningful use information can be accessed under the *Reports* tab. Figure 3.23 illustrates an example of a typical *Meaningful Use* report. Criteria may be calculated based on provider, year, attestation duration, and start and end dates.

You can also access the *Activity Feed* report on the *Reports* tab. The *Activity Feed* feature in the EHR Navigator tracks your access to various components in the system. Each time you log in or out, or each time you make updates or add data to a patient's chart, the activity is tracked. If you create an appointment or submit a prescription to the pharmacy, that activity will also appear in the *Activity Feed*. This report, shown in Figure 3.24, enables the administrator to get a longitudinal view of actions occurring in the healthcare facility.

The *Reports* feature in the EHR Navigator allows users of Northstar Medical Center, Northstar Physicians, and Northstar Skilled Nursing and Rehabilitation to convert the facility's data into information that can be analyzed. Reports may be run on clinical data or administrative information, or by provider and

Figure 3.23   Meaningful Use Report

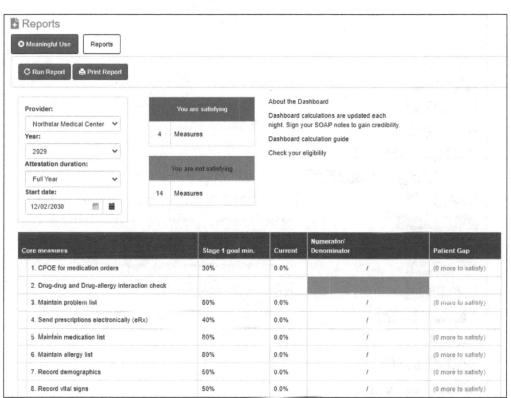

Core measures	Stage 1 goal min.	Current	Numerator/ Denominator	Patient Gap
1. CPOE for medication orders	30%	0.0%	/	(0 more to satisfy)
2. Drug-drug and Drug-allergy interaction check				
3. Maintain problem list	80%	0.0%	/	(0 more to satisfy)
4. Send prescriptions electronically (eRx)	40%	0.0%	/	
5. Maintain medication list	80%	0.0%	/	(0 more to satisfy)
6. Maintain allergy list	80%	0.0%	/	(0 more to satisfy)
7. Record demographics	50%	0.0%	/	(0 more to satisfy)
8. Record vital signs	50%	0.0%	/	(0 more to satisfy)

Figure 3.24   User Activity Report

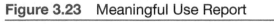

Provider	Activity	Date
Merck, Colotta	Scheduled Appointment	04/13/2030
Holzer, Gregory	Printed Document	02/27/2030
Corners, Bonnie	Printed Chart	04/12/2030
Romero, Peggy	Printed Bill	04/14/2030
Merck, Colotta	Logged Out	04/13/2030

Figure 3.25   List of Reports

Reports	
Title	**Description**
↻ Activity Feed	Displays the activities of logged in user or users
↻ Meaningful Use	Displays the Meaningful Use Dashboard
↻ Immunizations Due	Tracks the history of the patient's immunizations and screening tests
↻ Patient List Report	A list of patients generated grouped by specific conditions
↻ Canceled and No Show Appointments	
↻ Potential Duplicate Medical Record Number Assignment	A listing of Medical Record Numbers that may have been assigned to patients and need to be validated
↻ Remittance Advice	Displays the details about the provider's claims payment
↻ Diagnostic Test Report	This reports lists that patients that are more than one year past due on annual test/procedure
↻ Vaccine Effectiveness Report	
↻ Lab Values Report	This reports lists that patients with an abnormal HbA1C Test result with no FU HbA1C Test within 3 months
↻ Patient Aging Report	A patient's balance by age, date, and amount of last payment
↻ Billing Payment Status Report	Lists the status of all transactions with responsible insurance carriers who have paid and who have not been billed
↻ Day Sheet	
↻ Production by Provider Report	Incoming revenue for each provider
↻ Production by Procedure Report	Revenue for each procedure
↻ Production by Insurance Report	Revenue for each insurance carrier

date range. Figure 3.25 lists the various reports and descriptions available in the EHR Navigator.

The EHR Navigator *Reports* feature queries special reports based on particular criteria. An example of a query report might include generating a list of women aged 50 and older who have not yet scheduled mammography in the past year. Many of the reports will be covered in more depth in Chapter 11.

✉ Messages

The EHR Navigator messaging system allows you to communicate with other system users in your organization. Some EHR systems contain a HIPAA-compliant messaging feature that permits physicians, nurses, and other healthcare providers to communicate with medical colleagues outside their healthcare facilities. This feature is similar to a social media messaging system used to improve the collaboration and continuity of patient care.

The *Message* function allows you to send messages to patients, providers, and employees of the healthcare facilities using the EHR Navigator. The menu provides three options: *Inbox*, *Sent Messages*, and *Archived Messages*.

The *Inbox* lists messages received by the user or healthcare facility. Figure 3.26 illustrates the EHR Navigator Inbox. You may reply, forward, save, or delete messages. You may also send a new message, as illustrated in Figure 3.27. As shown in Figure 3.28, messages may be archived to allow you to document communication among healthcare providers, facilities, pharmacies, and the patient.

Figure 3.26   Messages—Inbox

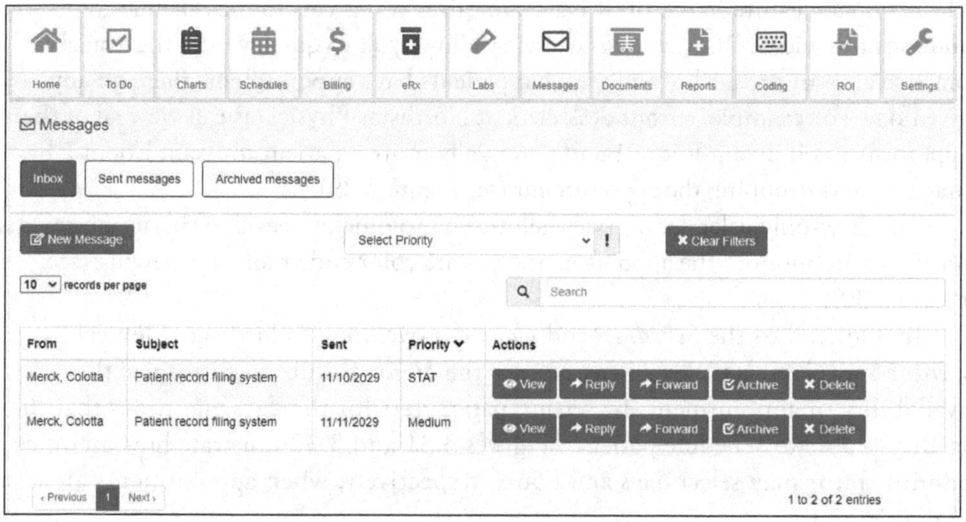

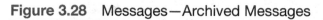

Figure 3.27   Messages—New Message

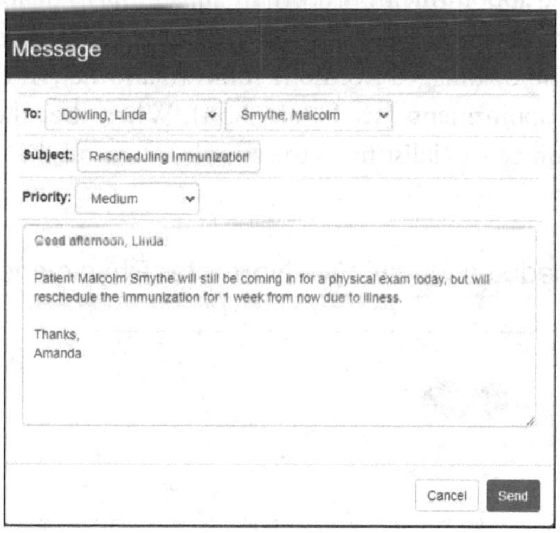

Figure 3.28   Messages—Archived Messages

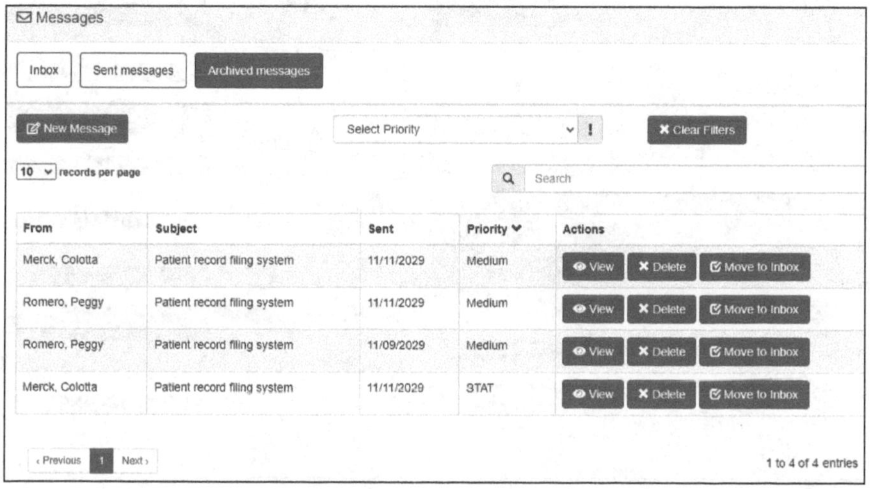

📅 Schedules

The *Schedules* feature in the EHR Navigator gives you access to the calendar in daily and monthly views. The *Schedules* overview allows you to quickly view the available practice areas at the facility and see what patients have appointments there on any given day. For example, a front desk clerk at Northstar Physicians can view all of the appointments in Exam Room 1 and potentially move a patient to Exam Room 2 by dragging and dropping the appointment (see Figure 3.29).

The view-only calendar overview allows you to quickly see all of the appointments for the entire month. The appointment types are color coded for easy viewing (see Figure 3.30).

In addition to the *Schedules* and *Calendar* overviews, Northstar Medical Center and Northstar Physicians can use the *Hours* feature to customize the availability of appointments by setting parameters for the days and times that the facility is able to schedule patients. Figures 3.31 and 3.32 illustrate how an office administrator may select days and hours, respectively, when appointments are available.

The *Schedules* tab is also where the medical office specialist adds and updates appointments. When adding an appointment, the user selects an available date, time slot, and room for the appointment. A *Schedule Appointment* dialog box opens, allowing the user to fill out the details of the patient appointment (see Figure 3.33). Appointments can also be dragged from one room to another, or they can be edited when you click the appointments (see Figure 3.34). When the scheduled patient arrives, the medical office specialist finds the appointment on the *Appointment List*.

Figure 3.29 Schedules Overview—Northstar Physicians

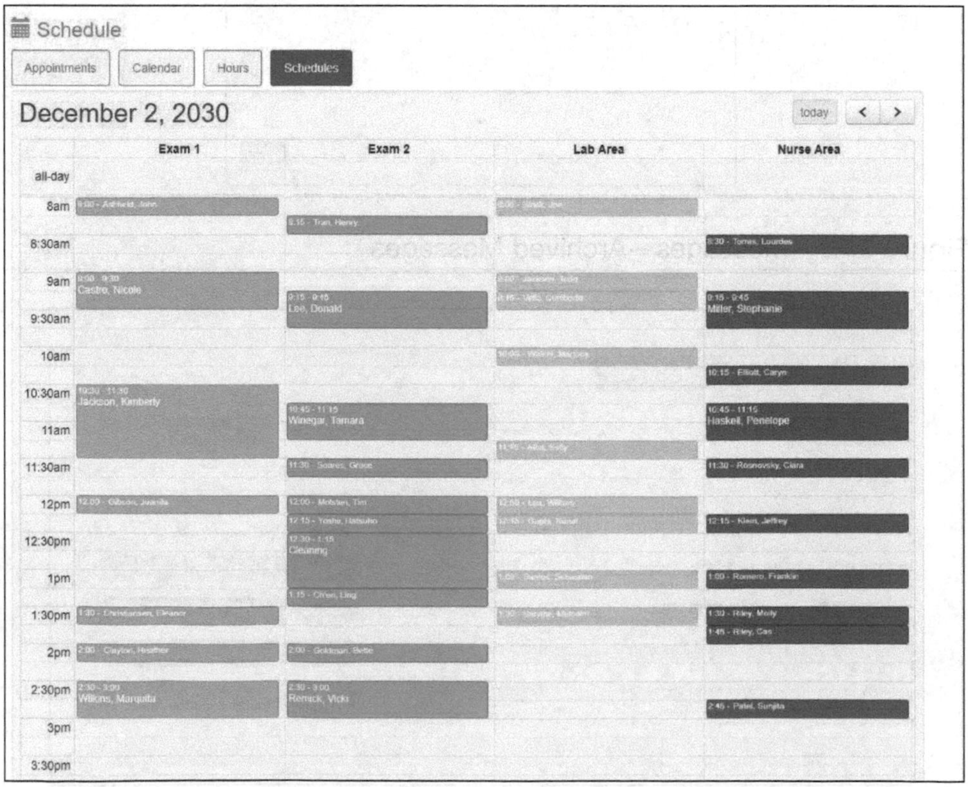

Figure 3.30   View Only Calendar—Northstar Physicians

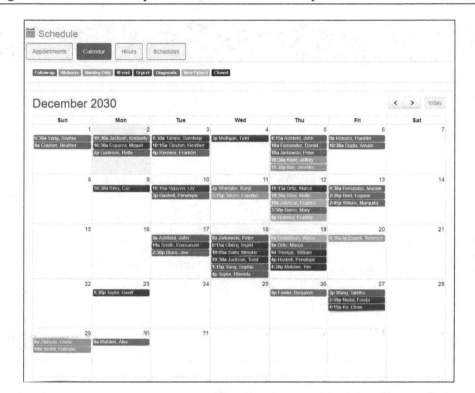

Figure 3.31   Facility Days and Hours

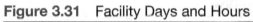

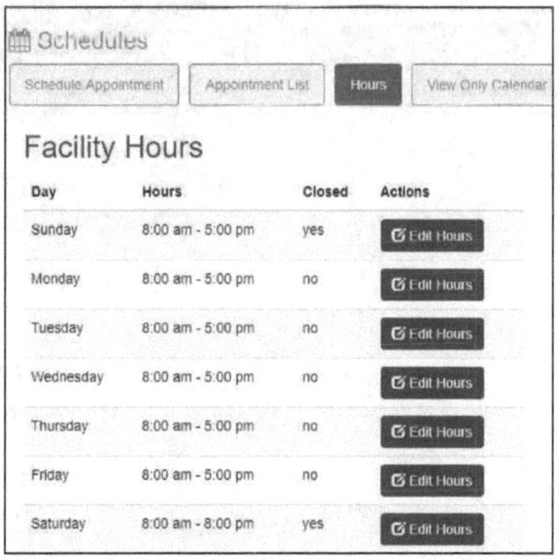

Facility Hours

Day	Hours	Closed	Actions
Sunday	8:00 am - 5:00 pm	yes	Edit Hours
Monday	8:00 am - 5:00 pm	no	Edit Hours
Tuesday	8:00 am - 5:00 pm	no	Edit Hours
Wednesday	8:00 am - 5:00 pm	no	Edit Hours
Thursday	8:00 am - 5:00 pm	no	Edit Hours
Friday	8:00 am - 5:00 pm	no	Edit Hours
Saturday	8:00 am - 8:00 pm	yes	Edit Hours

Figure 3.32   Customize Hours

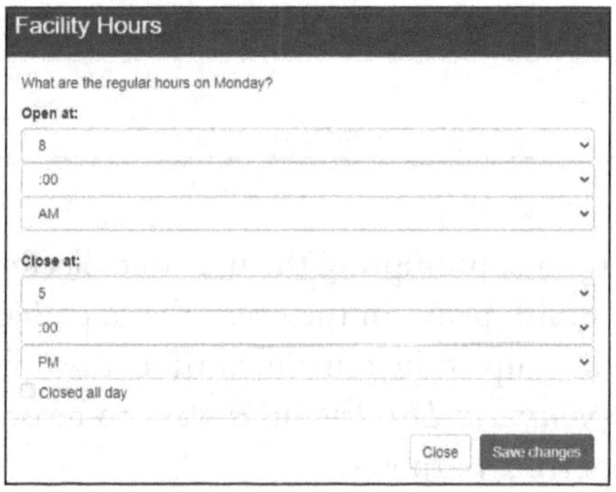

Facility Hours

What are the regular hours on Monday?

Open at:

8

:00

AM

Close at:

5

:00

PM

☐ Closed all day

Close   Save changes

Figure 3.33   Schedule Appointment Dialog Box

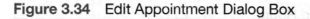

Schedule Appointment

Type		Date & Time
Appointment ▼		Dec 2, 2030 at 9:30 AM

Duration:

15m ▼

Provider:	Location:	Procedure:
Chaplin, Patrick ▼	Exam Room 2 ▼	Select procedure ▼

Patient:	Reason for Visit:	Preferred Contact:
Glazer, Aldjana ▼	Ill ▼	Cell Phone ▼

Notes:	Contact Information:
Patient has sore throat, possible strep.	513-555-7365

Cancel   Save

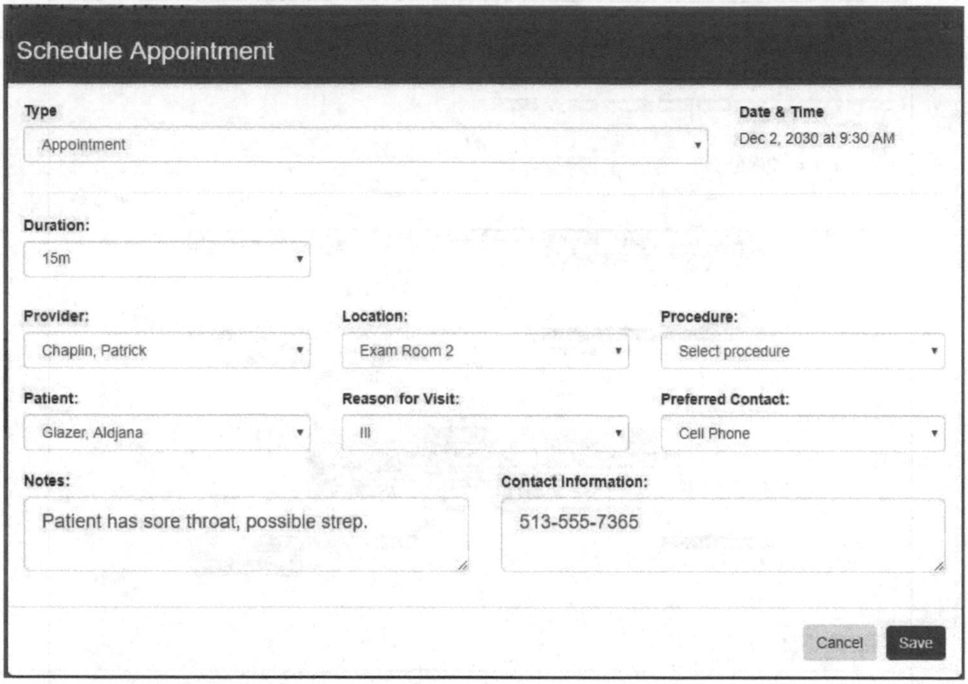

Figure 3.34   Edit Appointment Dialog Box

Edit Appointment:

Status:	Date:	Start Time:
Scheduled ▼	12/02/2030 📅	10 : 30 AM

Duration:

Time ▼

Provider:	Location:	Procedure:
Feltner, Alana ▼	Exam Room 1 ▼	Select procedure ▼

Patient:	Reason for Visit:	Preferred Contact:
	Follow-Up ▼	Home Phone ▼

Notes:	Contact Information:
	555-555-5555

Cancel   Save

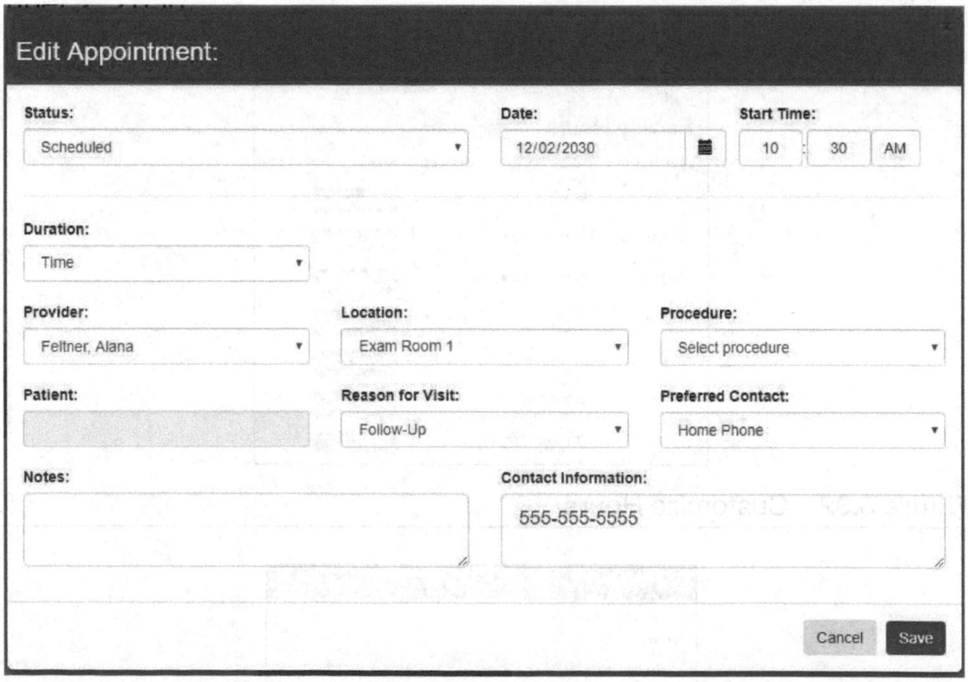

The Check In window appears, prompting the user to collect a copay amount if required by the patient's health plan. In the event that a patient has to cancel an appointment or fails to show up at the scheduled time, the office administrator can edit the status on the *Appointment List*. Facilities want to record cancellations and no-shows for practice reporting purposes.

$ Billing

Billing for treatment and services rendered is a main function of any healthcare organization. Figure 3.35 shows the main billing screen found in the EHR Navigator.

The main submenus of the *Billing* tab are *Electronic Superbill*, *Claims Management*, *Billed*, *Transmit Claims*, *Patient Bills*, *Patient Ledger*, and *Deposit Reports*.

On the *Electronic Superbill* submenu, a biller can view a superbill (a list of all charges relating to a patient visit), add charges, add payments, and add adjustments using the buttons in the *Actions* section. Figure 3.36 shows the *Add Superbill* dialog box.

Figure 3.35   Billing

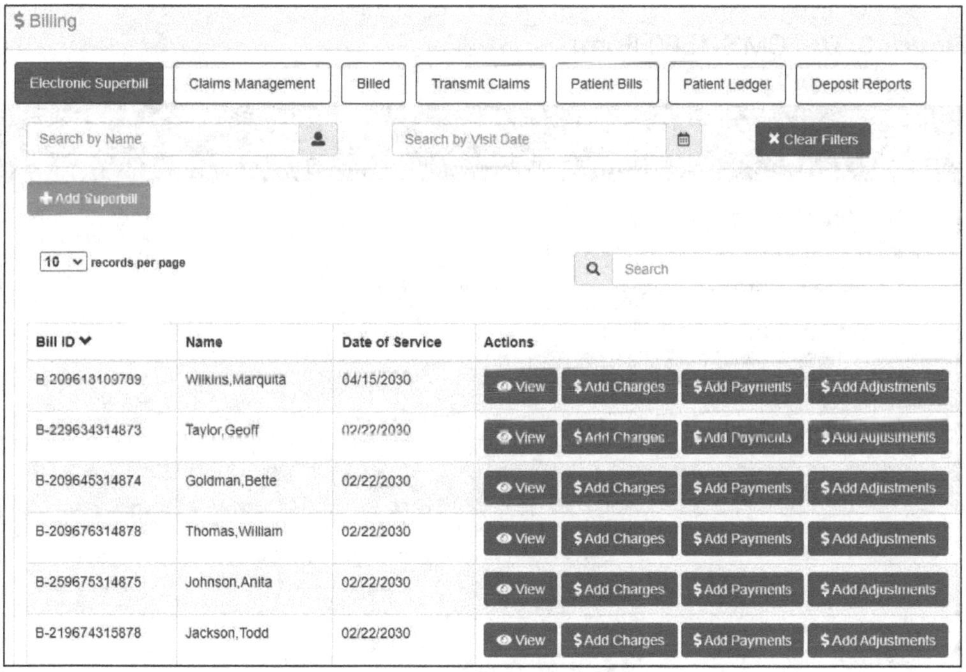

Figure 3.36   Add Superbill

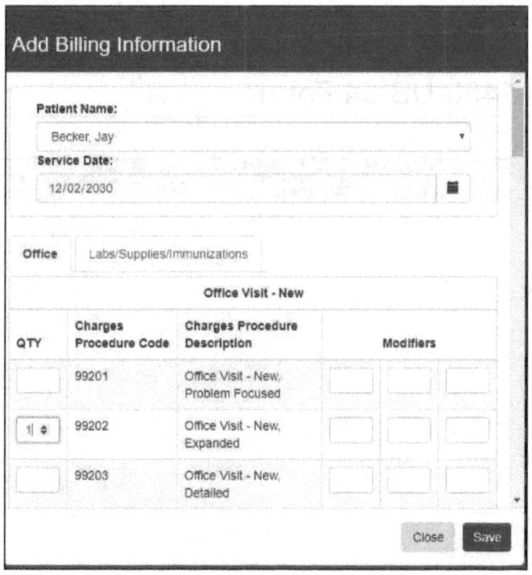

On the *Claims Management* submenu, a biller can view, edit, and bill for patient visits. You can also access the CMS-1500 form on this screen in Northstar Physicians and CMS-1450/UB-04 form in Northstar Medical Center. These are specialized billing forms that will be covered in more detail in Chapter 10. See Figures 3.37 and 3.38.

The *Billed* submenu shows the patient bills that have already been processed. The *Transmit Claims* submenu allows you to see the visits that are ready for review and transmit the claims (see Figure 3.39).

The *Patient Bills* submenu shows an archive of patient bills. The *Patient Ledger* submenu allows you to see a history of services, payments, and adjustments for a patient (see Figure 3.40).

You will experience the billing functions of the EHR Navigator in Chapter 10.

Figure 3.37   CMS-1500 Form

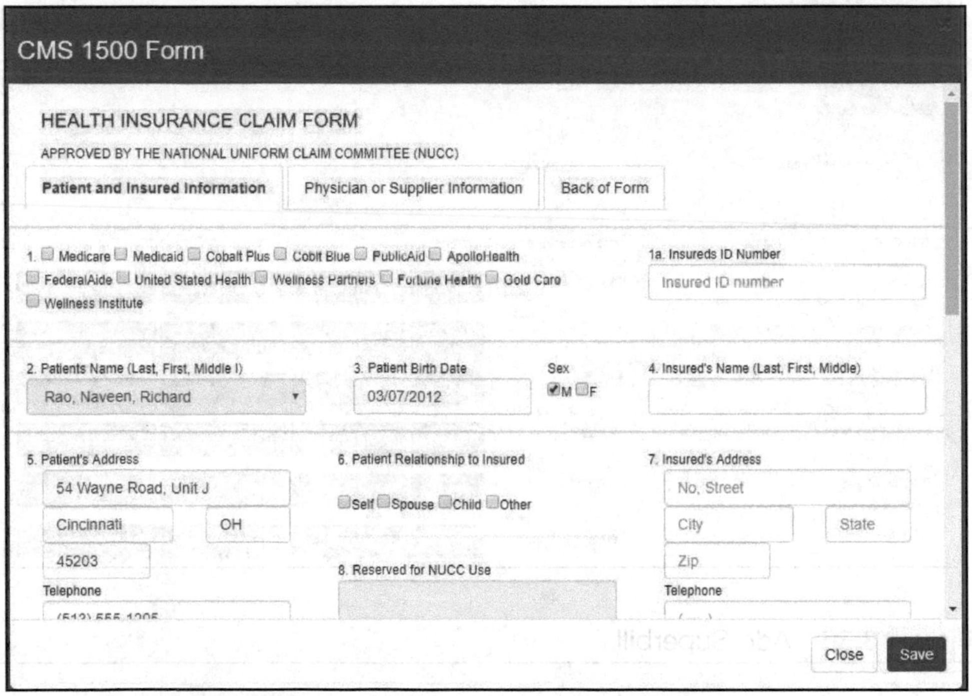

Figure 3.38   CMS-1450/UB-04 Form

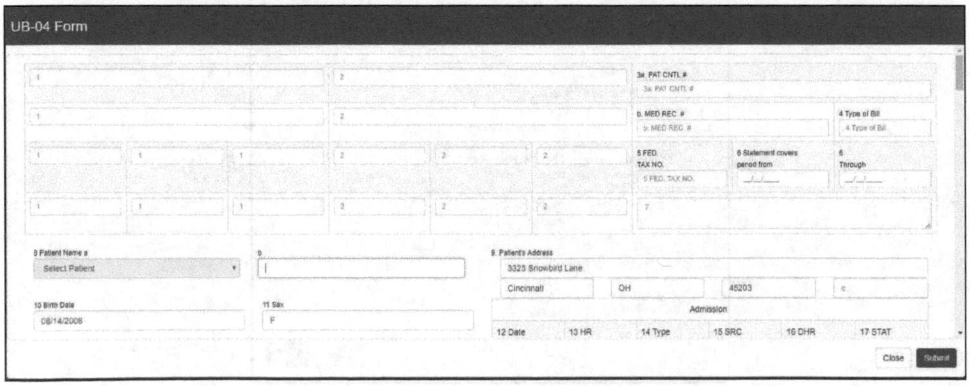

Figure 3.39   Transmit Claims

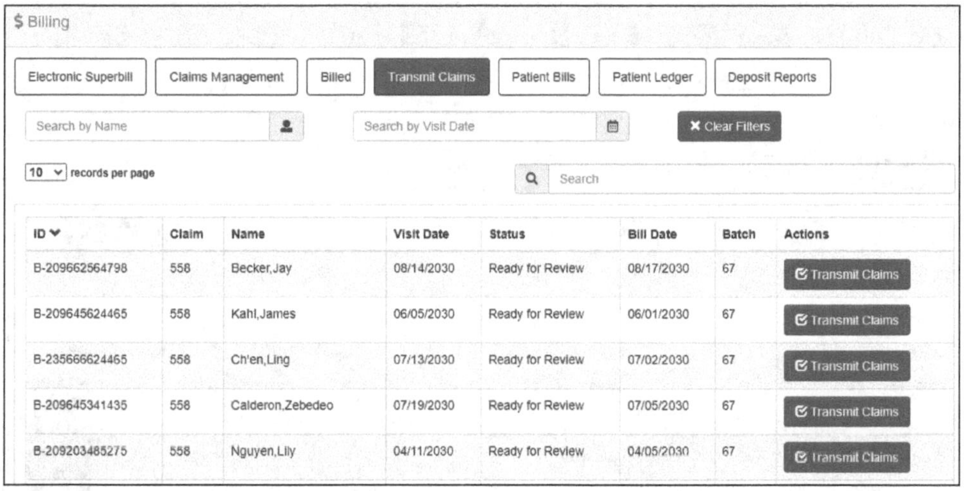

ID ∨	Claim	Name	Visit Date	Status	Bill Date	Batch	Actions
B-209662564798	558	Becker,Jay	08/14/2030	Ready for Review	08/17/2030	67	Transmit Claims
B-209645624465	558	Kahl,James	06/05/2030	Ready for Review	06/01/2030	67	Transmit Claims
B-235666624465	558	Ch'en,Ling	07/13/2030	Ready for Review	07/02/2030	67	Transmit Claims
B-209645341435	558	Calderon,Zebedeo	07/19/2030	Ready for Review	07/05/2030	67	Transmit Claims
B-209203485275	558	Nguyen,Lily	04/11/2030	Ready for Review	04/05/2030	67	Transmit Claims

Figure 3.40   Patient Ledger

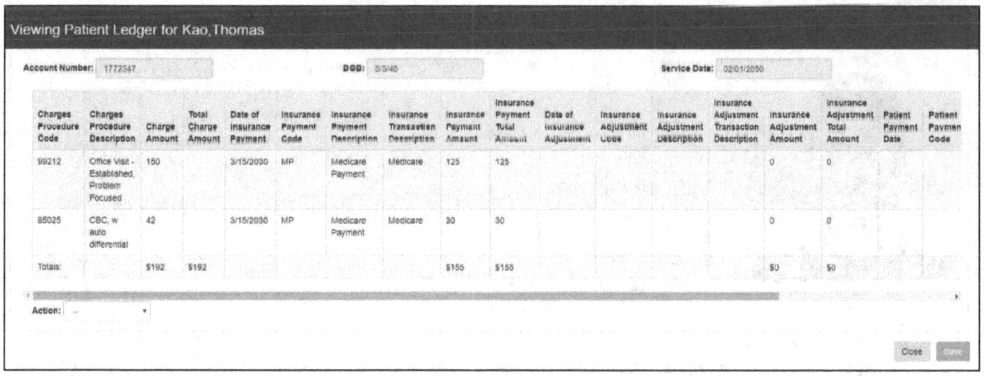

Viewing Patient Ledger for Kao,Thomas

Account Number: 1772547   DOB: 6/3/40   Service Date: 02/01/2030

Charges Procedure Code	Charges Procedure Description	Charge Amount	Total Charge Amount	Date of Insurance Payment	Insurance Payment Code	Insurance Payment Description	Insurance Transaction Description	Insurance Payment Amount	Insurance Payment Total Amount	Date of Insurance Adjustment	Insurance Adjustment Code	Insurance Adjustment Description	Insurance Adjustment Transaction Description	Insurance Adjustment Amount	Insurance Adjustment Total Amount	Patient Payment Date	Patient Payment Code
99212	Office Visit - Established, Problem Focused	150		3/15/2030	MP	Medicare Payment	Medicare	125	125							0	0
85025	CBC, w auto differential	42		3/15/2030	MP	Medicare Payment	Medicare	30	30							0	0
Totals:		$192	$192					$155	$155							$0	$0

Action: __

Close   Save

📋 Charts

The *Charts* feature in the EHR Navigator contains both administrative and clinical information. This section addresses only the administrative information; the clinical information will be discussed in the *Clinical Features* section. In the *Charts* feature, a list of patients treated at the healthcare facility appears. The user is able to find, filter, and add patients. The administrative features in the EHR Navigator contain patient demographics, insurance information, location, clinical information, and a list of appointments. Within the patient chart, the healthcare facility can enroll a patient in a personal health record, print a patient chart, send a referral or response letter, export a patient record, export an immunization registry, provide public health surveillance information, and update the patient's location and status via the Patient Tracker. Figures 3.41 and 3.42 provide examples of the patient list and patient chart found in the *Charts* feature.

Figure 3.41 Charts—List of Patients

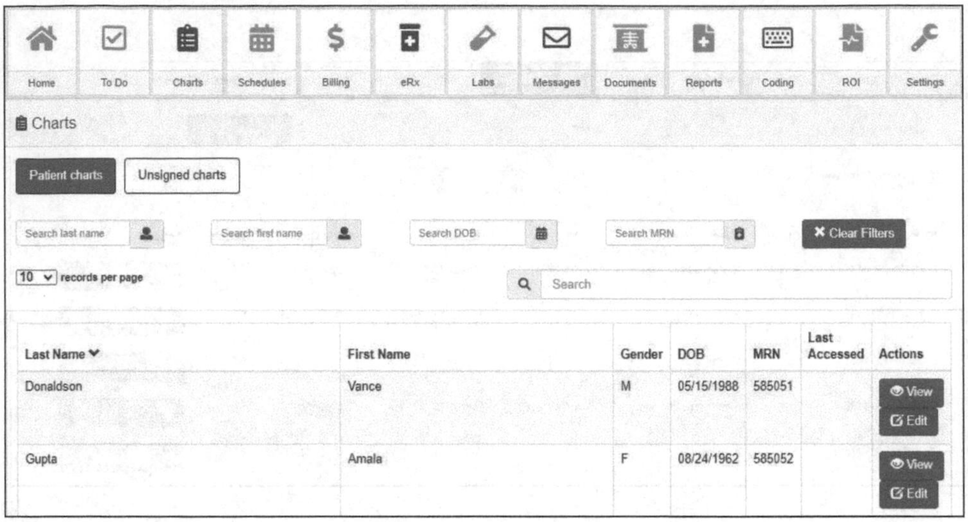

Figure 3.42 Charts—Patient Chart

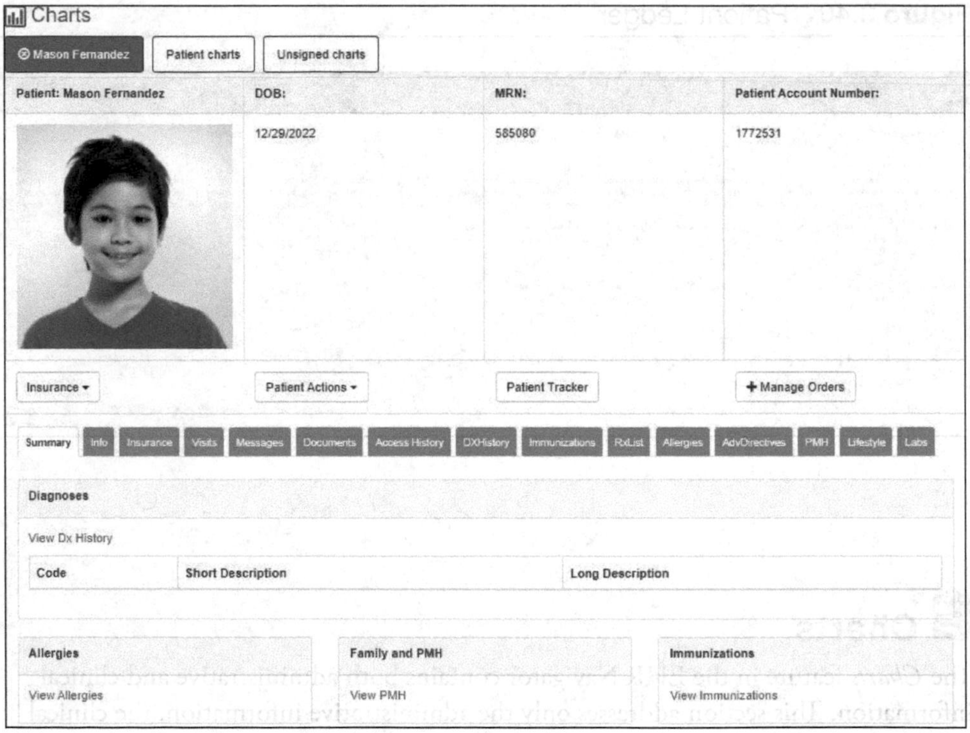

表 Documents

As part of the transition from paper to electronic records, paper documents may be scanned and saved in the EHR system as part of the patient record. To facilitate this, the EHR Navigator allows you to add documents from a predetermined list— Summary Report, Insurance Form, or a dictation—to a patient's chart. This action can be taken at the *Documents* tab or on the patient's chart. The system also allows you to make notations on a document before assigning the file to a patient's chart and to digitally sign documents. Figure 3.43 shows how to add a document.

Figure 3.43   Adding Documents

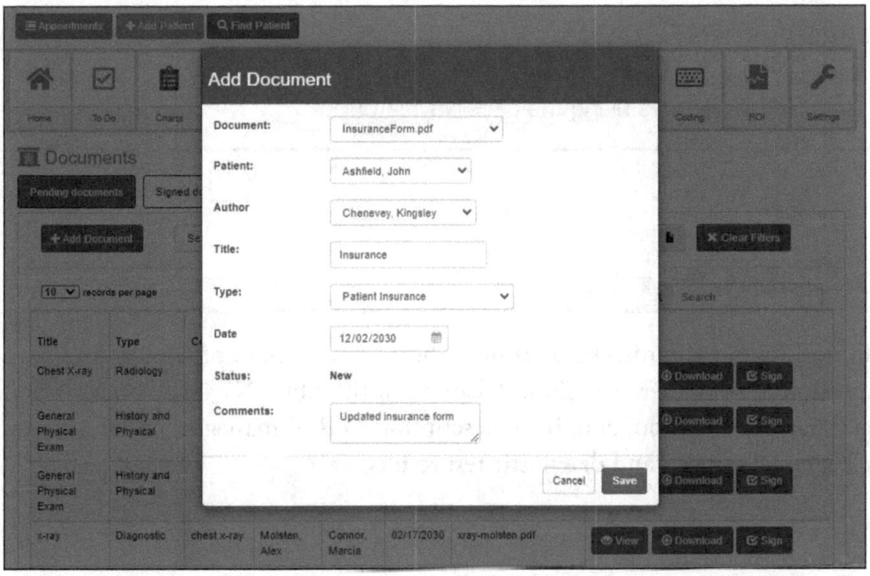

Figure 3.44   Pending Documents

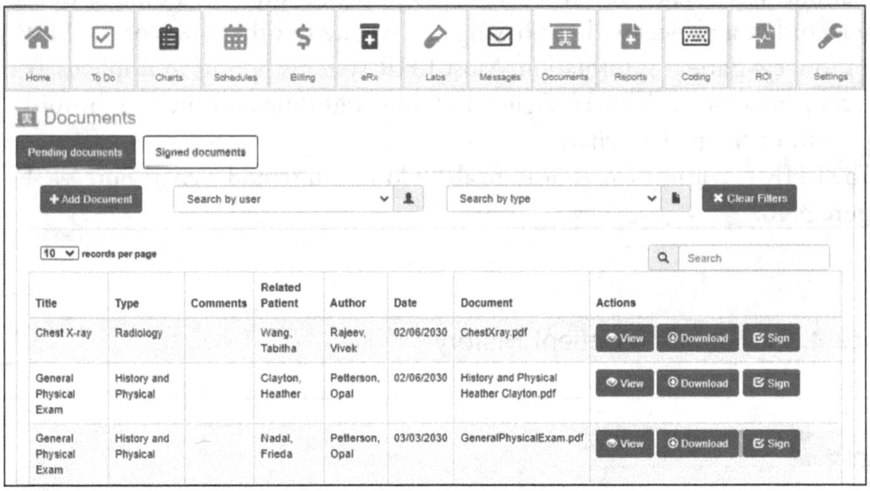

Documents can be viewed either as pending or signed, and they may be filtered by provider and document type. Figure 3.44 illustrates pending documents. For example, a pending document may be a physician order waiting for a doctor to authenticate.

CHECKPOINT 3.2

1. Explain why *Messages* is an important feature in an EHR system.

_____

_____

_____

2. Name two ways to view appointments in the *Schedules* tab.

a. _____

b. _____

Tutorial 3.3

Scheduling an Outpatient Appointment

Go to your online course to launch Tutorial 3.3. As a physician, practice the administrative features using the EHR Navigator.

3.6 Clinical Features

In addition to the administrative features, there are a number of clinical features available to an EHR user. The clinical features of the EHR Navigator include updating patient chart information, entering eprescriptions (eRx), managing physician orders, and viewing laboratory and diagnostic test results.

📋 Charts

The EHR Navigator *Charts* feature is the source for the patient's clinical data, including medical diagnoses, treatments, procedures, allergies, medical history, medications, test results, and reports. *Charts* provides you with a unique view of the entire record at a glance, without having to navigate to other areas of the EHR system to view patient information. Most EHR systems permit multiple users to have access to a patient's chart. Figure 3.45 illustrates the past medical history component of the patient chart.

The EHR Navigator *Charts* feature also allows you to add a chart note, as shown in Figure 3.46.

Figure 3.45   Charts—Patient History

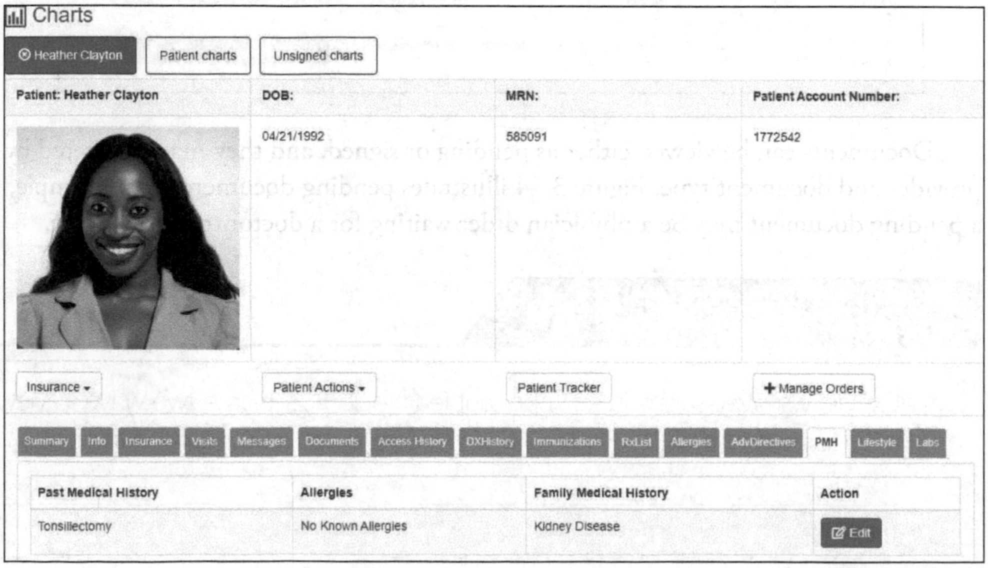

Past Medical History	Allergies	Family Medical History	Action
Tonsillectomy	No Known Allergies	Kidney Disease	Edit

Figure 3.46   Add Chart Note

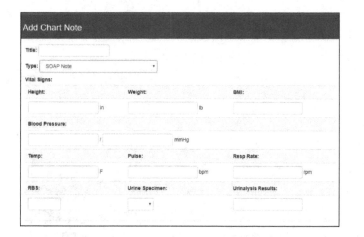

eRx

A typical EHR system has an electronic prescription (eRx) feature that enables the system to electronically submit prescriptions to pharmacies all across the United States. The use of e-prescribing helps to reduce medication errors, thus improving patient safety and increasing practice efficiency. An EHR system that integrates an e-prescribing function increases facility productivity and efficiency by allowing a healthcare provider to view the patient's medication history in the EHR rather than pulling a chart and writing a prescription by hand. Figure 3.47 shows the *eRx* screen in the EHR Navigator.

Figure 3.47   eRx

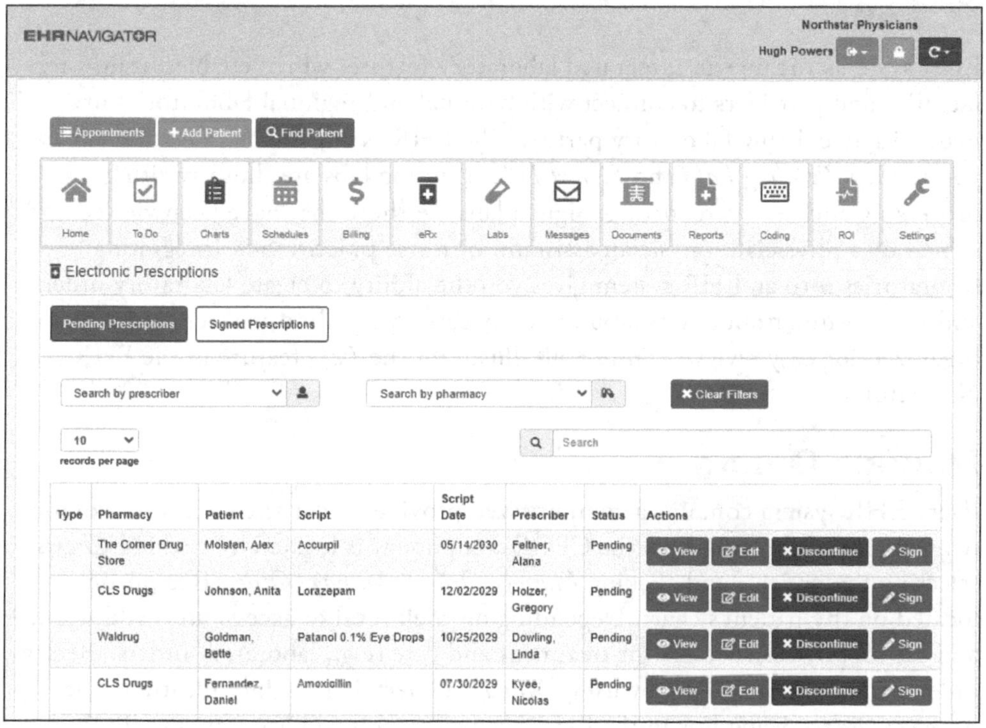

Type	Pharmacy	Patient	Script	Script Date	Prescriber	Status	Actions
	The Corner Drug Store	Molsten, Alex	Accurpil	05/14/2030	Feltner, Alana	Pending	View Edit Discontinue Sign
	CLS Drugs	Johnson, Anita	Lorazepam	12/02/2029	Holzer, Gregory	Pending	View Edit Discontinue Sign
	Waldrug	Goldman, Bette	Patanol 0.1% Eye Drops	10/25/2029	Dowling, Linda	Pending	View Edit Discontinue Sign
	CLS Drugs	Fernandez, Daniel	Amoxicillin	07/30/2029	Kyee, Nicolas	Pending	View Edit Discontinue Sign

Figure 3.48   Labs—Views

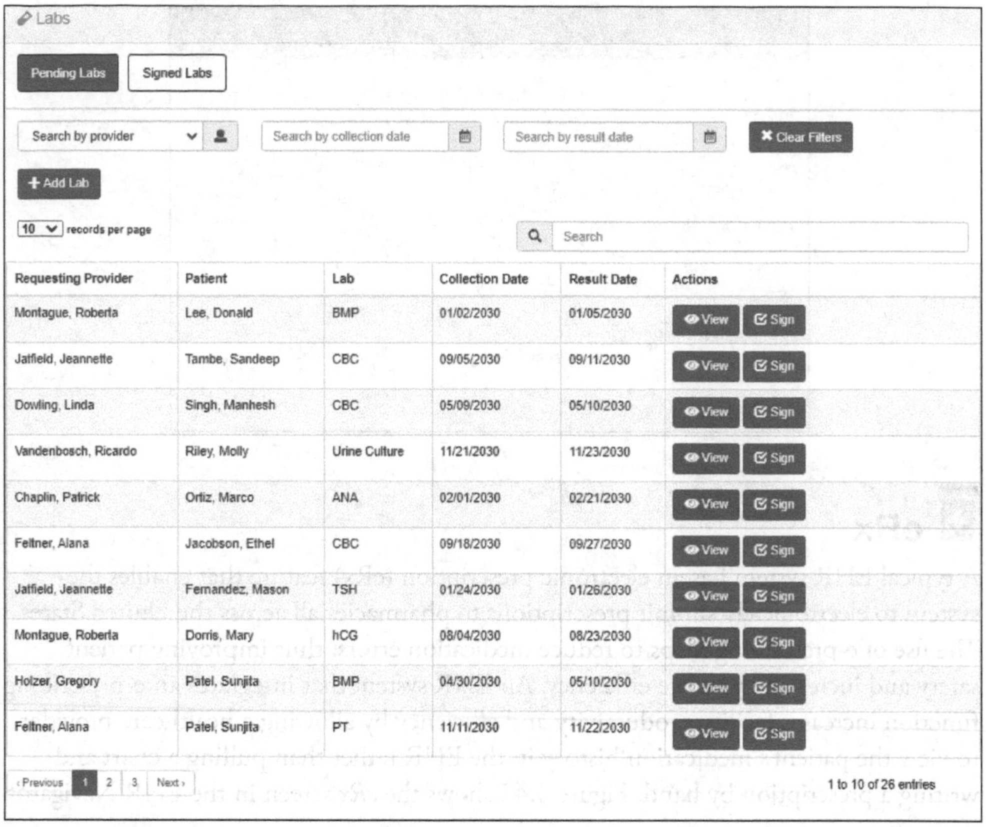

Labs

EHR systems include an integrated laboratory feature, which enables healthcare facilities and providers to connect with national and regional laboratories or maintain an existing laboratory partner. The EHR Navigator *Labs* feature allows you to view *Pending Labs* and *Signed Labs*. Pending labs are those awaiting test processing and results reporting. Signed labs are those that have been viewed and signed by a physician, physician assistant, or nurse practitioner. Integrating laboratories into an EHR system gives you the ability to create laboratory orders and view results from any computer at any time, with abnormal results flagged and organized for easy review. Figure 3.48 illustrates the *Labs* feature in the EHR Navigator.

Manage Orders

Every EHR system contains a computerized provider order entry (CPOE) component. In the EHR Navigator, the CPOE component is located by clicking *Charts*, selecting the patient, and clicking *Manage Orders*. *Manage Orders* is a button located on the patient's chart. Depending on their level of access, users add, view, and cancel physician orders for treatment and care (e.g., laboratory orders, dietary orders, and therapy orders) by using *Manage Orders*. Figure 3.49 illustrates the *Manage Orders* dialog box in the EHR Navigator. You will learn about CPOE in detail in Chapter 8.

Figure 3.49 Manage Orders

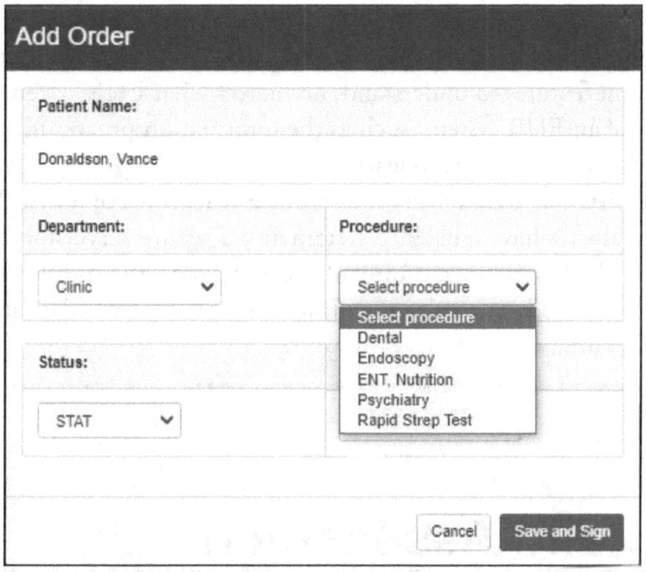

CHECKPOINT 3.3

1. Name four types of clinical information found in a patient's chart.

   a. _____

   b. _____

   c. _____

   d. _____

2. Explain the importance of an integrated laboratory feature.

   _____

   _____

   _____

Tutorial 3.4   **EHR**NAVIGAT✛R

Reviewing a Patient's Chart and Locking and Unlocking the EHR

Go to your online course to launch Tutorial 3.4. As a physician, practice reviewing patient clinical information using the EHR Navigator.

Chapter Summary

There are three primary healthcare settings—inpatient, outpatient, and skilled nursing and rehabilitation—and each setting requires its own features within an EHR system. Rather than learning one specific EHR system, mastering the knowledge behind an EHR system allows you the flexibility of working with a variety of EHR systems that you may encounter in the workplace. ONC-certified EHRs possess similar capabilities and functions as a result of standardized requirements for compliant EHRs.

With that in mind, the EHR Navigator provides you with the hands-on activities to help you master this basic knowledge. Assigning rights and permissions, managing and scheduling patients, reviewing medical documents, charting, reviewing laboratory results, sending eprescriptions, and sending secure messages are all important features to understand, no matter what EHR system you use. The structure of an EHR system, such as the information processing cycle, is also crucial background knowledge to learn.

Data security and accessibility are important features of an EHR system. EHRs should always have a backup system and a secure server location. Accessing the EHR system via mobile devices is becoming more commonplace as mobile technology becomes more affordable, secure, and adaptable to various EHR systems.

Review and Assessment

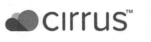

The following Review and Assessment activities are also available online in the Cirrus online course. Your instructor may ask you to complete these activities online. Cirrus also provides access to flash cards, a crossword puzzle, and practice quizzes to help strengthen your understanding of the chapter content.

Acronyms/Initialisms

Study the following acronyms discussed in this chapter. Go to the online course for flash cards of the acronyms and other chapter key terms.

CCHIT: Certification Commission for Health Information Technology

CPOE: computerized provider order entry

EIN: Employer Identification Number

HIPAA: Health Insurance Portability and Accountability Act

HITECH Act: Health Information Technology for Economic and Clinical Health Act

HL7: Health Level Seven International

IT: information technology

LAN: local area network

NPI: National Provider Identifier

PHI: protected health information

WAN: wide area network

Check Your Understanding

To check your understanding of this chapter's key concepts, answer the following questions.

1. Data storage in an electronic health record (EHR) may be handled by all of the following methods *except* a

   a. cloud server.

   b. vendor server.

   c. facility server.

   d. flash drive.

2. The four components of the information processing cycle are

   a. input, print, output, and save.

   b. input, output, print, and storage.

   c. input, processing, output, and storage.

   d. enter, print, save, and storage.

3. Which of the following is the organization that is responsible for certifying EHR vendors?

   a. Certified Commission for Health Information Technology

   b. American Medical Association

   c. Office of the National Coordinator for Health Information Technology

   d. Health Information Technology

4. Meaningful use provides

   a. incentives for a healthcare facility that meets established criteria for an EHR system.

   b. a report to the patient on their healthcare information.

   c. a measurement of the functionality of the EHR system.

   d. incentives for patients who use a personal health record.

5. Mobile devices include

   a. iPads.

   b. iPhones.

   c. Androids.

   d. All of the choices are correct.

6. True/False: Interoperability allows various healthcare facilities to communicate with each other.

7. True/False: A microphone is a type of input device.

8. True/False: A local area network is a computer connected to the internet.

9. True/False: All users of an EHR system have the right to access all components of the EHR.

10. True/False: EHR systems may be customized to meet the needs of the facility.

Go on the Record

To build on your understanding of the topics in this chapter, complete the following short-answer activities.

1. Discuss the importance of assigning passwords and rights to users of an EHR system.

2. Explain why it is important to lock an EHR system when not actively working with it.

3. Compare and contrast the advantages and challenges of using mobile devices with an EHR system.

4. Explain the advantage of using the e-prescribing feature of an EHR system.

Navigate the Field

To gain practice in handling challenging situations in the workplace, consider the following real-world scenarios and identify how you would respond to each.

1. You are the health information technology (HIT) training specialist at Northstar Medical Center, and you have been tasked with training new employees on the EHR Navigator. Prepare an outline you will follow for training employees.

2. After completing an overview of the EHR Navigator in this chapter, prepare a list of features that are most important to your job as the HIT training specialist at Northstar Medical Center. Explain why each feature is important and how each will help you complete your job more effectively and efficiently.

Think Critically

Continue to think critically about challenging concepts and complete the following activities.

1. Tabitha Iris Wang calls to schedule an appointment with Dr. Alana Feltner. List the steps that you must take to schedule this patient in the EHR system.

2. You are the information technology (IT) manager for your healthcare facility. A new employee will begin in the Health Information Management (HIM) department. Prepare a list of the steps you would take to add a new user and assign permissions to this new HIM employee.

Make Your Case

Consider the scenario and then complete the following project.

You are chairing a committee on selecting the EHR system for Cincinnati Grace Medical Center. The committee has decided to select a web-based EHR system because the facility does not have a large IT staff. You are in charge of researching Practice Fusion, a free, web-based EHR system. Create a presentation based on the instructions provided to you by your instructor.

Explore the Technology

EHRNAVIGAT♥R   *Complete the EHR Navigator practice assessments that align to each tutorial and the assessments that accompany Chapter 3 located in the online course.*

Chapter 4 Managing the Electronic Health Record

Field Notes

"From a front desk/receptionist perspective, electronic health records have greatly improved the standard of care we are able to provide to our patients. There is less duplication of charts, less paperwork, and less searching for information that is needed at check-in/registration. The ability to scan information (such as insurance card and photo ID) into electronic health records keeps the chart up to date and complete. Preparation of charts is simplified greatly. EHR-generated forms simply mainstream the process of obtaining signatures for consents. The ability to obtain information from outside physician offices for continuity of care is simplified through the EHR sharing capabilities."

– Tracy Clyburn, Clinical Intake Coordinator

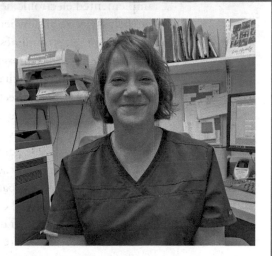

Learning Objectives

4.1 Differentiate between the two main healthcare setting categories and identify four types of healthcare settings.

4.2 Identify key elements of the patient entry process.

4.3 Identify the purpose, goals, and elements of the master patient index.

4.4 Explain the registration process for a patient requiring acute care.

4.5 Explain the registration process for a patient requiring ambulatory care.

4.6 Differentiate between a new and an established patient.

4.7 Identify the importance of insurance information in the administrative management process.

4.8 Describe document imaging and its importance in the EHR.

Healthcare providers create and maintain an individual health record for every patient. Each health record contains the reason for the visit, the services rendered, diagnoses, and recommended treatments. Regardless of whether a patient is treated in a clinic, hospital, physical therapy facility, or imaging clinic, their health records require administrative management. As most healthcare facilities have implemented electronic health record (EHR) systems, more administrative functions are being electronically performed. This technology changes the daily tasks of healthcare personnel, streamlines the workflow of health records, and improves the accuracy of documentation. For example, front desk personnel input patient appointments into the EHR system rather than entering the data on a physical calendar, thus reducing the chance of error. Staff directly input patient demographic data into the EHR instead of pulling it from a paper form. Billing specialists enter insurance data into the system and update the electronic record if the patient's insurance changes, thus ensuring accurate billing. These administrative functions also allow healthcare providers and other staff members easy access to a patient's medical record, providing them with a complete picture of the patient's health history.

Generally, the initial contact for a patient is the healthcare personnel at the admission or registration desk. This person, called a **registrar**, is often required to collect information before and at the time the patient is seen. Increasingly, healthcare facilities may refer to professionals performing the registration or admission process as *patient access specialists*.

At the initial visit, the patient provides **demographic information**, such as name, date of birth, home address, or other key information used to identify the patient, that connects the registrar to the correct record. If no record exists for the patient, the registrar must create a new record and add it to the master patient index (MPI). The MPI is also discussed in Chapter 5.

Depending on the nature of the appointment, patient information may be new or may require updating, such as insurance coverage, contact information, or demographic data. The Health Insurance Portability and Account-ability Act (HIPAA) Notice of Privacy Practices for Protected Health Information and the advance directives notice are also given at registration. Copayments or coinsurance for acute care and for outpatient services at a hospital are collected at the time of service. Collecting accurate information from the patient is a critical job requirement for the registrar who

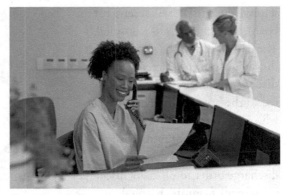

A registrar usually works at the front desk of a healthcare facility.

completes the admission and registration process for the patient. Accurate data entry is also crucial to ensuring patient safety and preventing communication problems among providers.

4.1 Different Types of Healthcare Settings

As discussed in Chapter 2, patient care is divided into two main setting categories: acute care and ambulatory care.

An acute care facility's goal is to care for patients who have short-term illnesses and require an overnight stay in a hospital. Acute care facilities provide round-the-clock diagnostic, surgical, and therapeutic care to patients.

An ambulatory care facility provides care to patients who do not require an overnight stay. Ambulatory care centers have grown within the past 30 years as technology has improved and fewer medical procedures require patients to stay overnight. In addition, health insurance has changed how patients pay for services and procedures, and many policies will not cover extended overnight care in a hospital if it is not medically necessary. There are times when a patient may go to an ambulatory care facility for a procedure and complications occur, requiring the patient to be admitted to an acute care facility. The patient would then be an acute care patient rather than an ambulatory care patient.

Patient care in the acute and ambulatory settings is different. The following sections examine the differences in these two care setting categories and identify additional types of healthcare settings that are differentiated by length of stay or specialty of care.

Patient Care in an Acute Care Setting

Hospital personnel provide acute care to patients who experience sudden health issues or illnesses and cannot be treated in an outpatient care facility. Patients requiring acute care are either admitted to a hospital through the emergency department or sent from an outpatient clinic or a physician's office.

Acute care can range from a minimum stay of 24 hours to a maximum stay of 30 days, although exceptions to this guideline may occur. For example, a patient whose postsurgical care and monitoring are expected to require a stay of one to two days may need extended acute care in the event of an infection.

The day and time the patient is admitted to the acute care facility is the **admission date**. The admission registrar is the initial contact with the patient, which is, in part, why this interaction is increasingly referred to as *patient access*. In the acute care setting, the patient will receive room, board, and care from the hospital. The day and time the patient leaves the facility are considered the **discharge date**. A patient is admitted to the hospital by the physician, who must document the admission order in the patient record. The physician must also document a discharge order to officially discharge the patient from the hospital.

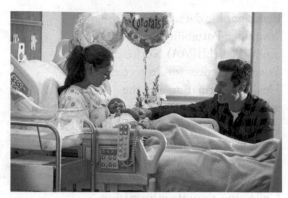

A hospital is an acute care facility.

Patient Care in an Ambulatory Care Setting

Ambulatory care includes services provided to the patient that do not require hospitalization or institutionalization. In most cases, the patient is discharged from the ambulatory care center in less than 24 hours. However, there are some exceptions to this rule, such as a patient who is placed on observation status.

Ambulatory care settings are numerous and include (but are not limited to):

- Birthing centers
- Cancer treatment centers
- Clinics
- Correctional facilities
- Dentist offices
- Dialysis clinics

- Emergency departments
- Home care
- Physician offices
- Surgery centers
- Therapeutic services
- Urgent care centers

Patient Data Management in Acute and Ambulatory Care Settings

Although gathering patient data is similar within an acute care or ambulatory care setting, there are some differences. Table 4.1 compares the types of patient data managed in the two healthcare delivery settings.

Table 4.1 Patient Data Managed in Acute and Ambulatory Care Settings

Data Category	Acute Care	Ambulatory Care
Patient Contact	Admit a patient	Schedule an appointment
Health Record Content	History and physical exam, diagnostic records, treatment records, and discharge summary	SOAP, progress, or chart note
Patient Care	Admission	Visit
Length of Stay	More than 24 hours	Length of appointment, or less than 24 hours
List of Patients	Master patient index (MPI)	Patient list
Completion of Patient Care	Discharge	Check out
SOAP = subjective, objective, assessment, plan		

Other Healthcare Settings

Other types of healthcare settings are identified either by length of stay or by specialty of care:

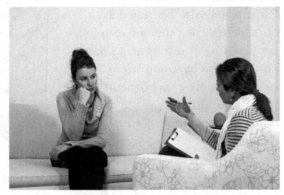

Behavioral health therapists may provide both acute care and ambulatory care.

- A **long-term care facility** typically has patients who reside for more than 30 days.

- A **behavioral health setting** provides care to patients with psychiatric diagnoses. The facility may offer a combination of acute care and ambulatory care for patients.

- A **rehabilitation facility** may also offer acute care and ambulatory care, typically serving patients recovering from accidents, injuries, or surgeries.

- **Hospice care** is short-term, palliative care provided to terminally ill patients within acute care or home care settings. The purpose of hospice care is to make patients comfortable until death and to support their families during this difficult time.

CHECKPOINT 4.1

1. Name four types of healthcare settings.

   a. _____

   b. _____

   c. _____

   d. _____

2. When may a patient transition from an ambulatory care to an acute care setting?

   _____

   _____

   _____

4.2 Patient Entry into the Healthcare System

Patients enter healthcare facilities for a number of reasons. For example, patients might be urgently admitted to a hospital via the emergency room, from a nursing home, or directly from home. A patient may also be admitted on an inpatient basis to an acute care facility for the delivery of a child, or for other medical or surgical treatment requiring an overnight stay in the hospital.

Patients might also be treated at a hospital as an outpatient. Outpatients treated at an acute care hospital might be treated in the emergency room and released to their home without the need to be admitted to the hospital. Patients may also be treated as outpatients when they are seen in a clinic setting or testing area. Many hospitals also have outpatient surgical centers where patients have minor surgery and are sent home without the need to spend the night.

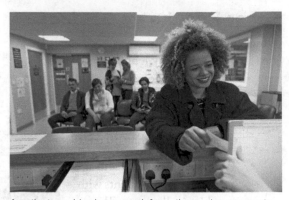

A patient provides insurance information and copayments when checking in for an appointment.

Patients may be treated in a variety of outpatient settings, including a physician's office, drug or alcohol treatment center, psychologist's office, or dialysis facility.

One thing that all of these patients have in common is that they need to be admitted or registered in the EHR prior to care and treatment. The next section will discuss the admission and registration processes.

Admission and Registration

Admission or registration begins when the patient or healthcare provider contacts the acute care or ambulatory care facility to make an appointment or schedule an admission in person or by telephone, email, or secure patient portal. Some ambulatory care facilities provide an opportunity for patients to register by using a self-service kiosk, which is a computer station located in the patient waiting area that connects newly entered patient information to the registration system. If the healthcare facility uses a combination of electronic and paper forms for registration, a patient may download forms from a healthcare facility website, or the forms may be provided by mail, email, or in person when the patient arrives. Registration clerks might also telephone the patient to collect information over the phone. All of these methods of data collection help streamline the registration process and reduce the amount of face-to-face time needed upon arrival of the patient to the inpatient admission area or an outpatient appointment. In addition to demographic information, the data collected also includes payer information. This information is used to determine patient benefits and any required approvals from the third-party payer. Figure 4.1 shows a sample of a patient registration form.

Check-In Process

When the patient arrives at a healthcare facility, a staff member must verify the patient's identity by copying or scanning the patient's insurance card and checking a driver's license or other proof of identification. Verification of identity is necessary to ensure proper rendering of patient care and to lessen the opportunities for insurance fraud.

Following the proof of identification, a copy of the patient's insurance is scanned into the EHR, and consents for treatment, billing, notice of privacy practices acknowledgement, and release of patient information for billing and continuity of care are signed. The patient's insurance is verified, and the copayment is collected from the patient.

Figure 4.1 Patient Registration Form

Northstar Physicians

Northstar Physicians
Patient Registration Form

For Office Use Only:
MRUN: ________
Registrar: ______

PATIENT INFORMATION

Patient's Last Name / First / Middle Initial		Type of Care: ❑ Inpatient ❑ Maternity ❑ Outpatient ❑ Same-Day Surgery ❑ Surgery	
Race / Marital Status / Religion / Primary Language		Date of Birth (mm/dd/yyyy)	Date of Scheduled Visit
Physician's Last Name / First Name		❑ Female ❑ Male	Social Security No.
Patient's Street Address / Apt. No.		City / State	ZIP
Home Phone ( ) / Work Phone ( ) / Cell Phone ( )		Visit Reason or Diagnosis	Admission Date
Temporary Address / Apt. No.		City / State	ZIP
Patient's Current Employer Name	Employer Address	City / State	ZIP
Employer Phone ( )	Patient's Occupation	Employment Status: ❑ Not Employed ❑ Full Time ❑ Part Time ❑ Student ❑ Retired and Date:	
Full Name of Emergency Contact	Relationship	Home Phone ( )	Work Phone ( )
Have you ever been a patient at EMC Medical Center? ❑ Yes ❑ No		If yes, when was your last visit?	Under what name?

Guarantor

Last Name / First / Middle Initial		Relationship	Date of Birth (mm/dd/yyyy)
Street Address / Apt. No.		❑ Female ❑ Male	Marital Status / Social Security No.
City / State / ZIP	Home Phone ( )	Work Phone ( )	Cell Phone ( )
Employer Name	Employer Address	City / State	ZIP
Employer Phone ( )	Occupation	Employment Status: ❑ Not Employed ❑ Full Time ❑ Part Time ❑ Student ❑ Retired and Date:	

Insurance Information

Primary Insurance Name		Name of Insured (exactly as it appears on card)	
Insurance Billing Address / City		State / ZIP	Phone No. ( )
Policy No. / Group No. / Plan Code		State / Effective Date	Expiration Date
Subscriber's Full Name	Subscriber's Soc. Sec. No.	Subscriber's Date of Birth (mm/dd/yyyy)	❑ Female ❑ Male
Subscriber's Employer Name (if self-employed, company name)	Relation to Insured	Subscriber's Employment Status: ❑ Not Employed ❑ Full Time ❑ Part Time ❑ Student ❑ Retired and Date:	
Subscriber's Employer Address / City		State / ZIP	Phone No. ( )

...on card	Effective Date (mm/dd/yyyy)	❑ Part A (Hospital Benefit) ❑ Part B (Medical Benefit)
...on card	Effective Date	State
	Name of Insured (exactly as it appears on card)	
City	State / ZIP	Phone No. ( )
...lan Code	State / Effective Date	Expiration Date
...ber's Soc. Sec. No.	Subscriber's Date of Birth (mm/dd/yyyy)	❑ Female ❑ Male
...n to Insured	Subscriber's Employment Status: ❑ Not Employed ❑ Full Time ❑ Part Time ❑ Student ❑ Retired and Date:	
City	State / ZIP	Phone No. ( )
	Date of Accident: (mm/dd/yyyy)	Claim No.
...ct Name	Phone No. ( )	Insurance Name
City	State / ZIP	Phone No. ( )

Advance Directive

Do you have an Advance Directive, such as a Living Will or Durable Power of Attorney for Health Care? ❑ Yes ❑ No

Please specify the type: ________________________________

*** *If yes, please bring a copy at the time of your admission.* ***

Self-Pay

* If insured but your procedure is not covered or verified by your plan, a deposit is required at the time of admission.

* If you do not have insurance, please call our *EMC Financial Services at (513)-555-1122* before your scheduled arrival date to discuss financial terms.

Additional Information

Do you need special accommodations, such as translation, visual aid, etc.? ❑ Yes ❑ No

*** *If yes, please specify so that prior arrangements can be made for the day of your visit.* ***

❑ Language Interpreter ______________ ❑ Sign Language Interpreter ❑ Visual Aid ❑ Other: ______________

Tutorial 4.1 EHRNAVIGATOR

Checking in a Patient

Go to your online course to launch Tutorial 4.1. As an admission clerk, practice checking in a patient using the EHR Navigator. After completing the tutorial, apply your skills with the Checking in a Patient practice assessments.

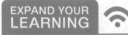

EXPAND YOUR LEARNING

The healthcare community is still debating the need to implement a unique patient identification system. To learn more on this controversy, visit https://EHR3.ParadigmEducation.com/PatientID.

4.3 Master Patient Index

Most acute care facilities that use an EHR system call their list of patients a **master patient index (MPI)** or a patient list. The MPI is a database created by a healthcare organization to assign a unique medical record number to each patient served, thus allowing easy retrieval and maintenance of patient information.

Patient Identifiers

Typically, the EHR system automatically generates and assigns a unique patient or medical record number, also known as the **patient identification number**. Figure 4.2 illustrates the dialog box used to add a new patient and generate the patient's medical record number in the EHR Navigator.

HIPAA established and required the implementation of a unique patient identification system. The patient identifier is truly unique to the patient, unlike a name or a date of birth. The patient identifier consists of a set of numeric or alpha characters and seamlessly connects a person to their healthcare information.

Figure 4.2 Generating a Patient Number

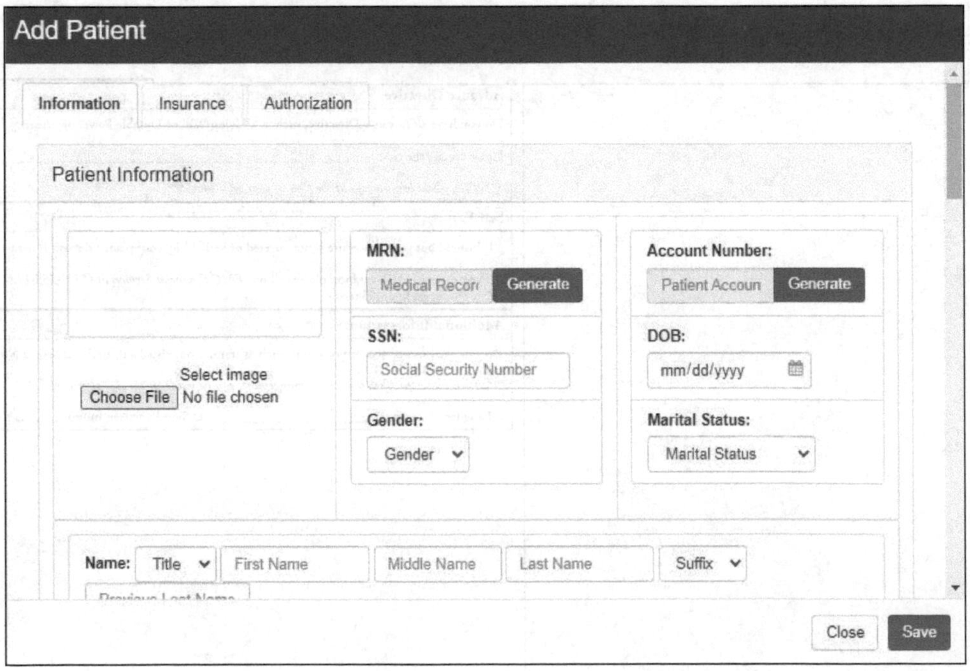

Add Patient
Information
Insurance
Authorization
Patient Information
Select image
Choose File
No file chosen
MRN:
Medical Recor
Generate
SSN:
Social Security Number
Gender:
Gender
Account Number:
Patient Accoun
Generate
DOB:
mm/dd/yyyy
Marital Status:
Marital Status
Name:
Title
First Name
Middle Name
Last Name
Suffix
Close
Save

It is crucial that healthcare providers use the MPI to verify that a patient has only one patient identifier (i.e., medical record number). If a patient has multiple identifiers, then providers may not see the true picture of a patient's health status because important healthcare information may be misplaced, lost, or duplicated.

> **WHY YOUR JOB MATTERS**
>
> By choosing to pursue a career in health information technology (HIT), you are at the start of something monumental. Health information specialist positions will grow much faster than the average for all occupations. Additionally, an estimated 23,000 new jobs will need to be filled to implement EHR systems.

Purpose and Goals of the Master Patient Index

The EHR system stores the MPI permanently (see Figure 4.3). The following are goals of the MPI:

- Match the patient with their MPI record
- Minimize duplication
- Retain lifelong health records

An efficient and effective MPI system makes it possible to meet these goals.

The MPI contains the patient medical record number, with each information field containing data about a patient. These data fields produce a unique record. Healthcare providers use the MPI to determine whether a patient record exists in the EHR system. If such a record exists, that same patient identifier is used each time a healthcare provider or facility sees the patient. In doing so, the patient identifier can be used to track all of the patient's encounters at the healthcare facility.

Figure 4.3 Master Patient Index

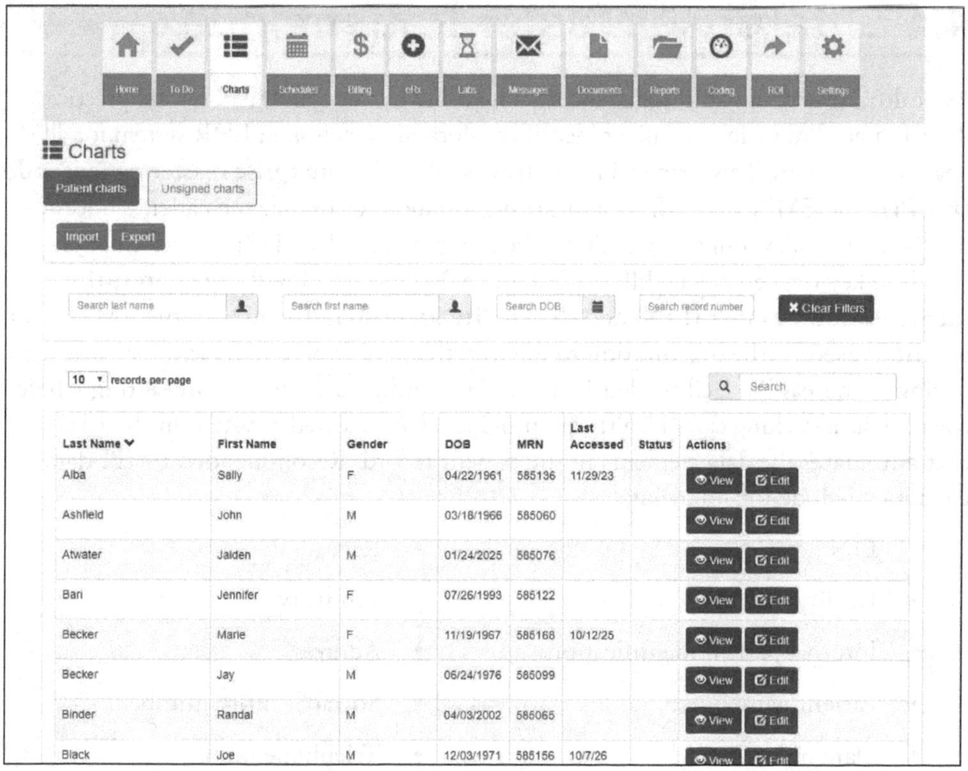
Home
To Do
Charts
Schedules
Billing
eRx
Labs
Messages
Documents
Reports
Coding
ROI
Settings
Charts
Patient charts
Unsigned charts
Import
Export
Search last name
Search first name
Search DOB
Search record number
Clear Filters
10 records per page
Search
Last Name | First Name | Gender | DOB | MRN | Last Accessed | Status | Actions
Alba | Sally | F | 04/22/1961 | 585136 | 11/29/23 | | View Edit
Ashfield | John | M | 03/18/1966 | 585060 | | | View Edit
Atwater | Jaiden | M | 01/24/2025 | 585076 | | | View Edit
Bari | Jennifer | F | 07/26/1993 | 585122 | | | View Edit
Becker | Marie | F | 11/19/1967 | 585168 | 10/12/25 | | View Edit
Becker | Jay | M | 06/24/1976 | 585099 | | | View Edit
Binder | Randal | M | 04/03/2002 | 585065 | | | View Edit
Black | Joe | M | 12/03/1971 | 585156 | 10/7/26 | | View Edit

Core Data Elements

The American Health Information Management Association (AHIMA) recommends searching for a patient based on core data elements for indexing. In an MPI, the **core data elements** of a patient record include the following:

- Medical record number
- Name
- Date of birth
- Sex
- Race
- Ethnicity
- Address

- Previous name
- Social Security number
- Facility identifier
- Account number
- Admission date
- Discharge date
- Service type

Optional Data Elements

AHIMA has identified the following **optional data elements** for the MPI:

- Marital status
- Telephone number
- Mother's maiden name
- Place of birth
- Advance directive decision making

- Organ donor status
- Emergency contact
- Allergies
- Problem list

4.4 Enterprise Master Patient Index

As healthcare systems continue to incorporate acute care and ambulatory care practices, there is a need to maintain patient identifier information across an EHR system for all healthcare settings. This systemwide database is called the **enterprise master patient index (EMPI)**. The EMPI allows the healthcare organization to compile the patient's information into one index, using registration, scheduling, financial, and clinical information.

Two key data elements differentiate the MPI from the EMPI: the **enterprise identification number (EIN)** and the **facility identifier**. The EIN in the EMPI is an identifier used by the organization to identify the patient across the various healthcare settings, whereas the facility identifier is used to indicate the healthcare setting where the patient is seeking care. Healthcare providers have created a system in the EHRs that automates the data elements in the patient record. Recommended EMPI data elements include the following:

- EIN
- Facility identifier
- Internal patient identification
- Patient name
- Date of birth
- Sex

- Race
- Ethnicity
- Address
- Social Security number
- Telephone number

Tutorial 4.2   **EHR**NAVIGAT⊕R

Searching for a Patient's Chart
Go to your online course to launch Tutorial 4.2. As an admission clerk, practice
the various ways to search for a patient using the EHR Navigator.

4.5 Collecting Patient Data

The patient registration and admission processes may be slightly different for acute care
and ambulatory care settings, but personnel in both settings focus on collecting accurate
patient information.

Acute Care Registration

As mentioned earlier, the registrar is typically the first person the patient approaches
upon arrival at the care facility. The registrar collects demographic and administrative
information from the patient. If the patient is already in the EHR system, then the
registrar will verify the accuracy of that information and update it as necessary.

Although similar to the registration process for ambulatory care, acute care
personnel must follow the **Uniform Hospital Discharge Data Set (UHDDS)** for
inpatient care. Developed by a committee in 1969, the UHDDS outlined a set of
patient-specific data elements. This protocol, revised by the National Committee on
Vital and Health Statistics (NCVHS) in 1984, was adopted by federal health programs
in 1986. Since then, the UHDDS has been revised several times.

The recommended **UHDDS core data elements** include the following:

- Patient identifier
- Date of birth
- Sex
- Ethnicity
- Address
- Healthcare setting identification
- Admission date
- Type of admission
- Discharge date
- Attending physician identification

- Surgeon identification
- Principal diagnosis
- Other diagnoses
- Qualifier for other diagnoses
- External cause of injury code
- Birth weight of neonate
- Significant procedures and dates
- Disposition of patient
- Expected source of payment
- Total charges

Ambulatory Care Registration

In an outpatient or a physician's office setting, the front office staff usually handles the
registration process. The information gathered in the outpatient setting should follow
the **Uniform Ambulatory Care Data Set (UACDS)** for outpatient services. The
primary purpose of using this data set is to ensure that all healthcare settings and
providers are gathering identical types of information on each patient and that the data
collected is defined consistently across all healthcare settings.

The NCVHS approved this data set in 1989. The UACDS is used in surgery centers, physician's offices, outpatient clinics, and emergency departments. The UACDS is not required but highly recommended.

Some of the recommended UACDS data elements include:

- Patient identification
- Address
- Date of birth
- Sex
- Ethnicity
- Provider identification
- Provider address
- Provider specialty
- Place of encounter
- Reason for encounter

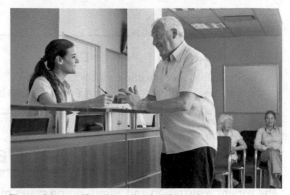
The registrar verifies the patient's information.

- Diagnostic services
- Problem, diagnosis, and assessment
- Therapeutic services
- Preventive services
- Disposition
- Source of payment
- Total charges

4.6 New versus Established Patients

After identifying the patient, you must determine if they are an established patient or a new patient. To make this determination, it is important to understand the differences between these types of patients.

New Patient

For the purposes of admission and registration, a **new patient** is defined as a patient who has not received any services from a provider or another provider in the group in the same specialty and subspecialty within the past three years. For instance, if the patient was seen two years and eleven months ago, then they are considered an established patient; however, if the patient was seen three years and one day ago, then they are considered a new patient.

To add a new patient to the system, the registrar must collect administrative information, including demographics used to identify the patient, report statistics, conduct research, and allocate resources. The demographic information gathered includes the following:

- First, middle, and last names
- Medical record number (if known by the patient)
- Address
- Telephone numbers: home, work, and cell

- Sex
- Date of birth
- Place of birth
- Marital status
- Ethnicity

- Social Security number
- Emergency contact
- Date of service

- Physician
- Dentist

Consider This

When a patient arrives at an emergency department (ED), he or she is neither a new patient nor an established patient. The patient may have a record in the EHR system, but patients in the ED are not identified as being new or established. The terms *new* and *established* are primarily used for patients in an ambulatory care setting.

Patients may have been to the ED for previous visits, but they would not be classified as established.

How would you handle a situation in which a patient states that they have been to Shoreview Emergency Department before and, consequently, should not have to provide their information again?

Tutorial 4.3   EHRNAVIGAT⊕R

Adding a New Patient

Go to your online course to launch Tutorial 4.3. As an admission clerk, practice preadmitting a patient using the EHR Navigator.

Established Patient

An **established patient** has received professional services from a healthcare provider or another provider in the same group in the same specialty and subspecialty within the past three years.

To determine if a patient is an established patient, the registrar begins by searching for the patient's record in the EHR Navigator. There are multiple ways to search for a patient using a variety of criteria, such as the following:

- The patient's full or partial name in the *Last Name* and *First Name* fields

- The patient's medical record or patient number in the *Patient Record* field

- The patient's date of birth in the *Date of Birth (DOB)* field

Healthcare staff members can also use a combination of these criteria to find an established patient. When searching for an established patient, search by different core data elements, such as patient name, patient record number, DOB, Social Security number, or admission date, to ensure that the patient record exists in the EHR system.

Figure 4.4 shows the Find Patient dialog box. Use this dialog box to determine if the patient is registered in the EHR Navigator.

If the patient is registered in the EHR system, the existing information needs to be confirmed with the patient. If the patient needs to edit or update any demographic information, select the patient record and click the *Edit Patient* button to display the *Edit Patient* dialog box, as shown in Figure 4.5, and then update any patient demographic

Figure 4.4 Dialog Box to Search for a Patient

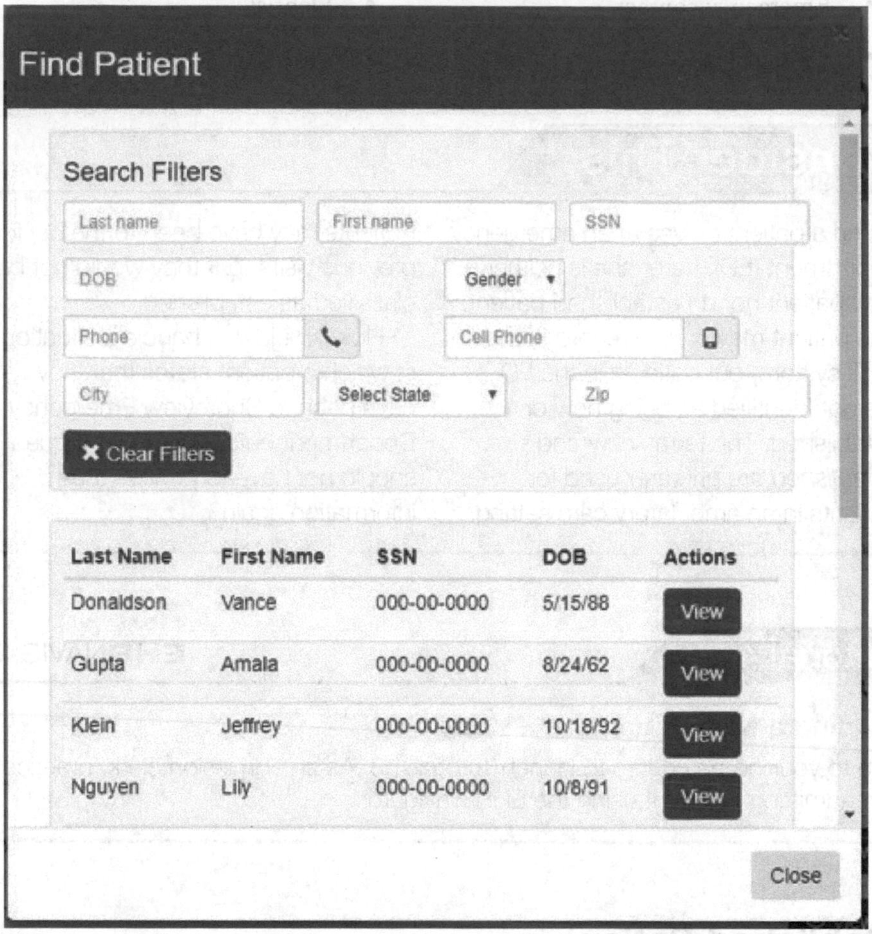

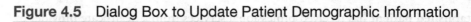

Figure 4.5 Dialog Box to Update Patient Demographic Information

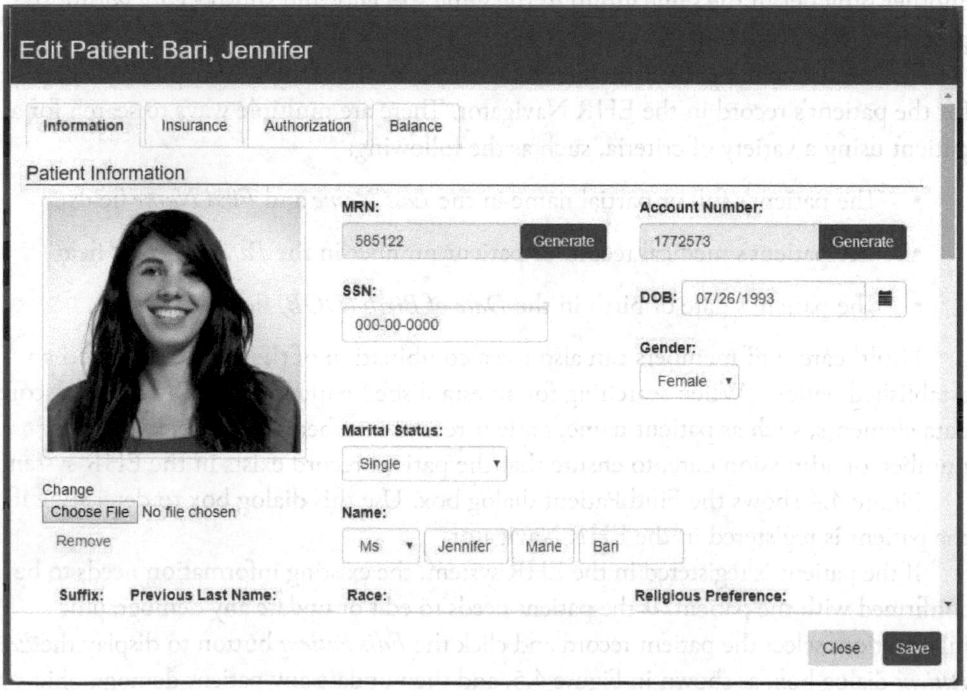

information required. To edit patient information, select the field and enter the appropriate data. Current demographic and insurance information is necessary in case the health care organization needs to contact the patient and to submit insurance claims for reimbursement.

Tutorial 4.4   **EHR**NAVIGAT**⊕**R

Editing a Record for an Established Patient

Go to your online course to launch Tutorial 4.4. As a front desk clerk, practice updating a record for an existing patient using the EHR Navigator.

4.7 Insurance Information

Insurance information includes details about the patient's insurance coverage, such as the insurance company, copay, and identification numbers, to assist with processing healthcare claims. Some patients may not have insurance or may not wish to use insurance and are considered cash payers. Figure 4.6 is an example of a typical insurance card a patient may provide to the healthcare facility. The insurance card contains the member name, member identification number, group number, and contact numbers for member services and claims and inquiries. A staff member will scan the insurance card and enter the scanned image and insurance coverage information into the EHR system.

Insurance Subscriber and Guarantor

When entering the patient's insurance and financial information into the EHR, you must identify the subscriber and the guarantor. The **subscriber** is the person whose insurance coverage is used for acute or ambulatory care. The subscriber may be the patient or a family member of the subscriber if they are on a shared insurance plan.

The **guarantor** is the person or financial entity that guarantees payment on any unpaid balances on the account. The guarantor may be the patient, another person, or a financial entity. Most patients older than 18 years are their own guarantors.

Figure 4.6 Insurance Card

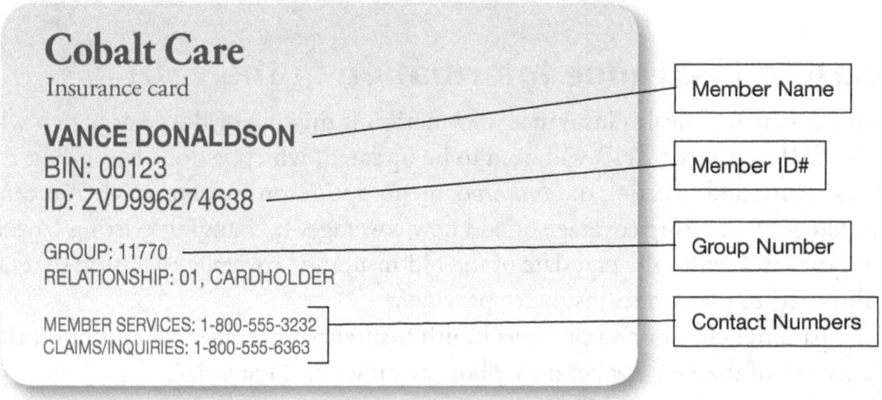

Cobalt Care
Insurance card

VANCE DONALDSON — Member Name
BIN: 00123
ID: ZVD996274638 — Member ID#

GROUP: 11770 — Group Number
RELATIONSHIP: 01, CARDHOLDER

MEMBER SERVICES: 1-800-555-3232 — Contact Numbers
CLAIMS/INQUIRIES: 1-800-555-6363

Table 4.2 Guarantor Types

Type	Description
Personal/Family	For general healthcare services, the guarantor is typically the subscriber of the primary insurance.
Workers' Compensation	The employer's workers' compensation insurance carrier is billed. If there are remaining charges, or injuries are deemed not work related, the patient is responsible for the charges.
Third-Party Liability	A third party, such as an insurance company, is responsible for payment.
Corporate	A company requires the patient to receive services from a healthcare facility or provider.
Research	The patient is involved in research or is a provider at the healthcare facility.

Minors usually have their parents or legal guardians as their guarantors. Any patient with decreased mental capacity typically has a guarantor.

Every patient must have at least one guarantor account prior to being admitted or checked in to a healthcare facility. When an acute or ambulatory healthcare facility sends a bill for a balance of a service or services not covered by insurance, the bill goes to the patient's guarantor. The **guarantor account** is a record that saves the information about the guarantor, including the guarantor's name and address. Various types of guarantor accounts are described in Table 4.2.

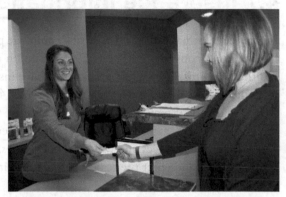

Upon arrival at the medical office, the patient provides the medical office specialist with their current insurance card.

Tutorial 4.5 　　　　　　　　　　　　　EHRNAVIGAT⊕R

Adding Insurance

Go to your online course to launch Tutorial 4.5. As a biller, practice adding insurance information using the EHR Navigator.

Updating Insurance Information in the EHR

If a patient's current health insurance information is missing or does not match what is in the EHR, then the EHR will need to be updated, which is done by finding the patient's record and selecting the *Insurance* menu option on the left panel. You can make changes to existing coverage or add new coverage. If changing existing coverage, it is important to enter the end date of the old insurance coverage to ensure that claims are submitted to the correct insurance provider.

The patient's current and previous health insurance coverage will appear on the *Insurance* tab of the *Edit Patient* dialog box, as shown in Figure 4.7.

Figure 4.7   Dialog Box to Review Patient's Insurance Information

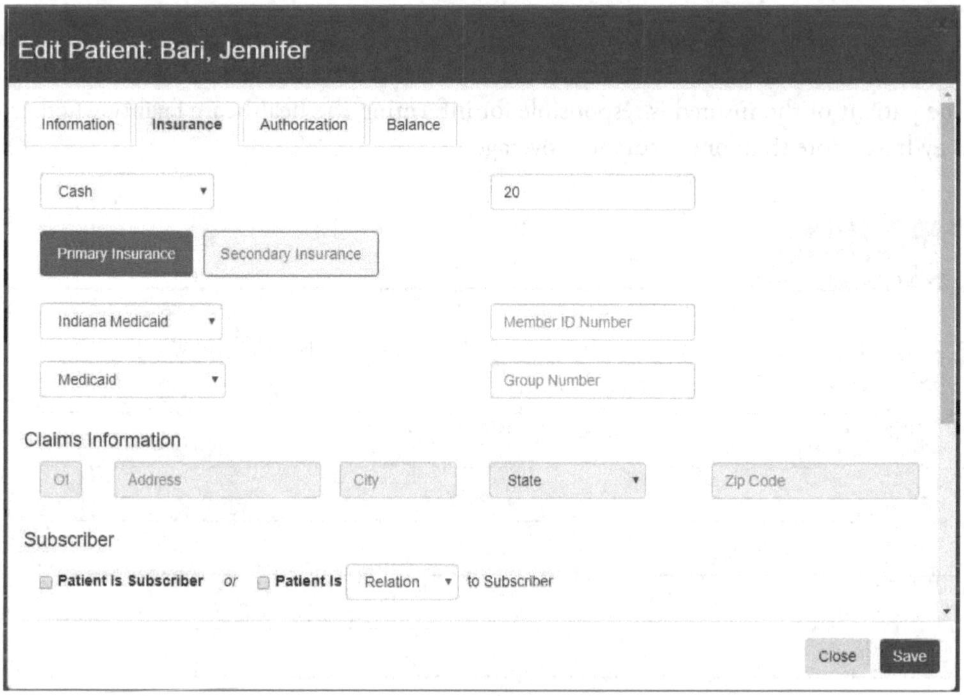

In most cases, a patient may be scheduled for appointments and receive care only after the EHR is updated with current patient insurance information.

Treatment Coverage

How insurance covers a patient's healthcare costs is based on the primary reason for the visit and a list of established insurance rules.

- If a patient is injured, the healthcare setting must determine how the injury occurred. If there was an accident, primary coverage may be provided by the company, property insurance, or accident insurance.

- If a service at an acute care or ambulatory care setting is not accident related, and each adult on the policy has their own insurance, then the patient's own insurance is primary.

- If a child is seen at an acute care or ambulatory care setting, and there are two insurance plans that cover the child, then the **birthday rule** is applied. The birthday rule specifies that the insurance of the parent whose birthday falls first in a calendar year will be the primary insurance. The ages of the separate cardholders have no bearing on this rule.

- If a patient has Medicare coverage and the services meet Medicare coverage guidelines, primary coverage is provided by Medicare.

- If a patient older than 65 years is being seen for something other than an injury, has two insurances (Medicare and a supplemental plan), is unemployed, and is not covered by a spouse's insurance, the primary insurance would be Medicare and the supplemental plan would be the secondary insurance. Typically, a supplemental plan pays the deductible, the copay, and any other charges not paid by Medicare.

- If a patient has Medicaid and a private insurance plan, the private insurance would be primary and Medicaid would be secondary.

For patients with insurance coverage through more than one provider, the primary coverage is determined by industry rules adopted by state insurance commissioners. The patient or the insured is responsible for informing the healthcare facility whether they have more than one insurance coverage.

CHECKP✚INT 4.2

1. Name the five different types of guarantors.

   a. _____

   b. _____

   c. _____

   d. _____

   e. _____

2. Explain the birthday rule. Why is it important?

   _____

   _____

   _____

   _____

   _____

4.8 Document Imaging

Billions of paper documents were created annually prior to the transition to EHRs. Document imaging is when a paper copy of medical information is converted to a digital format to attach to a patient's EHR. As healthcare organizations transitioned to EHRs, many organizations scanned paper records into current or new patient health records. Documents such as insurance cards, Notice of Privacy Practices, financial agreements, consent forms, advance directives authorizations, and living wills are examples of documents that may be scanned and added to a patient health record. It is important to audit documents, such as the consent form, release of information, or signature on file, to ensure the healthcare organization is in compliance with privacy and security requirements. Internal audits provide an opportunity for healthcare organizations to address areas of deficiency through training on privacy and security in the EHR.

Privacy Notices

The patient or the patient's representative must review and approve the Notice of Privacy Practices (NPP). The NPP informs patients of their rights and responsibilities and provides contact information for any questions they may have. The US Department of Health and Human Services requires the NPP as part of a rule that informs patients about the use and disclosure of information by the healthcare facility. An example of an NPP is shown in Figure 4.8. Each patient must receive a copy of the NPP at their first contact with the healthcare organization—for example, the first visit to a physician's office or first admission to a hospital. Either the patient or the patient's legal representative must sign the NPP. Some facilities use electronic patient signatures for these documents, while other facilities use paper copies, which need to be scanned after they are signed. A digital copy of the signed document must be saved in the patient's EHR.

Figure 4.8   Notice of Privacy Practices

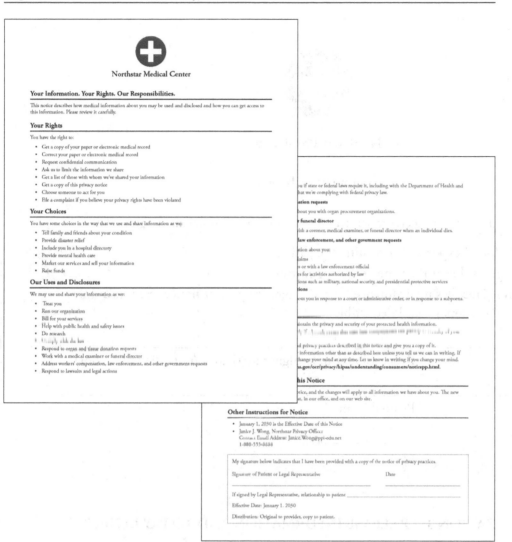

Financial Agreements

An example of a financial agreement that may be attached to a patient's EHR is the Assignment of Benefits form. The **Assignment of Benefits** form is an authorization by the patient to allow their health insurance or third-party provider to reimburse the healthcare provider or facility directly. A sample financial agreement is shown in Figure 4.9. If a healthcare facility requires patients to have a financial agreement on file, a staff member may ask for the patient's signature and then upload the signed document into the patient's EHR.

Consent Forms

A **general consent for treatment** form is used in acute care facilities. The patient or the patient's legal representative signs the general consent for treatment, giving the healthcare provider the right to treat them. The provider may require an informed consent form if the patient is having a specialty procedure. A sample consent form is provided in Figure 4.10. This consent may also request permission to bill the patient and/or the patient's insurance for services rendered.

Figure 4.9   Assignment of Benefits

Northstar Physicians

Assignment of Benefits

In consideration of the patient receiving services from Northstar Physicians, I agree that:

- I am responsible for all expenses for treating the patient.
- Payment of charges is due at the time of the appointment.
- If Northstar Physicians files my insurance for me, I agree to pay for noncovered insurance benefits, coinsurance, copays, and deductibles.

_____   _____
Patient Signature   Responsible Party's Signature (Parent/Guardian of Minor)

_____   _____
Printed Name   Printed Name

_____   _____
Date   Date

AUTHORIZATION TO RELEASE INFORMATION AND TO PAY BENEFITS

I authorize Northstar Physicians to release any of my medical information, including drug, alcohol, and HIV-positive test results, to my insurance company(s) as needed to process my insurance claim.

I authorize my insurance company to make payments directly to Northstar Physicians for covered medical and/or surgical services.

_____   _____
Patient's Signature   Responsible Party's Signature (Parent/Guardian of Minor)

_____   _____
Printed Name   Printed Name

_____   _____
Date   Date

Figure 4.10   Consent Form

Northstar Medical Center

Informed Consent for Invasive, Diagnostic, Medical, and Surgical Procedures

Patient's Name_____

Date of Birth_____

Medical Record #_____

I hereby authorize _____ and/or _____ and/or such assistants and associates as may be selected by him/her/they to perform the following procedure(s)/treatment(s) upon myself/the patient.

Procedure(s)/Treatment(s) _____

_____

The procedure has been explained to me, and I have been told the reasons why I need the procedure. The risks of the procedure
have also been explained to me. In addition, I have been told that the procedure may not have the results that I expect. I have also
been told about other possible treatments for my condition and what might happen if no treatment is received.

I understand that, in addition to the risks described to me about this procedure, there are risks that may occur with any surgical or
medical procedure. I am aware that the practice of medicine and surgery is not an exact science and that I have not been given any
guarantees about the results of this procedure.

I have had enough time to discuss my condition and treatment with my healthcare providers, and all of my questions have been
answered to my satisfaction. I believe I have enough information to make an informed decision, and I agree to have the procedure
performed. If something unexpected happens and I require additional or different treatment(s) from the treatment I expect, I agree
to accept any treatment necessary.

I agree to have transfusion of blood and other blood products that may be necessary in addition to the procedure I am having.
The risks, benefits, and alternatives have been explained to me, and all of my questions have been answered to my satisfaction. If I
refuse to have transfusions, I will cross out and initial this section and sign a Refusal of Treatment form.

I agree to allow this facility to keep, use, or properly dispose of tissue and parts of organs removed during this procedure.

_____   _____
Signature of Patient or Parent/Legal Guardian of Minor Patient   Date

If the patient cannot consent for himself or herself, the signature of either the healthcare agent or legal guardian acting on behalf
of the patient, or the patient's next of kin who is asserting to the treatment for the patient, must be obtained.

_____   _____
Signature of Patient or Parent/Legal Guardian of Minor Patient   Date

_____   _____
Signature and Relationship of Next of Kin   Date

Witness:

I, _____, am a facility employee who is not the patient's physician or authorized healthcare
provider named above, and I have witnessed the patient or other appropriate person voluntarily sign this form.

_____
Signature and Title of Witness

Interpreter/Translator (to be signed by the interpreter/translator if the patient required such assistance)

To the best of my knowledge, the patient understood what was interpreted/translated and voluntarily signed this form.

_____
Signature of Interpreter/Translator

Advance Directives

An **advance directive** is a document that provides information about how the patient would like to be treated if they are no longer able to make their own medical decisions. There are several types of advance directives. Figure 4.11 provides a sample of one type of document that may be attached to a patient's chart in the EHR system.

Figure 4.11 Advance Directive

ADVANCE DIRECTIVE

My Durable Power of Attorney for Health Care, Living Will, and Other Wishes

I, _____, write this document as a directive regarding my health care.

Put the initials of your name by the choices you want:

Part I. My Durable Power of Attorney for Health Care

As long as I can make my wishes known, my doctors will talk to me and I will make my own healthcare decisions.

_____ If there ever comes a time when I cannot make healthcare decisions about myself, I appoint this adult person to make decisions for me:

Name   Home Phone   Work Phone

Address

Email

_____ If the person above cannot or will not make decisions for me, I appoint a second person:

Name   Home Phone   Work Phone

Address

Email

_____ I understand that if I do not appoint a Durable Power of Attorney for Health Care, someone may be designated to make my healthcare decisions by law or by a court.

I want the person I have appointed, my doctors, my family, and others to be guided by my wishes described on the following pages.

... for it to be legal.

... the purpose and the effect of this document.

_____ Date_____

Your Witnesses' Signature

I believe the person who has signed this advance directive to be of sound mind, that he/she signed or acknowledged this advance directive in my presence, and that he/she appears not be acting under pressure, duress, fraud or undue influence. I am not related to the person making this advance directive by blood, marriage or adoption, nor, to the best of my knowledge am I named in his/her will. I am not the person appointed in this advance directive. I am not a health care provider or an employee of health care provider who is now, or has been in the past, responsible for the care of the person making this advance directive.

Witness #1

Name_____ Date_____

Address_____

Witness #2

Name_____ Date_____

Address_____

Figure 4.12 shows the documents that have been uploaded into the EHR system.

Figure 4.12 Patient Documents in the EHR Navigator

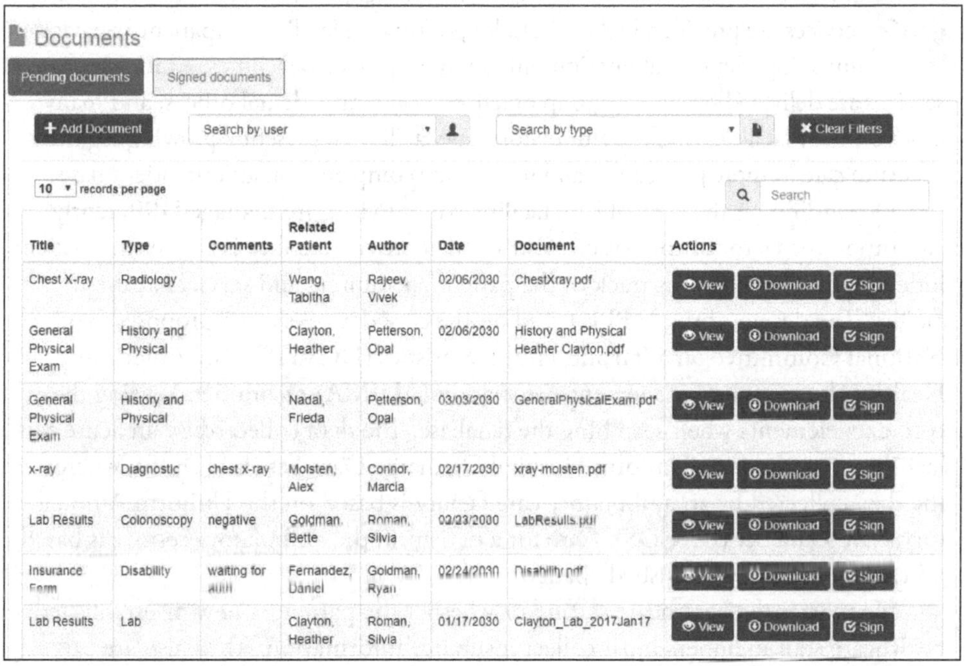

Title	Type	Comments	Related Patient	Author	Date	Document	Actions
Chest X-ray	Radiology		Wang, Tabitha	Rajeev, Vivek	02/06/2030	ChestXray.pdf	View Download Sign
General Physical Exam	History and Physical		Clayton, Heather	Petterson, Opal	02/06/2030	History and Physical Heather Clayton.pdf	View Download Sign
General Physical Exam	History and Physical		Nadal, Frieda	Petterson, Opal	03/03/2030	GeneralPhysicalExam.pdf	View Download Sign
x-ray	Diagnostic	chest x-ray	Molsten, Alex	Connor, Marcia	02/17/2030	xray-molsten.pdf	View Download Sign
Lab Results	Colonoscopy	negative	Goldman, Bette	Roman, Silvia	02/23/2030	LabResults.pdf	View Download Sign
Insurance Form	Disability	waiting for auth	Fernandez, Daniel	Goldman, Ryan	02/24/2030	Disability.pdf	View Download Sign
Lab Results	Lab		Clayton, Heather	Roman, Silvia	01/17/2030	Clayton_Lab_2017Jan17	View Download Sign

Tutorial 4.6

EHRNAVIGATOR

Attaching a Document to a Patient's Chart

Go to your online course to launch Tutorial 4.6. As an admission clerk, practice attaching a document to a patient's chart using the EHR Navigator.

Tutorial 4.7

EHRNAVIGATOR

Adding and Advance Directive

Go to your online course to launch Tutorial 4.7. As a nurse, practice adding an advance directive to a patient's chart.

Consider This

The *Documents* feature of an EHR system offers many benefits for healthcare personnel. For providers, this feature allows them to scan or upload documents, such as test results or handwritten notes, and attach them to a patient's chart. This feature also allows providers to sign the notes. For all healthcare staff members, the *Documents* feature allows them access to view the documents and helps prevent misplaced or misfiled paperwork. In short, the ability to attach documents in an EHR system increases efficiency, productivity, and quality of patient care. With all these benefits, do you think there are still opportunities for documentation errors? What types of errors may occur?

Chapter Summary

Patients seek health care at acute care and ambulatory care facilities. Acute care services are provided by hospitals, long-term care facilities, inpatient behavioral units, inpatient rehabilitation units, and hospice care facilities. Ambulatory care services are delivered by clinics, group practices, home care, dental offices, and many other types of facilities. In fact, ambulatory care facilities represent a growing segment of health care as more procedures and services are completed on an outpatient basis.

Depending on the type of care facility, patient visits are managed differently. An important factor of the patient visit in an acute care facility is the master patient index (MPI), which keeps track of the patient encounters and services at the facility. The design of the MPI is based on the core data elements proposed by the National Committee on Vital and Health Statistics (NCVHS). The American Health Information Management Association (AHIMA) recommends using the core data elements when searching the database. The data collected by an acute care facility is based on the Uniform Hospital Discharge Data Set (UHDDS), whereas the data collected by an ambulatory care facility is based on the Uniform Ambulatory Care Data Set (UACDS). Care for a patient in the ambulatory setting is based on the "new versus established" patient rule.

No matter the healthcare setting or whether the patient is new or established, healthcare staff members must collect insurance information. They also are required to gather and complete many documents during the patient's initial visit, including the Notice of Privacy Practices, assignment of benefits, consents, and advance directives. In an EHR system, these documents may be electronically signed and attached to the patient's record.

Review and Assessment

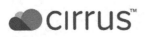

The following Review and Assessment activities are also available online in the Cirrus online course. Your instructor may ask you to complete these activities online. Cirrus also provides access to flash cards, a crossword puzzle, and practice quizzes to help strengthen your understanding of the chapter content.

Acronyms/Initialisms

Study the following acronyms discussed in this chapter. Go to the online course for flash cards of the acronyms and other chapter key terms.

AHIMA: American Health Information Management Association

EIN: enterprise identification number

EMPI: enterprise master patient index

HIPAA: Health Insurance Portability and Accountability Act of 1996

MPI: master patient index

NCVHS: National Committee on Vital and Health Statistics

UACDS: Uniform Ambulatory Care Data Set

UHDDS: Uniform Hospital Discharge Data Set

UPI: universal patient identifier

Check Your Understanding

To check your understanding of this chapter's key concepts, answer the following questions.

1. Demographic information includes

   a. date of birth.

   b. laboratory results.

   c. diagnostic history.

   d. immunizations.

2. The master patient index is a(n)

   a. spreadsheet of patient invoices.

   b. database of patients seen at the healthcare facility.

   c. index of patient telephone numbers.

   d. index of patient insurance coverage.

3. AHIMA recommends using which core data element when searching for a patient record in an EHR?

   a. Marital status

   b. Mother's maiden name

   c. Telephone number

   d. Patient identification number

4. The Uniform Hospital Discharge Data Set includes all of the following *except*

   a. date of birth.

   b. sex.

   c. reason for encounter.

   d. admission date.

5. If a child is covered by two insurance plans, the primary coverage is the insurance of the

   a. parent who is older.

   b. parent who is younger.

   c. parent whose birth date occurs first in a calendar year.

   d. parent who has the best coverage.

6. True/False: Long-term care facilities have patients who reside for more than 30 days.

7. True/False: There is only one type of ambulatory care facility.

8. True/False: Workers' compensation is a type of guarantor account.

9. True/False: Most EHR systems allow documents to be uploaded to a patient's chart.

10. True/False: EHR systems do *not* have the capability for a healthcare provider to electronically sign documents.

Go on the Record

To build on your understanding of the topics in this chapter, complete the following short-answer activities.

1. Compare the registration processes in acute care versus ambulatory care settings.

2. Describe the different types of ambulatory care settings.

3. Explain the differences between the Uniform Hospital Discharge Data Set (UHDDS) and the Uniform Ambulatory Care Data Set (UACDS).

4. Review the image of Vance Donaldson's Cobalt Care insurance card. Identify the different parts of the insurance card.

Cobalt Care
Insurance card

VANCE DONALDSON
BIN: 00123
ID: ZVD996274638

GROUP: 11770
RELATIONSHIP: 01, CARDHOLDER

MEMBER SERVICES: 1-800-555-3232
CLAIMS/INQUIRIES: 1-800-555-6363

5. Discuss how a patient is identified as either a new patient or an established patient.

Navigate the Field

To gain practice in handling challenging situations in the workplace, consider the following real-world scenarios and identify how you would respond to each.

1. You are part of the team from Lincoln County Hospital working with the EHR Savvy company on the design of the master patient index (MPI). What elements are required for the MPI? Create a table with the elements that must be included in the MPI.

2. You are the EHR training specialist with Lincoln County Hospital. You are meeting with the registration staff to review the appropriate procedures for searching for patients. What steps should those procedures contain? Create a checklist for the registrars to follow when determining whether a patient is new or established.

Think Critically

Continue to think critically about challenging concepts and complete the following activities.

1. A new patient calls the admissions desk at Northstar Medical Center to preregister for a surgery. Prepare a list of steps that you would take to add the new patient to the EHR system.

2. Identify common errors made in the registration process. How could these errors be avoided or minimized? What is the impact of these errors on patient care?

Make Your Case

Consider the scenario and then complete the following project.

You are a member of the Medical Records Department at Lincoln County Hospital. You are training the registration staff on the admission process. Prepare a presentation for your class that provides detailed guidelines to follow when collecting patient information.

Explore the Technology

Complete the EHR Navigator practice assessments that align to each tutorial and the assessments that accompany Chapter 4 located in your online course.

EHRNAVIGAT✛R

Chapter 5 Scheduling and Patient Management

Field Notes

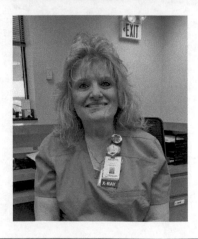

"Looking at electronic health records through the lens of a radiologic technologist improves the quality of care and communication among varied disciplines, streamlines the registration process for imaging, and enables imaging to be accessed and viewed by various healthcare providers. Maintaining an EHR improves patient care from start to finish."

– Collette Eisen, X-Ray Technologist

5.1 Explain the importance of using the scheduling feature in an EHR.

5.2 Customize a healthcare facility's schedule.

5.3 Describe the five types of scheduling methods.

5.4 Describe the benefits of allowing patients to schedule appointments using a patient portal.

5.5 List the information required to schedule an appointment.

5.6 Schedule, cancel, and reschedule an appointment in the EHR.

5.7 Generate a provider schedule from the EHR.

5.8 Transfer a patient in the EHR.

5.9 Check out or discharge a patient in the EHR.

5.10 Explain how the patient tracker can improve workflow.

Scheduling appointments is a common task among healthcare staff members, particularly in an ambulatory care setting. An electronic health record (EHR) system that includes a scheduling feature helps simplify the scheduling and billing processes in a healthcare facility. To facilitate scheduling, the EHR system is programmed to coordinate information from the facility's schedule with provider schedules and default appointment and visit times. After the visit, the EHR links the patient chart to the visit information for billing and follow-up purposes. You will learn how to schedule a visit in the EHR Navigator. Some systems will use a separate electronic program to handle scheduling and communicate with the EHR system via a Health Level 7 International (HL7) interface. The system's patient portal also includes scheduling and messaging features for the patient to choose the time and purpose of their visit and communicate with the healthcare staff.

Before scheduling any patient visits, however, the facility must set up a facility template showing its overall schedule of operations. Once these scheduling parameters have been set, healthcare staff members can schedule patient appointments in the *Schedules* tab of the EHR system (see Figure 5.1).

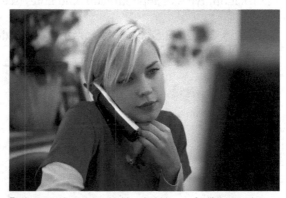

Patients make contact with a healthcare facility to make an appointment.

Figure 5.1 Scheduling Tab on the EHR Navigator

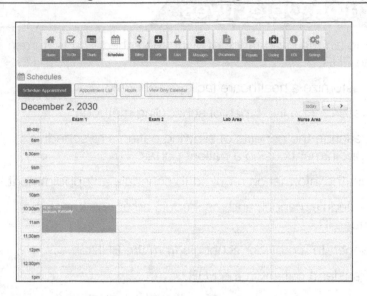

5.1 Healthcare Facility Schedule

A healthcare facility should create a matrix that shows available and unavailable appointment times. Unavailable times may include meetings, holidays, lunch hours, surgical schedules, physician rounds, or emergencies. The schedule may be viewed as daily, weekly, or monthly calendars, and it may be viewed by provider or facility. The scheduling tools are used to insert, edit, cancel, or clear an appointment from the schedule. When setting up the EHR system, the acute care or ambulatory care facility enters the parameters for scheduling patients. Typically, a practice administrator or a representative from the healthcare facility works with the EHR vendor to create available days, times, and types of appointments. Such parameters typically include available providers, available scheduling days and hours, and types of visits. A typical EHR schedule for an ambulatory care facility displays a calendar; lists of available providers, such as physicians, nurse practitioners, and physician assistants; and a list of open appointments, currently scheduled patients, contact information, types of appointments, and notes (see Figure 5.2).

Figure 5.2 EHR Schedule for an Ambulatory Care Facility

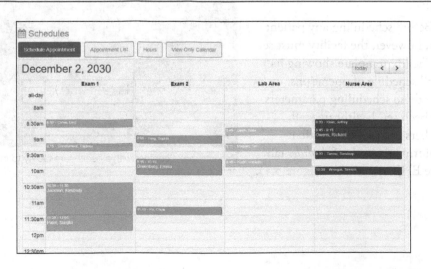

Figure 5.3   Blocked-Off Time in a Facility Schedule

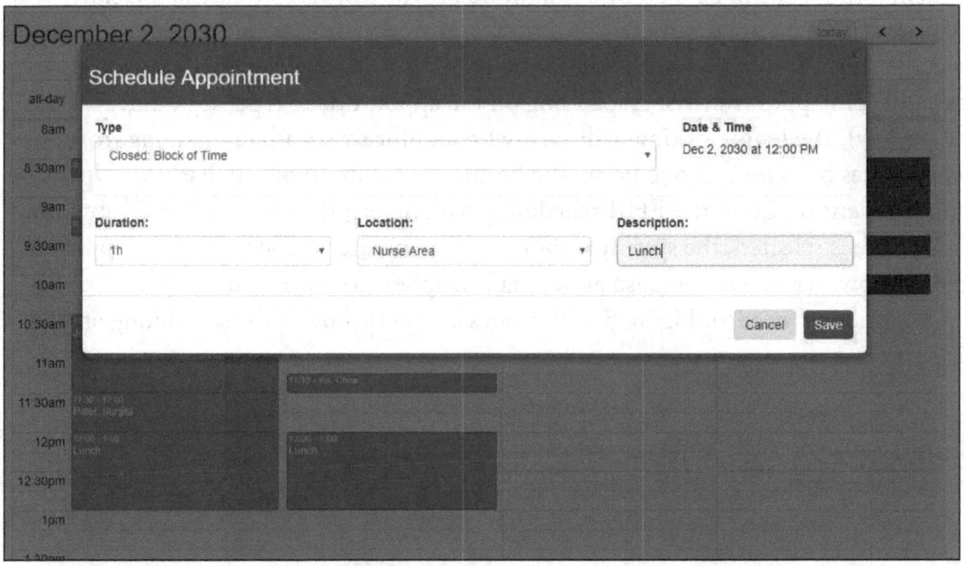

As mentioned earlier, the EHR scheduling system must block off time for holidays, lunch hours, vacations, personal time, and meetings, as necessary. These unavailable hours should be blocked off as soon as possible so patients are not scheduled during those times (see Figure 5.3). This can be accomplished by using the *Schedules* feature and adding the blocked off time directly to the calendar or by clicking *Hours* and adjusting the times or days the facility is open.

Tutorial 5.1	EHRNAVIGATOR

Blocking Time in the EHR Schedule

Go to the online course to launch Tutorial 5.1. As an office manager, practice closing the office and adjusting the hours for Northstar Physicians.

Printing a Provider's Schedule

The EHR must generate reports of clinical or administrative information. One example is to print the provider's schedule.

Tutorial 5.2	EHRNAVIGATOR

Printing a Provider's Schedule

Go to the online course to launch Tutorial 5.2. As a medical assistant, practice printing a provider's schedule using the EHR Navigator.

Appointment Scheduling Process

Patients who want to be seen by a healthcare provider or receive care at a facility typically make an appointment for a specific date and time. Most healthcare facilities use a fixed schedule, whereas others, such as urgent care clinics or after-hours clinics, take walk-in appointments. Depending on the appointment type (e.g., office visit or surgery), the length of time will vary, with an office visit usually ranging from 10 minutes to as long as one hour. The healthcare facility typically has each type of appointment set up in the EHR scheduling parameters; therefore, when an appointment type is selected, the system automatically populates the length of the appointment. However, the system also allows staff members to customize the length of an appointment if needed. Figure 5.4 illustrates a typical process for scheduling an appointment for an outpatient.

Figure 5.4 Scheduling an Outpatient Appointment

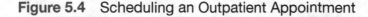

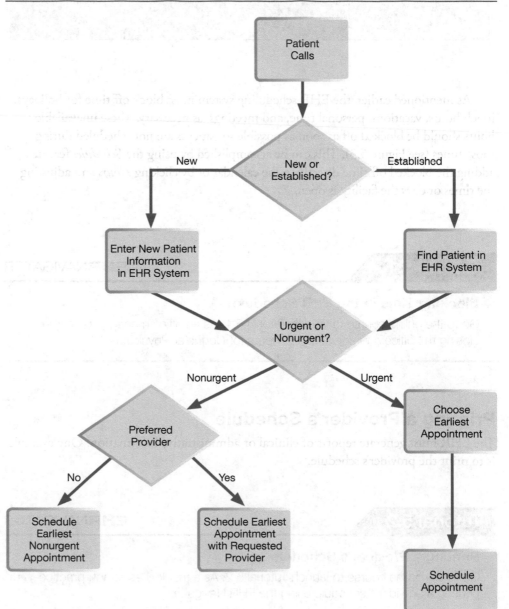

Scheduling Methods

There are several ways healthcare facilities choose to schedule appointments. No matter the type of scheduling method selected by the healthcare facility, the schedule must meet the needs of the facility's providers and patients. The types of scheduling methods that may be implemented include open hours, time specified, wave, modified wave, and cluster.

- **Open Hours:** Patients are seen throughout certain time frames or on a first-come, first-served basis. This type of scheduling is typically used in an urgent care setting.

- **Time Specified:** Patients are given a specific date and time to arrive at a facility. A time-specified schedule may be used in an acute care setting where the patient has a specific date and time for surgery.

- **Wave:** Patients are scheduled to arrive at the beginning of the hour (hence, the term *wave*), and the number of appointments is determined by dividing the hour by the length of an average visit or procedure. The expectation is that patient visits will average out the time usage during that hour. This type of scheduling may be used in a primary care office where a group of patients arrive at the top of the hour, and then no appointments are scheduled at the bottom of the hour.

- **Modified Wave:** Patients arrive at planned intervals in the first half hour, then, in the second half hour, the healthcare provider catches up. This type of scheduling may be used in an internal medicine office where the provider does not have to be in the room with the patient for the entire appointment.

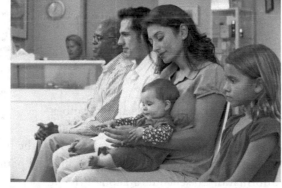

- **Cluster:** Similar appointments are scheduled together at specific times of the day. For example, in a pediatrician's office, well-child visits may be scheduled in the morning, and ill-child appointments may be scheduled in the afternoon.

In wave scheduling, all patients arrive at the beginning of the hour.

CHECKPOINT 5.1

1. What types of events are placed on a schedule as blocked-off time?

_____

_____

_____

2. List the five types of scheduling methods.

a. _____

b. _____

c. _____

d. _____

e. _____

5.2 Patient Appointment Scheduling

Once the facility schedule includes the necessary parameters, patient appointments may be scheduled. There are a few ways to schedule an appointment in the EHR scheduling system. A patient can schedule an appointment through a secure patient portal, which gives the patient the opportunity to request their preferred appointment. Or, more traditionally, patients can contact the healthcare facility to schedule their appointments.

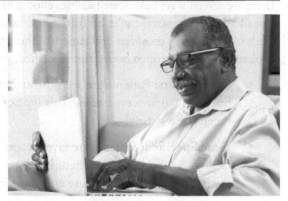

A patient can make an appointment from a home computer, using a patient portal.

Information Needed to Schedule an Appointment

When a patient, whether inpatient or outpatient, initiates an admission or appointment, specific patient information must be collected. For a new patient, this information includes the following:

- Patient's full name
- Telephone number
- Date of birth
- Chief complaint or reason for appointment
- Type of insurance
- Insurance identification number

- Referring physician
- Social Security number
- Sex
- Address
- Emergency contact
- Responsible party information
- Employer information

Using the master patient index (MPI), the healthcare facility may populate the admission or appointment for an established patient by collecting the following information to schedule an appointment:

- Patient's full name
- Date of birth
- Telephone number
- Chief complaint or reason for appointment

The patient information that already exists in the EHR must be verified and updated at the time of scheduling.

Using the Patient Portal to Schedule an Appointment

Many EHR systems contain either a patient portal or a personal health record (PHR) component. The **patient portal** provides a secure communication tool between patients and healthcare providers that complies with the Health Insurance Portability and Accountability Act of 1996 (HIPAA). Patient portals can also provide patients with information for their PHRs. Some patient portals are web based and provide 24-hour, self-service components for patients to use. The patient portal links to the facility's EHR system and thus allows the patient to view a provider's calendar of available dates and times and to schedule an appointment. This type of portal also allows the patient to update demographic, insurance, medical history, and current health information prior to an appointment. Patients who use the patient portal reduce the resources necessary from the healthcare facility.

The patient portal scheduling component is used only by established patients of an acute care or ambulatory care facility. The healthcare provider gives an established patient an access code that allows them to schedule an appointment, send a message, update information, view laboratory appointments, request prescription refills, and view their health record. See Figures 5.5 and 5.6 for examples of a patient portal. Chapter 14 will cover the personal health record and the patient portal in more detail.

The patient accesses the patient portal by entering a username and password. Once logged in, the patient can view upcoming appointments, schedule appointments, view past appointments, and request referrals.

To begin, the patient would select *Schedule an Appointment*. The patient can select a provider and appointment type. The patient is then able to see the available appointments based on the criteria they have selected. Once a patient selects an appointment, the information is sent to the healthcare facility, and then the healthcare facility sends an email message to the patient with a confirmation. Figure 5.7 shows an example of the *Inbox* area on the *Messages* tab of a patient portal.

Figure 5.5   Log-In Screen of a Patient Portal

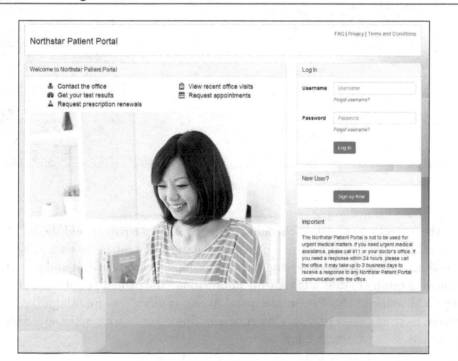

Figure 5.6   Dialog Box to Schedule an Appointment in a Patient Portal

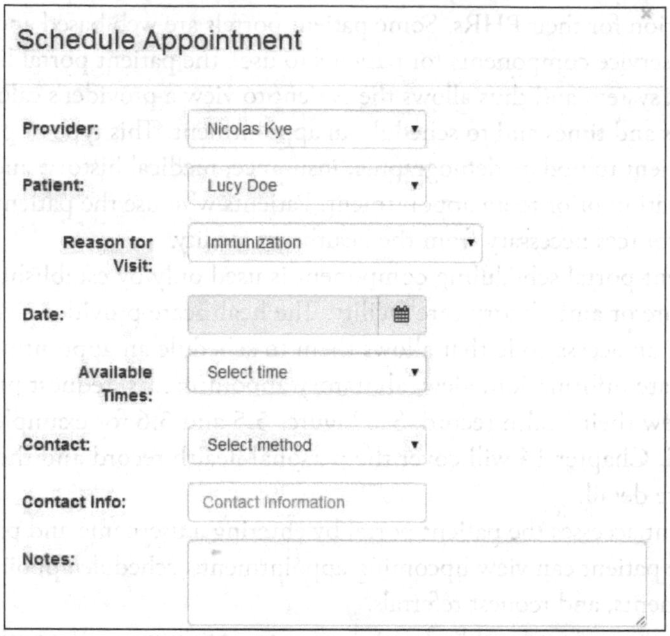

Figure 5.7   Messages in a Patient Portal

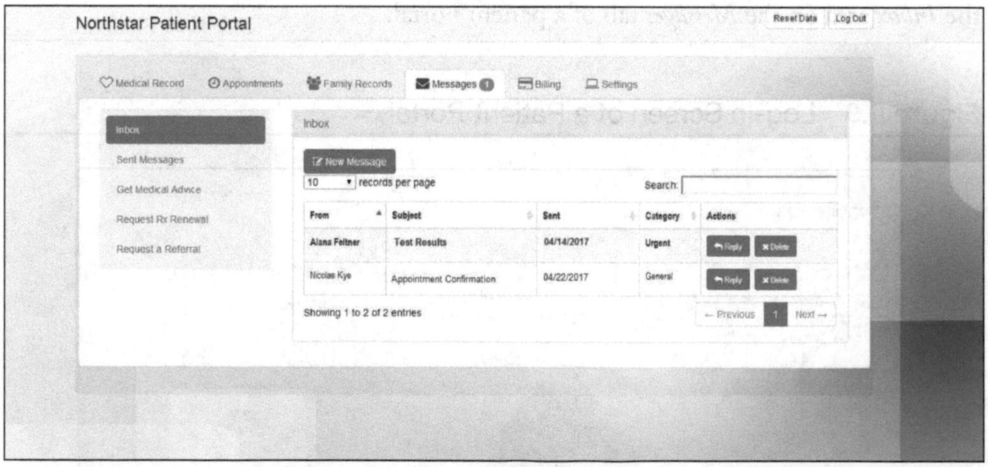

The patient portal makes scheduling convenient for the patient and the healthcare facility. Practices that implement a patient portal provide value to the patient by increasing patient access, enhancing the relationships between patients and providers, improving quality of care, and securing information. The patient portal was a goal of Stage 2 Meaningful Use, Patient Electronic Access. It meets four meaningful use criteria: electronic copy of health information, clinical summaries, appointment recalls, and timely access to health information.

Initiating an Appointment in the EHR System

When a patient telephones the healthcare facility or is present to schedule an appointment, there are two ways to initiate an appointment within the EHR Navigator scheduling feature.

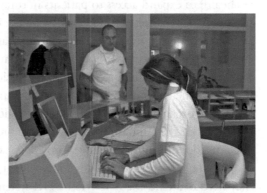

The healthcare worker searches for available appointments when a patient calls the facility.

- Select *Schedules*: This method is the easiest way to schedule an appointment, as it allows the user to see all the available time slots and facility areas at a glance (see Figure 5.8). Users click in an open time slot and can add the appointment details in the dialog box.

- Select *Appointment List* and then *Add Appointment*: This method allows the user to modify the traditional appointment times.

Both methods produce the same result: an appointment. The difference in the various ways to schedule appointments depends on user needs and preferences. The scheduling feature shows various colors that define the visit type or scheduled department.

Figure 5.8 Schedule an Appointment

Schedule Appointment

Type
Appointment

Date & Time
Dec 2, 2030 at 10:45 AM

Duration:
15m

Provider:
Chapman, Julie Ann

Location:
Lab Area

Procedure:
Select procedure

Patient:
Darnell, William

Reason for Visit:
Diagnostic

Preferred Contact:
Cell Phone

Notes:

Contact Information:

Cancel   Save

Scheduling Telehealth Appointments

In addition to traditional appointments and visits, EHR scheduling systems have been adapted to meet the demands of telehealth. Telehealth appointments are health visits conducted remotely with the assistance of technology. Healthcare organizations use telehealth to expand access to patients in rural areas and to provide healthcare services when a patient cannot or should not visit the facility in person. Due to the coronavirus pandemic, policies were changed to reduce barriers to telehealth access. Telehealth can be delivered synchronously or asynchronously, meaning the patient and the provider may or may not use the technology—such as a live video service or messaging application—at the same time. Telehealth visits require scheduling just like onsite appointments. A healthcare organization can assign one provider to all the telehealth visits on a specific day or divide the appointments among the providers. The healthcare organization may also consider limiting the services provided via telehealth visits.

On the day of the telehealth appointment, the patient receives the link or information they need to attend the visit. Most EHR systems ask the patient to log on 15 minutes early to make updates to their patient profile or insurance information and pay any copays before they are seen by a provider. At the end of the visit, the patient and provider end their session, and any follow-up communication is typically done in the PHR. Recent advancements in the technology used for telehealth appointments and the types of services conducted at these visits are discussed in Chapter 14.

Tutorial 5.3   **EHR**NAVIGAT⊕R

Scheduling an Inpatient Procedure

Go to the online course to launch Tutorial 5.3. As a unit clerk, practice scheduling an inpatient procedure using the EHR Navigator.

Tutorial 5.4   **EHR**NAVIGAT⊕R

Scheduling an Outpatient Appointment

Go to the online course to launch Tutorial 5.4. As a front desk clerk, practice scheduling an outpatient appointment using the EHR Navigator.

CHECKP⊕INT 5.2

1. Describe the benefits of scheduling using a patient portal.

   _____

   _____

   _____

2. What are two methods for scheduling an appointment in the EHR?

   a. _____

   b. _____

Canceling and Rescheduling Appointments

Many facilities struggle with patients who cancel appointments or those who do not show for their scheduled appointments (called **no-shows**). Patients cancel their appointments for a variety of reasons, including scheduling conflicts, emotional issues, financial concerns, and—for no-shows—forgetfulness. Regardless of the reason, each facility must set its own policy on cancellation fees, and each canceled appointment or no-show should be documented in the EHR system. Tracking these types of appointments will enable the healthcare facility to run reports and determine its rate of no-shows. See Figure 5.9 for a sample No-Show Report.

Confirming appointments decreases the incidences of no-shows, which in turn increases practice productivity and revenue. Healthcare staff can decrease the number of no-shows by setting up automated confirmation of appointments in the EHR system. To maximize the results of confirming appointments, patients can be given an option to receive a phone call, text message, or secure email reminder based on personal preference. Rescheduling may be the outcome of a canceled or no-show appointment.

EXPAND YOUR LEARNING

Most healthcare practices begin each day with the thought that all patients will show up and there will not be any no-shows. This is often not the case. Read the article on strategies for optimizing patient appointment scheduling at https://EHR3 .ParadigmEducation.com/ PatientAppointments.

Figure 5.9 No-Show Report

Select Date
From date:

11/01/2030	📅

Filter by Status:

No Show	▼

Status ❯	Canceled Date	Start	End	Duration	Provider	Patient
No Show	11/01/2030	8:00am	8:30am	30	Alana Feltner	Sebastian Santos
No Show	11/01/2030	12:15pm	12:30pm	15	Linda Dowling	Jeffrey Klein
No Show	11/01/2030	9:15am	9:30am	15	Ricardo Vanderbosch	Franklin Romero
No Show	11/01/2030	1:00pm	1:15pm	15	Linda Dowling	Lourdes Torres
No Show	11/01/2030	1:00pm	1:30pm	30	Avis Turrell	William Carreno
No Show	11/01/2030	11:00am	11:15am	15	Linda Dowling	Hannah Dam
No Show	11/01/2030	2:15pm	2:30pm	15	Patrick Chaplin	Mary Dorris
No Show	11/01/2030	11:30am	12:00pm	30	Jeannette Jatfield	Hallie Rooney
No Show	11/01/2030	10:00am	10:30am	30	Alana Feltner	Tim Molsten
No Show	11/01/2030	10:00am	10:15am	15	Ricardo Vanderbosch	Marquita Wilkins
No Show	11/01/2030	12:15pm	12:30pm	15	Alana Feltner	Ingrid Oberg
No Show	11/01/2030	9:30am	10:00am	30	Avis Turrell	Miguel Esparza
No Show	11/01/2030	4:30pm	5:00pm	30	Gregory Holzer	Amelia Fernandez
No Show	11/01/2030	2:00pm	2:15pm	15	Avis Turrell	Kenji Wantabe

Tutorial 5.5

EHRNAVIGAT✚R

Running a Report of No Shows

Go to the online course to launch Tutorial 5.5. As a front desk clerk, practice pulling a report of no-show patients, using the EHR Navigator.

Rescheduling an Appointment

Go to the online course to launch Tutorial 5.6. As a medical assistant, practice canceling and rescheduling an appointment using the EHR Navigator.

Consider This

No-shows affect a healthcare organization through lost revenue, jumbled employee work schedules, and increased expenses. A missed appointment, on average, costs the healthcare organization $120 per no-show. Due to the cost, many healthcare organizations charge patients for missed appointments. For a healthcare facility that has an average of 160 appointments per day with a 5% no-show rate, the cost for no-shows is $11,520. Healthcare organizations are using different technologies to reach patients to remind them of their appointments. In the past, healthcare organizations sent postcards that often went into the trash, made telephone calls that went unanswered, and sent emails that went to a patient's spam folder. However, 90% of all text messages are viewed within three minutes, making them an effective mode of communication. Text messages can create more engagement between patients and healthcare facilities, and they also save staff time.

5.3 Patient Transfers in the EHR System

While receiving care in a hospital, a patient may need to be transferred from one unit or room to another. Some of the reasons for a patient transfer include a change in patient condition, change in isolation status, or patient preference. All intrafacility transfers must be documented within the EHR system to ensure accuracy in patients' locations and hospital census data.

Consider This

In February 2017, the US Department of Defense (DoD) launched an inpatient and outpatient EHR called *MHS Genesis*. The EHR connects medical and dental information. MHS Genesis supports 9.4 million DoD beneficiaries and approximately 205,000 military personnel globally. The DOD plans to have MHS Genesis implemented by 2024. Why do you think it is taking the DoD approximately seven years to fully implement MHS Genesis?

Change in Patient Condition

During an inpatient stay, a patient's condition may improve or deteriorate to the point that they must be transferred to a nursing unit in the hospital that can more adequately address their needs. For example, a patient in a room on a postoperative hospital unit who experiences cardiac arrest will likely be transferred to a more intensive nursing unit, such as a cardiac intensive care unit. As the patient stabilizes and improves, they may be moved to a less intensive care unit.

Change in Isolation Status

Isolation status refers to the precautions that must be taken by healthcare staff and visitors to prevent the spread of bacterial or viral infections. Many hospital rooms are semiprivate, meaning there are two patients occupying a room. Patients can be admitted to the same room only if they have the same isolation status. For example, a patient infected with methicillin-resistant *Staphylococcus aureus* (MRSA) cannot be admitted to the room of a patient without the same infection, as there is a substantial risk that the other patient may also become infected with MRSA.

Patient Preference

Patients may ask to be transferred to another hospital room for many reasons, such as noise levels or roommate issues. All EHR systems should have a transfer patient function. In the EHR Navigator, this function is accessed through the *Admission/Discharge* tab.

Tutorial 5.7　　　　　　　　　　　　　**EHR**NAVIGAT⊕R

Transferring a Patient

Go to the online course to launch Tutorial 5.7. As a unit clerk, practice transferring a patient using the EHR Navigator.

5.4 Checkout and Discharge Procedures

The procedure for a patient leaving a medical facility varies depending on whether the patient is **checking out** at an outpatient facility or being **discharged** from an inpatient facility.

Outpatient Checkout

Following an outpatient visit, the patient will check out. The checkout procedure may include collecting payments, ordering tests, making referrals, or scheduling a future appointment for the patient. During the checkout process, all the necessary prescriptions and completed forms must be verified.

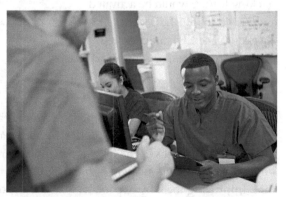

Before checking out of an outpatient facility, a patient may be asked to schedule a follow-up appointment.

Inpatient Discharge

The discharge of an inpatient from an acute care hospital is entered into the EHR Navigator via the *Admission/Discharge* tab. The date and time of the patient's discharge are automatically captured when the nurse or staff member enters the discharge into the EHR system. The **discharge disposition**, or the patient's destination following a stay in the hospital, is also entered. Examples of discharge dispositions include home, skilled nursing facility, rehabilitation hospital, and long-term acute care hospital. If an inpatient has died, the discharge disposition entered is "expired."

Discharge documents may be generated from the EHR system. These documents may include discharge instructions specific to the patient's diagnoses and the procedures performed. Discharge documents may also include information regarding recommended follow-up with the patient's surgeon or primary care physician. In addition, to comply with accreditation requirements, a current medication list should be provided from the EHR system to the patient at the time of discharge. At that time, the patient or patient representative should acknowledge and sign receipt of the discharge summary and instructions.

Tutorial 5.8   EHRNAVIGAT⊕R

Discharging a Patient
Go to the online course to launch Tutorial 5.8. As a unit clerk, practice discharging a patient using the EHR Navigator.

5.5 Electronic Patient Tracker

An EHR system has an **electronic patient tracking (EPT)** function to track a patient's location from admission to discharge (for inpatients) or from check-in to checkout (for outpatients). This feature offers a real-time, at-a-glance view of a patient's current status and location. For example, when a patient checks in at Northstar Physicians, the patient tracking feature would be activated and would follow the patient until checkout. The EPT function replaces the traditional use of a whiteboard.

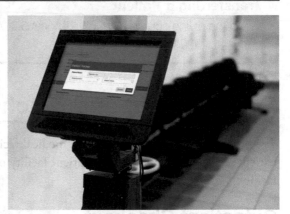

Workstations in the waiting room can be used to check in a patient and begin tracking their location.

EXPAND YOUR LEARNING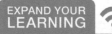

As value-based care models expand, the importance of patient wait times is now more important than ever to healthcare organizations. A value-based payment program is often tied to the patient satisfaction scores and reimbursement. If the patient satisfaction score is low because of wait time, the reimbursement to the healthcare organization may be reduced. To learn more about how a healthcare organization may decrease patient wait times, read the following article:

https://EHR3
.ParadigmEducation
.com/PatientWait.

Benefits of Electronic Patient Tracking

Knowing the location and status of all patients at all times is the obvious benefit of an EPT system. Other benefits of EPT include real-time monitoring of patient wait times and bottlenecks in the flow of patient care, room and provider utilization statistics for analysis, and identification of opportunities for improvement in patient flow and care. Improving the flow of patients with the use of EPT results in operational cost savings for the healthcare organization and increased patient satisfaction because of a reduction in wait times. Busy hospital emergency departments benefit greatly from the use of EPT, because patients in the most serious conditions can be identified, located, and triaged much faster. Patient families may also benefit from EPT. Have you ever waited for news about a family member undergoing a surgical procedure? Many hospitals and surgical centers have HIPAA-compliant electronic displays that update as a patient is moved from preop to surgery, postop, and the recovery room.

Simple and Complex Electronic Patient Tracking Systems

The functionality of EPT can be simple or complex. EPT, at its simplest, is represented by an outpatient checking in for a scheduled appointment. The staff member indicates the patient's arrival in the EPT system, the medical assistant enters the patient's location as the patient is taken back to an exam room, and then a staff member enters the patient's departure at the time of checkout. To locate a patient, a staff member has to access one of the office's computers.

A more complex EPT functionality might have patients check in via a kiosk. The kiosk prints a wristband that contains a computer chip that tracks the patient via the organization's secure wireless internet. Authorized users of the healthcare organization can determine a patient's location via the organization's computers and their authorized mobile devices. Consider the time savings for providers and staff who are able to quickly determine whether a patient is in his or her hospital room, CT scanning room, surgery, or somewhere else. The EHR Navigator's *Patient Tracker* feature is illustrated in Figures 5.10 and 5.11.

Figure 5.10   Dialog Box to Update the Patient's Location

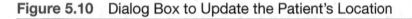

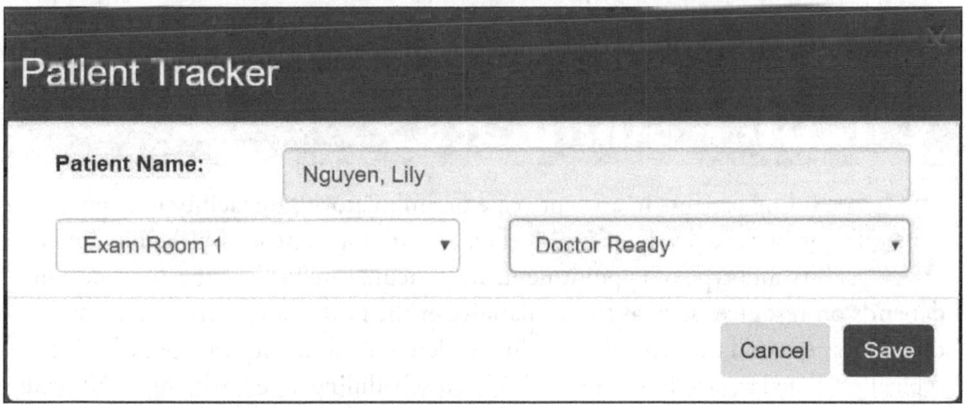

Figure 5.11   Patient Status Summary

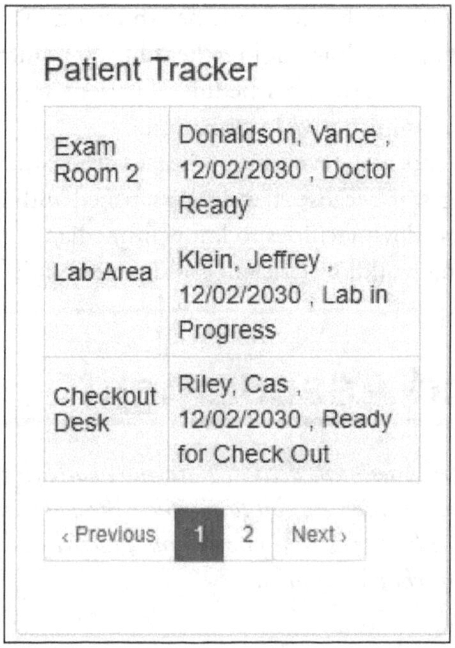

Tutorial 5.9

EHRNAVIGAT✛R

Using the Patient Tracker

Go to the online course to launch Tutorial 5.9. In this activity, practice using the EHR Navigator Patient Tracker to follow the patient from arrival to checkout. You will log in as several different staff members of Northstar Physicians.

CHECKP✛INT 5.3

1. List three reasons a patient might be transferred.

a. _____

b. _____

c. _____

2. Describe the purpose of a patient tracker system.

_____

_____

Chapter Summary

Scheduling patients in an acute care or ambulatory care facility is a key factor in the delivery of health care. Scheduling depends on the type of facility and type of appointment. In an acute care facility, the appointment depends on resources such as the availability of the healthcare provider and/or the equipment and the type of procedure ordered. Ambulatory care patients are typically labeled as new or established. When scheduling a new patient, healthcare staff must gather demographic and financial information.

There are five scheduling methods, each designed to meet the specific needs of the facility. The scheduling methods include open hours, time specified, wave, modified wave, and cluster. The electronic health record (EHR) system provides features for scheduling, canceling, and rescheduling appointments.

An EHR system must display a schedule of patient appointments and generate reports of clinical or administrative information.

Transferring patients may be necessary because the patient's condition or isolation status changes or because they are dissatisfied with the room.

Tracking patients allows facilities to know immediately the location and status of a patient, increasing workflow efficiency and patient satisfaction.

Review and Assessment

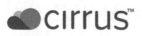

The following Review and Assessment activities are also available online in the Cirrus online course. Your instructor may ask you to complete these activities online. Cirrus also provides access to flash cards, a crossword puzzle, and practice quizzes to help strengthen your understanding of the chapter content.

Acronyms/Initialisms

Study the following acronyms discussed in this chapter. Go to the online course for flash cards of the acronyms and other chapter key terms.

EPT: electronic patient tracking

PHR: personal health record

Check Your Understanding

To check your understanding of this chapter's key concepts, answer the following questions.

1. Scheduling an appointment requires that the scheduler collect all the following pieces of information *except*

   a. health insurance information.

   b. patient demographics.

   c. reason for the visit.

   d. means of arrival.

2. An electronic health record (EHR) contains unavailable times for scheduling appointments. Unavailable times may include all of the following *except*

   a. holidays.

   b. hospital rounds.

   c. lunch.

   d. pharmaceutical sales visits.

3. A healthcare facility may choose one of the following scheduling methods to create its appointment schedule.

   a. modified cluster

   b. wave

   c. open wave

   d. cluster time

4. A patient portal is

   a. owned and controlled by a patient, may contain additional information not in the medical record, and is used for managing health information.

   b. generated by a healthcare provider to document a patient's medical and health information and is not directly accessed by a patient.

   c. a secure website that allows patients to access a personal health record (PHR) to communicate with healthcare providers, request prescription refills, review laboratory test results, or schedule appointments.

   d. a nonsecure website that allows patients to access a PHR to communicate with healthcare providers, request prescription refills, review laboratory test results, or schedule appointments.

5. Which of the following is *not* an appropriate reason for a patient transfer?

   a. The patient's condition has changed.

   b. The patient does not like their roommate.

   c. The patient is in isolation status.

   d. A nurse does not like the patient.

6. True/False: Scheduling is used to insert, edit, delete, or remove an appointment.

7. True/False: The patient tracker feature in an EHR follows the patient from admission or check-in to discharge or checkout.

8. True/False: Time-specified appointment scheduling requires the patient to be seen on a first-come, first-served basis.

9. True/False: A patient may request a transfer because they find the room too noisy.

10. True/False: A patient portal provides the patient with an opportunity to schedule their own appointments.

Go on the Record

To build on your understanding of the topics in this chapter, complete the following short-answer activities.

1. Why would a healthcare facility choose to use a specific type of scheduling?

2. There are times when a schedule should be blocked from appointments. Explain the different types of activities of a healthcare facility or provider that would necessitate blocked schedule time.

3. What are the different reasons that a patient's appointment may need to be adjusted?

4. Why is it important to track a patient during their stay at a healthcare facility?

5. Describe how the patient tracker feature may improve the healthcare facility's workflow and patient satisfaction.

Navigate the Field

To gain practice in handling challenging situations in the workplace, consider the following real-world scenarios and identify how you would respond to each.

1. You receive an appointment request from Ms. Ying through the patient portal. She is requesting an appointment time already filled by another patient. You contact Ms. Ying, and she informs you that when she requested the appointment, the time was available and she needs to be seen right away. How should you handle this situation?

2. You are preparing the 2030 calendar for Northstar Physicians. You are working with the physicians, staff, and IT manager to create the schedule in the EHR Navigator. What are the steps you would take to prepare the calendar to be customized for the EHR Navigator? What would be the best

way to communicate this to the IT manager so that the EHR Navigator calendar may be customized?

Think Critically

Continue to think critically about challenging concepts and complete the following activities.

1. A new patient calls to schedule an appointment. Describe the process you would follow to schedule the initial appointment.

2. Dr. Nelson's office contacts the Scheduling Department at St. Francis Hospital to schedule Mr. Yadav's double bypass surgery. Mr. Yadav will have to stay a minimum of three days in the hospital. Prepare a list of steps you would follow to schedule the surgery for Dr. Nelson's patient.

Make Your Case

Consider the scenario and then complete the following project.

You work for Pleasant Valley Urgent Care, which is implementing a new electronic health record (EHR) system. You are responsible for working with the EHR vendor to determine the scheduling parameters of the system and must provide the vendor with a presentation on the type of scheduling Pleasant Valley Urgent Care will use. Include in the presentation the urgent care days, times, a list of healthcare providers, number of examination rooms, necessary equipment, any nonpatient times, and any additional resources that will be used for scheduling. You will be presenting to the vendor and the director of Pleasant Valley Urgent Care.

Explore the Technology

Complete the EHR Navigator practice assessments that align to each tutorial and the assessments that accompany Chapter 5 located in the online course.

EHRNAVIGAT✚R

Chapter 6 Privacy, Security, and Legal Aspects of the EHR

Field Notes

"I worked in a busy physical therapy clinic treating 24 patients per day. When a physician wrote an order that was illegible, we would have to take time away from treating patients to place a call for clarification, many times waiting until the provider had a chance in their schedule to speak with us. With an EHR, we have accurate information. We have access to diagnostic results with a mouse click. The EHR saves time, as we do not have to place a call and wait for information to be faxed. The EHR also allows for the use of prompts built into the system, which allow us to document and bill more effectively, maximizing reimbursement. We also have the ability to customize useful keyboard shortcuts that can be shared among clinicians. In big clinics, a patient may see more than one therapist, and our notes help us to achieve continuity of care."

– Kim Shearer, Physical Therapy Assistant

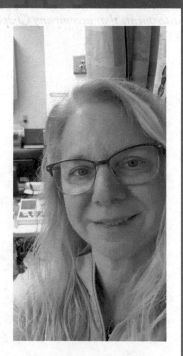

Learning Objectives

6.1 Define Health Insurance Portability and Accountability Act of 1996 (HIPAA), specifically the Administrative Simplification provisions and the date enacted.

6.2 Identify who is and who is not considered to be a covered entity under HIPAA.

6.3 Identify the basic principles of the Privacy Rule and differentiate between when disclosure of protected health information is permitted and when it is not permitted.

6.4 Demonstrate release of information (ROI) functions carried out by health information management (HIM) staff in the electronic health record (EHR) environment.

6.5 Demonstrate how to produce an accounting of disclosures log.

6.6 Discuss the concept of "minimum necessary" as it relates to the release of health information.

6.7 Explain the enforcement and penalty process for violations of HIPAA privacy and security regulations.

6.8 Discuss the HIPAA Breach Notification Rule.

6.9 State the two primary purposes for the development of the security standards of HIPAA.

6.10 List the major sections of the standards of the HIPAA Security Rule and provide safeguard examples that apply to each section.

6.11 Discuss the difference between required and addressable implementation specifications.

6.12 Explain why the 21st Century Cures Act is one of the most significant acts regarding EHR use and exchange.

6.13 Discuss the purpose of the United States Core Data for Interoperability (USCDI) and give examples of the data classes and data elements.

6.14 Define *information blocking* and give examples of what is and is not considered information blocking.

As you have already learned, privacy and confidentiality of health information is a major focus when implementing an electronic health record (EHR) system. As a user of an EHR system, you must understand and follow the laws and regulations regarding privacy, safety, and security of health information. Federal legislation that revolutionized the release and security of health information includes the HIPAA Privacy and Security Rules published in 2000, which were subsequently updated in 2010 and 2013. These rules provide guidance about the release and security of protected health information (PHI) as documented in paper health records, as well as the release and security of identifiable EHR patient information, known as electronic protected health information (ePHI). In addition, there are procedures for safeguarding health information that are not mandated by law but should be considered when implementing and using EHRs.

6.1 Health Insurance Portability and Accountability Act of 1996

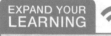

EXPAND YOUR LEARNING

Locate a website sponsored by the US government, such as https://EHR3 .ParadigmEducation .com/HIPAAindex, that provides information and resources regarding HIPAA.

The **Health Insurance Portability and Accountability Act of 1996 (HIPAA)** was enacted on August 21, 1996. HIPAA includes many provisions that affect all healthcare facilities. For example, HIPAA allows for health insurance to be "portable"—in other words, the insurance can be moved from one employer to another without denial or restrictions. HIPAA mainly addresses the confidentiality of patients' medical records, including the safeguards that need to be implemented by a healthcare facility to protect the privacy and security of patient information. In addition to setting standards for health information privacy and security, HIPAA also addresses standards to improve the efficiency and effectiveness of healthcare systems. For example, Sections 261–264, known as the Administrative Simplification Provisions, required the US Department of Health and Human Services (HHS) to adopt national standards for electronic healthcare transactions and code sets, unique health identifiers, and security. To gain a broad picture of the tenets of HIPAA, see Figure 6.1. This chapter will specifically focus on the HIPAA provisions for the electronic exchange, privacy, and security of health information.

Figure 6.1 HIPAA Administrative Simplification Provisions

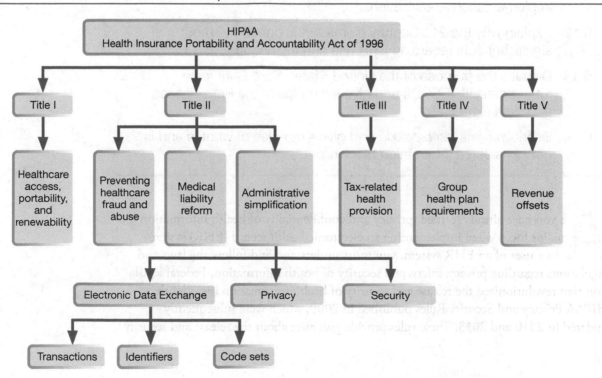

6.2 HIPAA Privacy Rule

In response to HIPAA legislation, the HHS secretary published the **Privacy Rule** in December 2000, with the intent to define protected health information and the entities and circumstances in which it may be used or disclosed by covered entities, which are defined in the next section. HHS modified the HIPAA Privacy, Security, and Enforcement Rules in January 2013, to align with the provisions of the Health Information Technology for Economic and Clinical Health (HITECH) Act, particularly with regard to EHRs. Healthcare providers, health plans, and healthcare clearinghouses were required to be in complete compliance with HIPAA, including these modifications, by September 2013.

In December 2020, the Office for Civil Rights (OCR) and the HHS proposed changes to the HIPAA Privacy Rule to support individuals' engagement in their care, remove barriers to coordinated care, and reduce regulatory burdens on the health care industry. Although these proposed changes to the HIPAA Privacy Rule had not been finalized at the time of publication, they are discussed in this chapter. See Figure 6.2 for a timeline of modifications to and expansions of HIPAA.

Covered Entities

The Privacy and Security Rules apply to healthcare providers, health plans, and healthcare clearinghouses transmitting health information in an electronic format. These entities are called **covered entities** (see Table 6.1). Individuals, organizations, and agencies meeting the definition of a covered entity under HIPAA must comply with the rules' requirements to protect the privacy and security of health information, and they must provide individuals with certain access rights with respect to their health information.

EXPAND YOUR LEARNING

The Final HIPAA Privacy Rule published on December 28, 2000, can be viewed at the following website: https://EHR3.ParadigmEducation.com/PrivacyRule.

Modifications made to HIPAA on January 25, 2013, can be viewed at the following website: http://EHR3.ParadigmEducation.com/HIPAAModifications.

And the proposed changes to the HIPAA Privacy Rule published on December 10, 2020, can be viewed at the following website: https://EHR3.ParadigmEducation.com/HIPAAProposedChanges.

Table 6.1 Covered Entities

Healthcare Provider	Health Plan	Healthcare Clearinghouse
The term *healthcare provider* refers to a provider who transmits health information in an electronic format and includes the following professionals and organizations. • Physicians • Clinics • Psychologists • Dentists • Chiropractors • Nursing homes • Pharmacies • Hospitals	The term *health plan* refers to the following entities: • Health insurance companies • Health maintenance organizations • Company health plans (some self-administered company health plans with fewer than 50 participants are not covered) • Government programs that pay for health care, such as Medicare, Medicaid, and military and veterans' healthcare programs	The term *healthcare clearinghouse* refers to public or private entities, including billing services, repricing companies, community health management information systems, community health information systems, or value-added networks and switches, that do either of the following functions: • Process or facilitate the processing of health information received from another entity in a nonstandard format or containing nonstandard data content into standard data elements or a standard transaction • Receive a standard transaction from another entity and process or facilitate the processing of health information into nonstandard format or nonstandard data content for the receiving entity

Figure 6.2 HIPAA Timeline

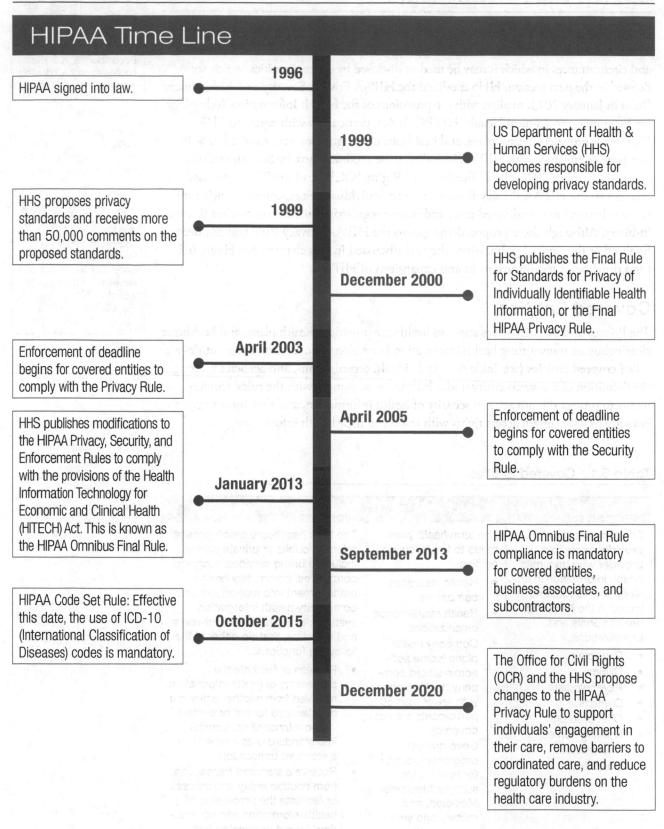

HIPAA Time Line

1996
HIPAA signed into law.

1999
US Department of Health & Human Services (HHS) becomes responsible for developing privacy standards.

1999
HHS proposes privacy standards and receives more than 50,000 comments on the proposed standards.

December 2000
HHS publishes the Final Rule for Standards for Privacy of Individually Identifiable Health Information, or the Final HIPAA Privacy Rule.

April 2003
Enforcement of deadline begins for covered entities to comply with the Privacy Rule.

April 2005
Enforcement of deadline begins for covered entities to comply with the Security Rule.

January 2013
HHS publishes modifications to the HIPAA Privacy, Security, and Enforcement Rules to comply with the provisions of the Health Information Technology for Economic and Clinical Health (HITECH) Act. This is known as the HIPAA Omnibus Final Rule.

September 2013
HIPAA Omnibus Final Rule compliance is mandatory for covered entities, business associates, and subcontractors.

October 2015
HIPAA Code Set Rule: Effective this date, the use of ICD-10 (International Classification of Diseases) codes is mandatory.

December 2020
The Office for Civil Rights (OCR) and the HHS propose changes to the HIPAA Privacy Rule to support individuals' engagement in their care, remove barriers to coordinated care, and reduce regulatory burdens on the health care industry.

Business associates of a covered entity must also follow the Privacy and Security Rules if they perform services for the covered entity involving the use or disclosure of individually identifiable health information.

Noncovered Entities

If an entity is not considered a covered entity, it does not have to comply with HIPAA Privacy and Security Rules. Some examples of **noncovered entities** include workers' compensation carriers, employers, marketing firms, life insurance companies, pharmaceutical manufacturers, casualty insurance carriers, pharmacy benefit management companies, and crime victim compensation programs.

Health Information and the Privacy Rule

Certain types of health information are classified under the HIPAA Privacy Rule. These types include protected health information, individually identifiable health information, and deidentified health information.

Protected Health Information

The Privacy Rule defines **protected health information (PHI)** as all individually identifiable health information held or transmitted by a covered entity or its business associate, in any form or medium, whether electronic, paper, or oral.

PHI is information, including demographic data, that identifies the individual, or for which there is a reasonable basis to believe that the information can be used to identify the individual, and that relates to at least one of the following:

- The individual's past, present, or future physical or mental health condition
- The provision of health care to the individual
- The past, present, or future payment for the provision of health care to the individual

There are 18 types of information that qualify as PHI according to guidance from the HHS Office of Civil Rights, which includes:

1. Name
2. Address
3. Any dates (except years that are directly related to the individual, such as birth date)
4. Telephone number
5. Fax number
6. Social Security number
7. Medical record number
8. Health plan beneficiary number
9. Account number
10. Certificate/license number

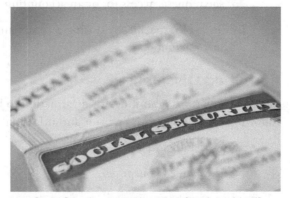

Your Social Security number is a type of common identifier.

11.   Vehicle identifiers

12.   Device identifiers or serial numbers

13.   Email address

14.   Digital identifiers, such as website URLs

15.   IP addresses

16.   Biometric elements, including finger, retinal, and voice prints

17.   Full face photographic images

18.   Other identifying numbers or codes

Deidentified Health Information

The term **deidentified health information** was first used and identified in the Privacy Rule and is health information that neither identifies an individual nor provides a reasonable basis to identify an individual. Therefore, the Privacy Rule does not restrict the use of deidentified health information. Healthcare staff primarily use deidentified health information for summary purposes, as illustrated by the following scenarios:

- The marketing department of a healthcare provider wants to know how many patients are from each ZIP code.

- A dentist's office wants to know the number of patients who recently had a cavity filled to determine if the office's use of dental supplies is appropriate.

- A home care agency wants to know the number of physical therapy home care visits made last year to determine whether additional physical therapists should be hired.

Basic Principles of the Privacy Rule

A major purpose of the Privacy Rule is to define and limit the circumstances in which an individual's PHI may be used or disclosed by covered entities. A covered entity may not use or disclose PHI except either (1) as the Privacy Rule permits or requires or (2) as the individual who is the subject of the information (or the individual's personal representative) authorizes in writing.

Required Disclosures

A covered entity *must* disclose PHI in only two situations:

1.   To an individual (or their personal representative), specifically when he or she requests access to, or an accounting of disclosures of, their PHI

2.   To HHS, specifically during a compliance investigation, review, or enforcement action

Permitted Disclosures

HIPAA regulations permit health information to be used and/or disclosed in the following scenarios without a prior authorization signed by the patient:

- To the individual patient

- For treatment purposes

- For payment purposes

- For healthcare operations

- Incidental to an otherwise permitted use or disclosure

- For public interest and benefit activities

- As a limited data set for purposes of research, public health, or healthcare operations

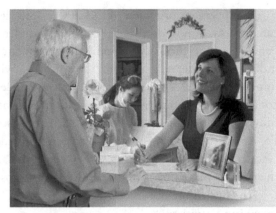

A patient is often asked to sign a HIPAA disclosure asking if it is acceptable to release their health information in certain situations.

To learn more about these specific provisions for the disclosure of health information, refer to the following sections.

Individual Patient   A patient has the right to view and receive a copy of their health information. The covered entity must release the health information in the format requested by the patient (e.g., paper electronic storage device). As a result of the HIPAA Omnibus Final Rule, patients also now have the right to download and transmit their health information electronically.

TPO Clause   Three types of permitted disclosures are commonly known in the healthcare industry collectively as **treatment, payment, healthcare operations (TPO)**. When health information managers, compliance officers, or administrators are asked questions related to the appropriate release of healthcare information and reply with, "Yes, you can release the health information under the TPO clause," they are referring to these permitted disclosures.

The treatment provision of the TPO clause applies to the application, coordination, or management of health care and related services for an individual by one or more healthcare providers, including consultation among providers regarding a patient and referral of a patient by one provider to another.

HIPAA has made it easier and faster for providers to release information for patient care purposes because written patient authorization is not necessary. This HIPAA provision is particularly important for EHRs, allowing healthcare practitioners to obtain health information within minutes or seconds. In comparison, a written authorization could take hours or days.

Consider This

A teenage patient brought to the emergency department (ED) of a hospital drifts in and out of consciousness. The ED physician suspects an adverse event from a medication the patient is taking or a possible drug overdose. The ED physician learns that the patient takes medications that have been prescribed by the patient's primary care physician.

Because the patient's EHR is interoperable with the hospital's EHR, the ED physician is able to access the medications prescribed for the patient. How does permitted disclosure of health information in the Privacy Rule allow the patient to receive the necessary care? What could happen if the patient needs to wait while the hospital seeks authorization to release her information?

The payment provision of the TPO clause allows the health plan to review healthcare information to determine premiums, to identify coverage responsibilities and benefits, and to furnish or obtain reimbursement for health care delivered to an individual. Under this provision, healthcare providers are allowed to release health information to receive payment for services rendered. In addition, health insurance companies can obtain health information to identify a subscriber's coverage and provision of benefits, as well as to offer reimbursement for healthcare services provided. For example, a nursing home is allowed to provide health information to an ambulance transportation company so that the ambulance company can be reimbursed for the transfer of a nursing home resident to the hospital.

The healthcare operations provision of the TPO clause applies to any of the following activities:

- Quality assessment and improvement, including case management and care coordination

- Competency assurance activities, including providers of health plan performance evaluation, credentialing, and accreditation

- Conducting or arranging for medical reviews, audits, and legal services, including fraud and abuse detection and compliance programs

- Specified insurance functions, such as underwriting, risk rating, and reinsuring risk

- Business planning, development, management, and administration

- Business management and general administrative activities of the entity, including—but not limited to—deidentifying PHI, creating a limited data set, and certain fundraising for the benefit of the covered entity

A covered entity is allowed to use health information for its own facility or the company's internal operations. The specific activities allowed by HIPAA are listed in the previous definition of healthcare operations. Some specific examples of permitted use and disclosures of health information under this provision are as follows:

- Health insurance companies want to contract for healthcare services from only the best providers, which are those providing the highest quality of care and services for the lowest cost. To select these high-quality, low-cost providers, the insurance company reviews specific health information, and HIPAA permits the use and disclosure of health information for this purpose.

- Healthcare providers conduct internal quality assessments to identify policies and procedures needing changes to provide higher-quality care. The HIPAA healthcare operations clause allows providers to use health information for these assessments.

It is important to note that covered entities may choose to require a signed patient authorization for any and all disclosures of patient health information, even in circumstances in which HIPAA does not require a patient's written authorization. For example, most healthcare providers request that patients sign an authorization to release healthcare information to insurance companies or other payers prior to rendering healthcare services. A good rule for a healthcare provider to follow is to obtain a written patient authorization prior to the release, disclosure, or use of an individual's health information. The authorization form should be HIPAA compliant and depict certain elements required by law.

Incidental to a Permitted Use or Disclosure The Privacy Rule does not require that every risk of an incidental use or disclosure of PHI be eliminated. A use or disclosure of this information that occurs as a result of, or as "incident to," an otherwise permitted use or disclosure is permitted as long as the covered entity has adopted reasonable safeguards as required by the Privacy Rule. For example, a hospital visitor may overhear a provider's confidential conversation with another provider, or a patient may glimpse another patient's information on a sign-in sheet or nurses' station whiteboard.

Public Interest and Benefit Activities The Privacy Rule permits the use and disclosure of PHI without an individual's authorization or permission for 12 national priority purposes, including subpoenas and court orders, certain law enforcement purposes, approved research purposes, public health purposes, organ donations, use by coroners or funeral homes, or compliance with workers' compensation laws.

Limited Data Set Use A **limited data set** is PHI from which certain specified direct identifiers of individuals and their relatives, household members, and employers have been removed. A limited data set may be used and disclosed for research, health-care operations, and public health purposes, provided the recipient enters into a data use agreement promising specified safeguards for the PHI within the limited data set.

When patient authorization is required or optionally used, specific core elements and required statements must be included in the authorization, including the date the authorization expires and a statement that the authorization is revocable. Covered entities should use a standard patient authorization form drawn up by legal counsel that includes all of the elements required by law.

Release of Information

Typically, health information management (HIM) professionals, in conjunction with compliance and information technology professionals, ensure that all healthcare staff members are educated in the organization's release of information (ROI) policies and procedures.

Rules and regulations related to the release of PHI are the same whether you are releasing information from a paper record or an EHR. However, the ROI process is significantly more streamlined in an EHR environment for many reasons, including the following:

- Physical records do not need to be located, resulting in significant time savings for HIM staff.

- Records can be printed on paper, saved to a digital storage medium, or emailed directly from the EHR rather than being copied or scanned by hand, resulting in significant time savings for HIM staff.

- Records can be released faster because the process takes less time.

The ROI workflow process follows these steps:

1. A requestor submits a written ROI request.

2. For verbal requests, the HIM staff completes a Verbal Request for Information.

3. The HIM staff logs the request into the EHR system or other designated ROI software.

4. A staff member scans the request, along with other pertinent documents, such as patient authorization, into the patient's EHR or ROI software.

5. A staff member reviews the request to verify the legitimacy for release of information. They look at items such as identification of the patient whose information is being requested, types of documents requested, and service dates.

6. The HIM staff produces the records in the format requested (paper or electronic).

7. An HIM staff member generates a correspondence letter to accompany the records.

8. The HIM staff mails or sends the records.

Tutorial 6.1   **EHR**NAVIGAT⊕R

Releasing Patient Information

Go to the online course to launch Tutorial 6.1. As a Registered Health Information Technician (RHIT), practice releasing patient information using the EHR Navigator.

Accounting of Disclosures

As you learned earlier in this chapter, the Privacy Rule states that a patient has the right to receive an accounting of disclosures of their PHI made by the covered entity. These accountings of disclosure are provided by the covered entity. ROI software that is either part of the EHR system or interfaces with the EHR system makes the release of an accounting of disclosures relatively simple because the ROI software automatically produces these documents on paper or electronically.

A sample accounting of disclosures log is found in Figure 6.3.

Figure 6.3 Accounting of Disclosures Log

NORTHSTAR MEDICAL CENTER

Accounting of Disclosures Log

Patient Name: _____

Medical Record Number: _____

Date Requested	Name of Requestor	Address	Authorization or Written Request (Y/N)	Purpose	PHI Disclosed	Date Disclosed	Disclosed By

Tutorial 6.2	**EHR**NAVIGAT✛R

Printing an Accounting of Disclosures Log

Go to the online course to launch Tutorial 6.2. As an RHIT, practice printing an accounting of disclosures log using the EHR Navigator.

Privacy Rule and State Laws

State laws that contradict the Privacy Rule are overruled by the federal requirements, unless an exception applies. Examples of exceptions are when the state law:

- provides greater privacy protections or rights with respect to individually identifiable health information;

- allows for the reporting of injury, illness, child abuse, birth, or death, or for public health surveillance, investigation, or intervention; and

- requires health plan reporting—for example, for management or financial audits.

In these examples, a covered entity is not required to comply with a contrary provision of the Privacy Rule.

CHECKP✛INT 6.1

1. True/False: A healthcare provider may not release patient health information without a specific authorization or consent signed by the patient.

2. True/False: HIPAA regulations cover only health information documented on paper.

3. The HIPAA Privacy and Security Rules apply only to health plans, healthcare clearinghouses, and healthcare providers who transmit health information in electronic format. What term is used for these plans, clearinghouses, and providers?

_____

Minimum Necessary Concept

Covered entities must make reasonable efforts to limit the use of, disclosure of, and requests for the minimum amount of PHI necessary to accomplish the intended purpose. This concept is called **minimum necessary** and is required by the Privacy Rule.

An example of a covered entity *not following* the minimum necessary concept is as follows. An insurance company needs to determine whether physical therapy services were necessary for a patient residing in a nursing home. One of its representatives requests a copy of the patient's entire medical record, including physician progress notes, laboratory and radiology results, medical history and physical examination findings, physical therapy progress notes, nutrition progress notes, and case management reports. This is more information than is needed. The insurance company representative should be able to determine whether physical therapy was necessary based on the history and physical examination, physician's orders, and physical therapy progress notes.

An example of a covered entity that *adheres to* the minimum necessary concept is as follows. A new patient is scheduled for a hemodialysis run tomorrow at an outpatient dialysis clinic. The hospital where the patient had hemodialysis discharged the patient yesterday. The outpatient dialysis clinic needs a copy of the last hemodialysis run sheet to plan the patient's hemodialysis run for tomorrow. The dialysis clinic requests only the last dialysis run sheet from the hospital.

6.3 HIPAA Privacy Rule Enforcement

As with any law, there are consequences when the HIPAA Privacy and Security Rules are not followed. Within HHS is the **Office for Civil Rights (OCR)**, which is responsible for enforcing the HIPAA Privacy and Security Rules. The enforcement process begins with a complaint and follows through to a resolution with the Department of Justice when violations are criminal or with the OCR when violations are civil, as illustrated in Figure 6.4.

Violations of the Privacy Rule fall into one of two categories: civil or criminal violations. The major difference between civil and criminal violations involves the intent behind the violation.

Civil Violations

If a person *mistakenly* obtained or disclosed individually identifiable health information in violation of HIPAA, and the covered entity corrected the violation within 30 days of when it knew or should have known of the violation, then a penalty is not imposed, as per the HITECH Act. Since the HITECH Act, civil monetary penalties of $100 to $50,000 per failure may be imposed on a covered entity failing to comply with a Privacy Rule requirement. The cumulative penalties may not exceed $1.5 million per year.

Criminal Violations

If a person *knowingly* obtains or discloses individually identifiable health information in violation of HIPAA, this is considered a criminal violation, and the person can be

Figure 6.4 HIPAA Privacy and Security Rules Complaint Process

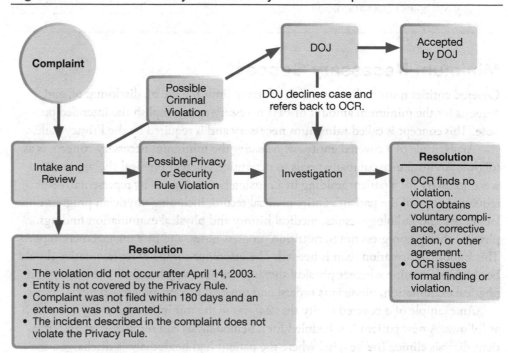

penalized with a fine of $50,000 and one year of imprisonment. Criminal penalties increase to $100,000 and up to five years of imprisonment if the wrongful conduct involves false pretenses. The penalties increase up to $250,000 and up to 10 years of imprisonment if the wrongful conduct involves the intent to sell, transfer, or use PHI for commercial advantage, personal gain, or malicious harm.

In addition to monetary penalties and imprisonment, the federal government can also require a **resolution agreement** with a covered entity, which is a contract signed by the federal government and a covered entity in which that entity agrees to perform certain obligations (e.g., staff training regarding privacy and confidentiality or audits of all releases of health information to ensure compliance) and to send reports to the federal government for a certain time period (typically three years). During this period, the federal government monitors the compliance of the covered entity with the obligations it has agreed to perform.

6.4 Breach Notification Rule

Implemented in August 2009, breach notification regulations require covered entities and their business associates to provide notification to affected individuals following a breach of unsecured PHI. Gener-

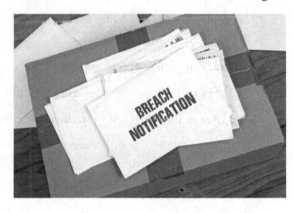

ally speaking, a **breach** is an impermissible use or disclosure under the Privacy Rule that compromises the security or privacy of PHI such that the use or disclosure poses a significant risk of financial, reputational, or other harm to the affected individual.

Following a breach of unsecured PHI, covered entities are required to provide notification of the breach to affected individuals, to the federal government (specifically HHS), and, in certain circumstances, to the media. In addition, business associates must notify covered entities that a breach has occurred.

Notice to Individuals Requirement

Covered entities must notify affected individuals following the discovery of a breach of unsecured PHI and must provide individual written notifications within 60 days following the discovery of a breach. These notifications must include the following items:

1. A description of the breach

2. A description of the types of information involved in the breach

3. The steps affected individuals should take to protect themselves from potential harm

4. A brief description of what the covered entity is doing to investigate the breach, mitigate the harm, and prevent further breaches

5. Contact information for the covered entity

Notice to the Media Requirement

Covered entities experiencing a breach affecting more than 500 residents of a state or jurisdiction are required to notify the affected individuals and provide notice to prominent media outlets serving the state or jurisdiction. Covered entities will likely provide this notification in the form of a press release to appropriate media outlets serving the affected area. Like individual notices, they must provide this media notification within 60 days following the discovery of a breach and must include the same information required for the individual notice.

From the HIPAA compliance date in April 2003 through May 2019, the federal government received 208,797 HIPAA privacy complaints. OCR resolved 98% of these complaints, with 69% resulting in no violation or no need for investigation. OCR resolved 31% of these cases by requiring covered entities to make changes in their privacy practices or to take corrective actions or by providing technical assistance to the covered entities or their business associates. Less than 1% (65) of the complaints resulted in monetary settlements or civil money penalties totaling $102,681,582. Many different types of entities, including national pharmacy chains, major medical centers, group health plans, hospital chains, and small provider offices, were part of the cases investigated.

The most often investigated compliance issues are listed below in order of frequency:

1. Impermissible uses and disclosures of PHI

2. Lack of safeguards of PHI

3. Lack of patient access to their PHI

4. Lack of administrative safeguards of ePHI

5. Uses or disclosures of more than the minimum necessary PHI

The most common types of covered entities required to take corrective action are listed below in order of frequency:

1. Private practices

2. General hospitals

3. Outpatient facilities

4. Pharmacies

5. Health plans (group health plans and health insurance issuers)

As patients and the public at large have become more familiar with HIPAA privacy rights, there has been a steady increase in the number of complaints made to OCR.

Cases of Protected Health Information Breaches

In recent years, several high-profile cases of enforcement of HIPAA Privacy and Security Rules have included significant monetary penalties and resolution agreements.

One of the largest HIPAA violation penalties, $16 million, was paid by Anthem, Inc., the largest US health insurance company in 2018, and resolved an investigation into its 78.8 million record data breach that was discovered in 2015. Anthem reported that, in February 2015, an unknown hacker had accessed a database containing personal information, including names, birth dates, Social Security, addresses, email addresses, and employment and income information. The $16 million penalty, paid to the federal government, was not the only monetary payment resulting from the data breach as Anthem also settled a class action lawsuit filed on behalf of victims of the breach in 2018 for $115 million and a multi-state lawsuit that resulted in Anthem's paying $48.2 million in penalties. Anthem also implemented a corrective action plan to address the areas of noncompliance with HIPAA rules.

In March 2015, Premera Blue Cross, the largest health insurance plan in the Pacific Northwest, filed a data breach report with the OCR when the company realized that hackers had accessed the information of over 10 million individuals. As a result of this breach, Premera Blue Cross paid a financial penalty of $6,850,000 to the federal government, a $10 million settlement for a multi-state lawsuit, and $74 million to the victims of the data breach. Premera implemented a corrective action plan to address all areas of noncompliance.

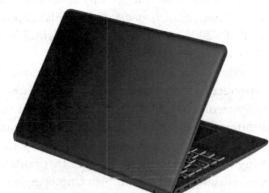

A laptop should not contain healthcare information unless it is encrypted.

Data breaches and fines are not experienced only by health insurance companies. In February 2017, Lifespan Health System in Rhode Island, a nonprofit healthcare system, experienced a data breach when an unencrypted laptop computer was stolen from an employee's vehicle. The laptop contained the ePHI of 20,431 patients. Lifespan paid a $1,040,000 penalty and implemented a corrective action plan to address all areas of noncompliance (i.e., data encryption on laptops).

In 2016, Athens Orthopedic Clinic, a Georgia-based healthcare provider, experienced a cyberattack in which a PHI database of over 200,000 patients was stolen. The hacker demanded a ransom to not release the data, and when payment was not received, the hacker published the database. The Athens Orthopedic Clinic paid a $1.5 million penalty and adopted a corrective action plan to address all areas of noncompliance.

Although major cases with high-dollar penalties receive considerable media attention, they are the exception rather than the rule.

While the penalties consider the nature and breadth of the data breach, they are more closely tied to an organization's failure to address and/or implement HIPAA policies and requirements. For example, an organization may have failed to conduct a risk analysis or worse: failed to implement systems and policies to negate the risks identified by the risk analysis.

EXPAND YOUR LEARNING

Describe two recent breaches of the Privacy or Security Rules. A list can be found at the following website: https://EHR3.ParadigmEducation.com/Breaches.

CHECKP◆INT 6.2

1. What is the difference between a civil violation and a criminal violation of the Privacy Rule?

_____

_____

_____

2. Name three of the top five investigated compliance issues.

a. _____

b. _____

c. _____

6.5 HIPAA Security Rule

Privacy of health information is one of the main subjects addressed by HIPAA. Another important component of HIPAA is the security of health information. Just as the Privacy Rule was developed to address the privacy provisions of HIPAA, the **Security Standards for the Protection of Electronic Protected Health Information** were developed to address the security provisions of HIPAA and are commonly known as the **Security Rule**. Security Rule provisions pertain exclusively to electronic health information. The Security Rule required all HIPAA-covered entities (the same covered entities discussed earlier in this chapter) to reach compliance no later than April 20, 2005, with the exception of small health plans, which had until April 20, 2006, to comply with the rule.

Prior to HIPAA, no national security standards or general requirements existed to protect health information. With healthcare delivery systems moving away from paper records and toward electronic systems to process claims, manage health information, and document clinical and administrative activities, it became clear that federal guidance was necessary to protect patient information. Covered entities are using web-based applications and other portals that give physicians, clinical staff, administrative staff, health plan employees, and pharmaceutical companies greater access to electronic health information. In addition to web-based products, an increasing number of healthcare providers use internal EHR software to varying degrees. As the United States moves toward its goal of a **Nationwide Health Information Network (NHIN)** and a greater use of EHRs, protecting the confidentiality, integrity, and availability of **electronic protected health information (ePHI)** becomes even more critical. The security standards in HIPAA were developed for two primary purposes: (1) to protect certain electronic healthcare information that may be at risk and (2) to promote the use of electronic health information in the healthcare industry.

Protecting an individual's health information, while permitting appropriate access and use of that information, ultimately promotes the use of electronic health information in the healthcare industry.

Objectives of the Security Rule

Although HIPAA established the two broad purposes of health information security standards as just noted, the Security Rule was adopted to more specifically define the objectives that covered entities would need to attain to comply with HIPAA. In the General Rules section of the Security Rule, the four major objectives include the following:

1. Each covered entity must ensure the confidentiality, integrity, and availability of ePHI that it creates, receives, maintains, or transmits.

2. Each covered entity must protect against any reasonably anticipated threats and hazards to the security or integrity of ePHI.

3. Each covered entity must protect against reasonably anticipated uses or disclosures of such information that are not permitted by the Privacy Rule.

4. Each covered entity must ensure compliance by the workforce.

Major Differences between the Privacy and Security Rules

When HHS developed the Security Rule, it chose to closely align it with the provisions in the Privacy Rule. Because both rules were developed in response to HIPAA, it made sense to ensure that the two rules were in sync. Therefore, it is easier for covered entities to implement the provisions of both rules and achieve the goals of HIPAA. Although the two rules are closely aligned, there are two areas of distinction:

1. The Privacy Rule applies to all forms of patient PHI, whether that information is in electronic, written, or oral format. In contrast, the Security Rule covers only PHI in electronic form, including ePHI that is created, received, maintained, or transmitted. For example, ePHI may be transmitted over the internet or stored on a server, computer, disc, flash drive, magnetic tape, or electronic storage media. The Security Rule does not cover PHI transmitted or stored on paper or provided in oral form.

2. The Privacy Rule contains minimum security requirements for the protection of PHI, whereas the Security Rule provides comprehensive security requirements.

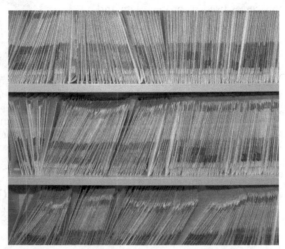

The Privacy Rule applies to all forms of patients' PHI, including paper records. The Security Rule covers PHI that is in electronic form.

Sections of the Security Rule

The standards of the Security Rule are divided into six main sections: General Rules, Administrative Safeguards, Physical Safeguards, Technical Safeguards, Organizational Requirements, and Policies and Procedures and Documentation Requirements.

General Rules

The General Rules section includes general requirements that all covered entities must meet. This section establishes the flexibility of approach that covered entities have when implementing and identifying the standards required and those that are addressable. Information in this section also addresses the required maintenance of security measures to continue reasonable and appropriate protection of ePHI.

Administrative Safeguards

Generally speaking, the Administrative Safeguards section includes the assignment or delegation of security responsibility to an individual and the need for security training for employees and users. Employees must be trained in security, and covered entities must have appropriate policies and procedures for security (e.g., a disaster backup plan or incident reporting of security breaches).

Physical Safeguards

The Physical Safeguards section includes mechanisms necessary to protect electronic systems and the data they store from threats, environmental hazards, and unauthorized intrusion. These safeguards include restricting access to ePHI and retaining off-site computer backups.

Technical Safeguards

The Technical Safeguards section primarily covers the automated processes used to protect data and control access to data. These processes include the use of authentication control to verify that the person signing onto a computer is authorized to access that ePHI or encryption and decryption of data as it is being stored, transmitted, or both.

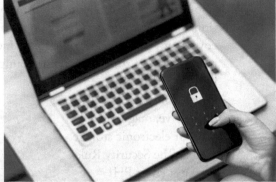

One example of a technical safeguard is the use of multi-factor authentication, which sometimes requires a user to enter their password and then verify their identity on another device.

Organizational Requirements

The fifth major section of the Security Rule, the Organizational Requirements, includes standards for business associate contracts and other arrangements and the requirements for group health plans.

Policies and Procedures and Documentation Requirements

The section titled Policies and Procedures and Documentation Requirements addresses the implementation of reasonable and appropriate policies and procedures to comply with the Security Rule standards. The covered entity must maintain written documentation and records that include policies, procedures, actions, activities, or assessments required by the Security Rule.

CHECKPOINT 6.3

1. List the six main sections of the Security Rule.

   a. _____

   b. _____

   c. _____

   d. _____

   e. _____

   f. _____

2. Encryption of healthcare data before transmission is an example of which type of security safeguard?

   _____

3. Security training of employees is an example of which type of security safeguard?

   _____

Security Standards Matrix

The Centers for Medicare & Medicaid Services (CMS) created a Security Standards Matrix, which is Appendix A of the Security Rule, to assist covered entities in the assessment of their compliance with the Security Rule (see Figure 6.5).

Note that the first column is a description of the Security Standard. The second column lists the section of the Security Rule published within the *Federal Register*. The third and fourth columns list a more specific reference to a portion of the security

Figure 6.5 The Security Standards Matrix

1 Security 101 for Covered Entities

Security Standards Matrix (Appendix A of the Security Rule)

ADMINISTRATIVE SAFEGUARDS			
Standards	**Sections**	**Implementation Specifications (R)= Required, (A)=Addressable**	
Security Management Process	164.308(a)(1)	Risk Analysis	(R)
		Risk Management	(R)
		Sanction Policy	(R)
		Information System Activity Review	(R)
Assigned Security Responsibility	164.308(a)(2)		(R)
Workforce Security	164.308(a)(3)	Authorization and/or Supervision	(A)
		Workforce Clearance Procedure	(A)
		Termination Procedures	(A)
Information Access Management	164.308(a)(4)	Isolating Health Care Clearinghouse Functions	(R)
		Access Authorization	(A)
		Access Establishment and Modification	(A)
Security Awareness and Training	164.308(a)(5)	Security Reminders	(A)
		Protection from Malicious Software	(A)
		Log-in Monitoring	(A)
		Password Management	(A)
Security Incident Procedures	164.308(a)(6)	Response and Reporting	(R)
Contingency Plan	164.308(a)(7)	Data Backup Plan	(R)
		Disaster Recovery Plan	(R)
		Emergency Mode Operation Plan	(R)
		Testing and Revision Procedures	(A)
		Applications and Data Criticality Analysis	(A)
Evaluation	164.308(a)(8)		(R)
Business Associate Contracts and Other Arrangements	164.308(b)(1)	Written Contract or Other Arrangement	(R)

CMS CENTERS for MEDICARE & MEDICAID SERVICES Volume 2 /Paper 1 10 11/2004:rev. 3/2007

Implementation Specifications (R)= Required, (A)=Addressable	
ontingency perations	(A)
acility Security Plan	(A)
ccess Control and alidation Procedures	(A)
aintenance Records	(A)
	(R)
	(R)
isposal	(R)
edia Re-use	(R)
ccountability	(A)
ata Backup and orage	(A)
Implementation Specifications (R)= Required, (A)=Addressable	
nique User entification	(R)
mergency Access rocedure	(R)
utomatic Logoff	(A)
ncryption and ecryption	(A)
	(R)
echanism to Authenticate Electronic rotected Health Information	(A)
	(R)
tegrity Controls	(A)
ncryption	(A)

CMS CENTERS for MEDICARE & MEDICAID SERVICES Volume 2 /Paper 1 11 11/2004:rev. 3/2007 standards along with a designation of *R* (required) or *A* (addressable). A **required standard** must be met, while an **addressable standard** should be met if it is a reasonable and appropriate safeguard in the entity's environment. Addressable standards should not be considered merely optional.

Because HIPAA is applicable to a variety of organizations classified as covered entities, HIPAA includes flexibility that allows covered entities to tailor security measures to their own situations while still keeping health information secure. Determining whether an addressable portion of the standard is applicable to a particular covered entity can be challenging. It involves analyzing the standard in reference to the likelihood of protecting the entity's ePHI from reasonably anticipated threats and hazards.

If the covered entity does not implement an addressable standard based on its assessment, the covered entity must document the reason that the implementation of the standard is not appropriate or reasonable. For example, a solo practitioner without any employees would likely not need to implement the Administrative Safeguards of the Security Rule. This specification states that employees should be sent security reminders about potential security threats via email, newsletters, and so on. Because there are no employees to be notified, this safeguard is not applicable.

Every covered entity is responsible for complying with the required and addressable standards or documenting why it does not need to comply with certain addressable elements. Covered entities should conduct an internal review of their compliance with the security standards.

EHR System Security

Because electronic data can be changed with a keystroke, EHR systems can track and record user activity. Consequently, once clinical documentation has been entered and authenticated (i.e., the author's signature is applied, confirming the accuracy of the data to the best of the author's knowledge), documented entries cannot be modified. Attempts to change a health record can easily be identified by an administrator by viewing the activity log.

Tutorial 6.3   **EHR**NAVIGAT◆R

Denying Access

Go to the online course to launch Tutorial 6.3. As a lab technician, you will experience what happens when you try to access a restricted area in the EHR Navigator.

Tutorial 6.4   **EHR**NAVIGAT◆R

Changing an Email

Go to the online course to launch Tutorial 6.4. As an office manager, practice changing a staff member's email address using the EHR Navigator.

Tutorial 6.5   **EHR**NAVIGAT✛R

Reviewing a User Activity Log

Go to the online course to launch Tutorial 6.5. As an IT administrator, practice reviewing a user activity log using the EHR Navigator.

HIPAA Security Rule Enforcement

Enforcement of the Security Rule follows the same process as enforcement of the Privacy Rule. The OCR has the responsibility for the enforcement, and the enforcement process starts with a complaint and follows through to a resolution with the Department of Justice when violations are criminal or the OCR when violations are civil.

Reported security breaches have led other organizations to bolster their efforts in the following ways:

- Reducing risk through network or enterprise data storage as an alternative to local devices. **Enterprise data storage** is a centralized system (online or offline) that businesses use for managing and protecting data.

- Encrypting ePHI on any desktop or portable device

- Maintaining clear and well-documented administrative and physical safeguards on the storage devices and media that handle ePHI

- Raising employee awareness of security and good data stewardship. **Data stewardship** can be defined as the authority and responsibility associated with collecting, using, and disclosing health information in its identifiable and aggregate forms. The principles of data stewardship apply to all the personnel, systems, and processes engaging in health information storage and exchange within and across organizations.

Consider This

An employee of the State Department of Health and Social Services left a portable electronic storage device (USB drive) in a car that was later stolen. The USB drive contained ePHI, so the State Department of Health and Social Services submitted a report to the OCR, as all covered entities are required to do when a breach of health information security has occurred. When the OCR investigated, it found evidence that the department did not have adequate policies and procedures in place to safeguard ePHI. In addition, the department had not completed a risk analysis, implemented sufficient risk management measures, completed security training for its workforce members, implemented device and media controls, or addressed device and media controls or encryption, as required by the HIPAA Security Rule.

Does the State Department of Health and Social Services have to follow the HIPAA Security Rule? Why? Is there a possibility that the department would be fined in this scenario? What do you think the findings of the OCR should be?

6.6 21ˢᵗ Century Cures Act and Final Rule

As you learned in Chapter 1, the 21ˢᵗ Century Cures Act, passed in 2016, was one of the most significant acts to address patient access to electronic medical records and the exchange and use of health information. The Final Rule sets the standards for interoperability to promote patient access and control of their ePHI. Using their own electronic devices, such as smartphones and computers, patients will have fuller access to their records, which include clinical notes, test results, and medications. The Final Rule includes provisions that require support and development of tools, such as apps, to facilitate the patient's access to their record. Having access to their own records should enable patients to take an active role in their care. The access and transparency will also allow patients to shop for care by comparing costs for treatments.

Similar to the data sets discussed in Chapter 4, the United States Core Data for Interoperability (USCDI) is a required, standardized set of health data for nationwide, interoperable health information exchange. The first version of the USCDI was published in May 2020 and the second version was published in July 2021. See Figure 6.6 for an excerpt. Data classes and elements were added to the second version, and more are expected to be added with each subsequent version of the USCDI, with the goal of continually expanding the data available to patients, providers, and researchers.

Information Blocking

The 21ˢᵗ Century Cures Act further protects patient interest and access to their ePHI by defining and disallowing information blocking. In general, **information blocking** is a practice by a health IT developer of certified health IT, health information network, health information exchange, or healthcare provider that, except as required by law or specified by the Secretary of HHS as a reasonable and necessary activity, is likely to interfere with access, exchange, or use of ePHI.

EHI, or *electronic health information*, as defined by the 21ˢᵗ Century Cures Act, means electronic protected health information. The acronyms *EHI* and *ePHI*, as published in any federal legislation (i.e., HIPAA, HITECH, or the 21ˢᵗ Century Cures Act), all mean the same thing and are afforded all the protection outlined in these regulations.

Examples of certain practices that could constitute information blocking include:

Practices that restrict authorized access, exchange, or use under applicable state or federal law of such information for treatment and other permitted purposes under such applicable law, including transitions between certified health information technologies (health IT);

o   Implementing health IT in nonstandard ways that are likely to substantially increase the complexity or burden of accessing, exchanging, or using EHI;

o   Implementing health IT in ways that are likely to:
   •   restrict the access, exchange, or use of EHI with respect to exporting complete information sets or in transitioning between health IT systems; or

   •   lead to fraud, waste, or abuse, or impede innovations and advancements in health information access, exchange, and use, including care delivery enabled by health IT.

This part of the Cures Act prevents healthcare providers, health organizations, and individuals who work in health IT from restricting access to or abusing EHI.

Figure 6.6   USCDI Version 2

USCDI v2 Summary of Data Classes and Data Elements

Allergies and Intolerances
- Substance (Medication)
- Substance (Drug Class)
- Reaction

Assessment and Plan of Treatment
- Assessment and Plan of Treatment
- SDOH Assessment

Care Team Member(s)
- Care Team Member Name
- Care Team Member Identifier
- Care Team Member Role
- Care Team Member Location
- Care Team Member Telecom

Clinical Notes
- Consultation Note
- Discharge Summary Note
- History & Physical
- Procedure Note
- Progress Note

Clinical Tests
- Clinical Test
- Clinical Test Result/Report

Diagnostic Imaging
- Diagnostic Imaging Test
- Diagnostic Imaging Report

Encounter Information
- Encounter Type
- Encounter Diagnosis
- Encounter Time
- Encounter Location
- Encounter Disposition

Goals
- Patient Goals
- SDOH Goals

Health Concerns
- Health Concerns

Immunizations
- Immunizations

Laboratory
- Tests
- Values/Results

Medications
- Medications

Patient Demographics
- First Name
- Last Name
- Previous Name
- Middle Name (including Middle Initial)
- Suffix
- Sex (Assigned at Birth)
- Sexual Orientation
- Gender Identity
- Date of Birth
- Race
- Ethnicity
- Preferred Language
- Current Address
- Previous Address
- Phone Number
- Phone Number Type
- Email Address

Problems
- Problems
- SDOH Problems/Health Concerns
- Date of Diagnosis
- Date of Resolution

Procedures
- Procedures
- SDOH Interventions

Provenance
- Author Time Stamp
- Author Organization

Smoking Status
- Smoking Status

Unique Device Identifier(s) for a Patient's Implantable Device(s)
- Unique Device Identifier(s) for a Patient's Implantable Device(s)

Vital Signs
- Diastolic Blood Pressure
- Systolic Blood Pressure
- Body Height
- Body Weight
- Heart Rate
- Respiratory Rate
- Body Temperature
- Pulse Oximetry
- Inhaled Oxygen Concentration
- BMI Percentile (2 - 20 Years)
- Weight-for-length Percentile (Birth – 36 Months)
- Head Occipital-frontal Circumference Percentile (Birth - 36 Months)

There are eight exceptions that are not considered information blocking.

1. Preventing Harm Exception: It will not be information blocking for an actor to engage in practices that are reasonable and necessary to prevent harm to a patient or another person, provided certain conditions are met. This exception recognizes that the public interest in protecting patients and other persons against unreasonable risks of harm can justify practices that are likely to interfere with access, exchange, or use of EHI.

2. Privacy Exception: It will not be information blocking if an actor does not fulfill a request to access, exchange, or use EHI to protect an individual's privacy, provided certain conditions are met. This exception recognizes that if an actor is permitted to provide access, exchange, or use of EHI under a privacy law, then the actor should provide that access, exchange, or use. However, an actor should not be required to use or disclose EHI in a way that is prohibited under state or federal privacy laws.

3. Security Exception: It will not be information blocking for an actor to interfere with the access, exchange, or use of EHI to protect the security of EHI, provided certain conditions are met. This exception is intended to cover all legitimate security practices by actors but does not prescribe a maximum level of security or dictate a one-size-fits-all approach.

4. Infeasibility Exception: It will not be information blocking if an actor does not fulfill a request to access, exchange, or use EHI due to the infeasibility of the request, provided certain conditions are met. This exception recognizes that legitimate practical challenges may limit an actor's ability to comply with requests for access, exchange, or use of EHI. An actor may not have—and may be unable to obtain—the requisite technological capabilities, legal rights, or other means necessary to enable access, exchange, or use.

5. Health IT Performance Exception: It will not be information blocking for an actor to take reasonable and necessary measures to make health IT temporarily unavailable or to degrade the health IT's performance for the benefit of the overall performance of the health IT, provided certain conditions are met. This exception recognizes that for health IT to perform properly and efficiently, it must be maintained, and in some instances improved, which may require that health IT be taken offline temporarily. Actors should not be deterred from taking reasonable and necessary measures to make health IT temporarily unavailable or to degrade the health IT's performance for the benefit of the overall performance of health IT.

6. Content and Manner Exception: It will not be information blocking for an actor to limit the content of its response to a request to access, exchange, or use EHI or the way it fulfills a request to access, exchange, or use EHI, provided certain conditions are met. This exception provides clarity and flexibility to actors concerning the required content (i.e., scope of EHI) of an actor's response to a request to access, exchange, or use EHI and the way the actor may fulfill the request. This exception

supports innovation and competition by allowing actors to first attempt to reach and maintain market-negotiated terms for the access, exchange, and use of EHI.

7. Fees Exception: It will not be information blocking for an actor to charge fees, including fees that result in a reasonable profit margin, for accessing, exchanging, or using EHI, provided certain conditions are met. This exception enables actors to charge fees related to the development of technologies and provision of services that enhance interoperability, while not protecting rent seeking, opportunistic fees, and exclusionary practices that interfere with access, exchange, or use of EHI.

8. Licensing Exception: It will not be information blocking for an actor to license interoperability elements for EHI to be accessed, exchanged, or used, provided certain conditions are met. This exception allows actors to protect the value of their innovations and charge reasonable royalties to earn returns on the investments they have made to develop, maintain, and update those innovations.

The ONC has a system of reporting and enforcement in place for information blocking. If an individual believes that a HIPAA covered entity or business associate violated their (or someone else's) health information privacy rights or committed another violation of the HIPAA Privacy, Security, or Breach Notification Rules, they can file their complaint online. Individuals may include contact information or may submit a claim anonymously.

> **EXPAND YOUR LEARNING**
>
> Refer to this website for more information about reporting a complaint of information blocking: https://EHR3 .ParadigmEducation .com/InformationBlocking.

Chapter Summary

Privacy and security of health information is a major focus of healthcare entities implementing and using EHRs. As a user of an EHR system, you must understand and follow the laws and regulations regarding privacy, safety, and security of health information. Federal legislation that revolutionized the release and security of health information includes the HIPAA Privacy and Security Rules published in 2000, which were subsequently updated in 2010 and 2013. These rules provide guidance about the release and security of protected health information (protected health information) as documented in paper health records, as well as the release and security of identifiable EHR patient information, known as electronic protected health information (ePHI).

Healthcare entities must carefully follow all of the Privacy and Security Rules when selecting and installing EHR systems, and they must remain vigilant in monitoring the use of PHI and ePHI in their organizations. In addition to setting standards for health information privacy and security, HIPAA also addresses standards to improve the efficiency and effectiveness of healthcare systems.

The Privacy Rule was published in December 2000 and later modified to yield the HIPAA Privacy, Security, and Enforcement Rules in January 2013, to comply with the provisions of the Health Information Technology for Economic and

Clinical Health (HITECH) Act, particularly with regard to EHRs. The Privacy and Security Rules apply to healthcare providers, health plans, and healthcare clearinghouses transmitting health information in an electronic format. These entities are called *covered entities*.

The types of health information classified under the HIPAA Privacy Rule include PHI and deidentified health information. The Privacy Rule defines PHI as all individually identifiable health information held or transmitted by a covered entity or its business associate, in any form or medium, whether electronic, paper, or oral. The term *deidentified health information* was first introduced by the Privacy Rule. It is health information that neither identifies an individual nor provides a reasonable basis to identify an individual.

A major purpose of the Privacy Rule is to define and limit the circumstances in which an individual's PHI may be used or disclosed by covered entities. The Privacy Rule generally requires covered entities to take reasonable steps to limit the use or disclosure of, and requests for, PHI to the minimum necessary to accomplish the intended purpose.

Workers must receive initial and ongoing training in the proper use and release of PHI and ePHI, as well as the importance of keeping healthcare data safe and secure.

Violations of the Privacy Rule fall into one of two categories: civil or criminal violations. The major difference between civil and criminal violations involves the intent behind the violation. A breach is an impermissible use or disclosure under the Privacy Rule that compromises the security or privacy of PHI such that the use or disclosure poses a significant risk of financial, reputational, or other harm to the affected individual.

Another important component of HIPAA is the security of health information. The Security Standards for the Protection of Electronic Protected Health Information were developed to address the security provisions of HIPAA and are commonly known as the Security Rule. The standards of the Security Rule are divided into six main sections: General Rules, Administrative Safeguards, Physical Safeguards, Technical Safeguards, Organizational Requirements, and Policies and Procedures and Documentation Requirements. The privacy and security of health information is the responsibility of all healthcare providers and breaches of such are reportable as outlined in the Security Rule.

The 21ˢᵗ Century Cures Act Final Rule sets the standards for interoperability to promote patient access and control of their ePHI. Having access to their own records should enable patients to take an active role in their care.

The United States Core Data for Interoperability (USCDI) is a required, standardized set of health data for nationwide, interoperable health information exchange. The second version was published in July 2021. Data classes and data elements will be added continually with the goal of expanding the data available to patients, providers, and researchers.

Information blocking is a practice by a health IT developer of certified health IT, health information network, health information exchange, or healthcare provider that, except as required by law or specified by the Secretary of HHS as a reasonable and necessary activity, is likely to interfere with access, exchange, or use of ePHI. The Cures Act prevents healthcare providers, health organizations, and individuals who work in health IT from restricting access to or abusing EHI.

Review and Assessment

The following Review and Assessment activities are also available online in the Cirrus online course. Your instructor may ask you to complete these activities online. Cirrus also provides access to flash cards, a crossword puzzle, and practice quizzes to help strengthen your understanding of the chapter content.

cirrus™

Acronyms/Initialisms

Study the following acronyms discussed in this chapter. Go to the online course for flash cards of the acronyms and other chapter key terms.

CMS: Centers for Medicare & Medicaid Services

ePHI: electronic protected health information

HHS: US Department of Health & Human Services

HIPAA: Health Insurance Portability and Accountability Act of 1996

HITECH Act: Health Information Technology for Economic and Clinical Health Act

NHIN: Nationwide Health Information Network

OCR: Office for Civil Rights

PHI: protected health information

ROI: release of information

TPO: treatment, payment, healthcare operations

Check Your Understanding

To check your understanding of this chapter's key concepts, answer the following questions.

1. What is an example of a noncovered entity?

   a. nursing home

   b. workers' compensation carrier

   c. military healthcare program

   d. healthcare clearinghouse

2. The acronym *TPO* stands for

   a. treatment, protection, organization.

   b. transmission, privacy, operations.

   c. treatment, payment, healthcare operations.

   d. type, patient, officials.

3. A breach is

   a. the transmission of health information in an electronic format.

   b. an impermissible use or disclosure under the Privacy and Security Rules.

   c. a data set used for healthcare research.

   d. a punishment enforced by the OCR.

4. After a Privacy Rule breach, _____ must be notified.

   a. the individual, the federal government, and in certain circumstances, the media

   b. the individual, the healthcare organization, and the insurance company

   c. the healthcare organization and the federal and state governments

   d. the federal and state governments and the media

5. Deidentified health information

   a. can never be used in marketing or research.

   b. neither identifies an individual nor provides a reasonable basis to identify an individual.

   c. does not directly identify an individual, but it may provide information that could be used to identify an individual.

   d. cannot be electronically transmitted.

6. True/False: Users of electronic health records are not required to follow the laws and regulations of the Health Insurance Portability and Accountability Act of 1996 (HIPAA).

7. True/False: If an entity does not meet the definition of *covered entity*, then it does not have to comply with the Privacy and Security Rules.

8. True/False: The Office for Civil Rights (OCR) has the responsibility for the enforcement of the HIPAA Privacy and Security Rules.

9. True/False: The major difference between criminal and civil punishments and penalties involves the intent behind the violation.

10. True/False: As patients and the public at large have become more familiar with HIPAA privacy rights, the number of complaints made to the OCR has steadily increased.

Go on the Record

To build on your understanding of the topics in this chapter, complete the following short-answer activities.

1. What is the major purpose of the Privacy Rule?

2. What are the two situations in which disclosure of protected health information is required?

3. Describe a limited data set for purposes of research, public health, or healthcare operations.

4. Describe the differences between civil and criminal acts in violation of the Health Insurance Portability and Accountability Act of 1996 (HIPAA).

5. List the top five compliance issues that have been investigated by the federal government since HIPAA went into effect.

Navigate the Field

To gain practice in handling challenging situations in the workplace, consider the following real-world scenarios and identify how you would respond to each.

1. Hans Frank, office manager of Mountainview Surgical Clinic, was working on year-end reports at his home over the weekend. He spent several hours on Sunday compiling reports related to the 3,000 surgical patients who received treatment from Mountainview Surgical Clinic during the previous year. Unfortunately, while on his way to work on the subway on Monday, he inadvertently left his work laptop under his seat. In a panic, Mr. Frank tried to locate his laptop but was unsuccessful. Because this is clearly a breach of unsecured protected health information, what notification processes must Mountainview Surgical Clinic initiate?

2. Green Hills Valley Hospital has hired you to be the electronic health records security officer. As you tour the hospital during your first week of employment, you notice that many of the nurses and other staff members are sharing user IDs and passwords to log onto the EHR system. As the security officer, what actions should you take to resolve this situation?

Think Critically

Continue to think critically about challenging concepts and complete the following activities.

1. Interview a privacy or security officer at an acute care hospital to learn about the challenges of complying with the Health Insurance Portability and Accountability Act of 1996 (HIPAA) in a hospital that uses an EHR system.

2. Nearly everyone has seen news reports of cyberattacks against nationwide utility infrastructures or the information networks of the Pentagon. Healthcare providers may believe that if they are small and low profile, they will escape the attention of the criminals running these attacks. Yet, every day, new attacks are specifically aimed at small and mid-size organizations, because they are low profile and less likely to have fully protected themselves. Criminals have been highly successful at penetrating these smaller organizations, carrying out their activities while their victims remain unaware until it is too late. Review the Office of the National Coordinator for Health Information Technology's cybersecurity checklist and discuss five best practices for a small healthcare environment to protect an EHR system. The checklist can be found at the following website: https://EHR3.ParadigmEducation.com/SecurityChecklist.

Make Your Case

Consider the scenario and then complete the following project.

Describe the main components of the Privacy Rule and create a presentation with your findings.

Explore the Technology

Complete the EHR Navigator practice assessments that align to each tutorial and the assessments that accompany Chapter 6 located in the online course.

EHRNAVIGAT✚R

Chapter **7** Clinical Documentation

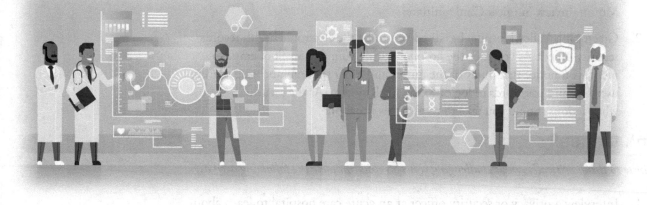

Field Notes

" I use a tablet to document my patients' diagnoses and the treatment I provide. This has enabled me to remain present when I am providing care and helps ensure that my documentation is timely and accurate. "

– Sarah Foltz, CNP

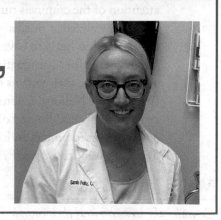

7.1 Differentiate between *structured* and *unstructured* data and identify examples of each.

7.2 Explain manual and automated methods of data collection.

7.3 Explain the clinical documentation cycle and give examples of its use in inpatient, outpatient, and long-term care settings.

7.4 Identify the elements of a history and physical examination.

7.5 Discuss the use of templates in the EHR.

7.6 Discuss documentation in inpatient, outpatient, and skilled nursing provider settings.

7.7 Identify the concerns related to cloned notes.

7.8 Define *e-prescribing,* including its benefits and challenges.

7.9 Modify an eprescription and override a drug allergy notification in the EHR.

7.10 Describe the benefits of computerized provider order entry (CPOE), portable medical orders, and the electronic medication administration record (eMAR).

7.11 Demonstrate how to enter progress notes, modify patients' eprescriptions, and override drug allergy notifications in the EHR system.

7.12 Discuss the purpose of the Minimum Data Set (MDS) in a skilled nursing and rehabilitation provider setting.

The implementation of the EHR has streamlined data entry and encouraged interoperability of data and information. Depending on compatibility of the clinical system interface with other systems such as radiology, laboratory, pharmacy, and transcription services, healthcare staff members enter patient and clinical data either automatically or manually to create the EHR. Examples of clinical data include the history and physical examination (H&P), progress notes by all clinicians, immunization information, laboratory test results, and medications. The clinical input of medication information via the e-prescribing feature of EHR systems has improved the safety and efficiency of drug administration. While this textbook has explored many of the scheduling, administrative, and health information management data activities in an EHR system, this chapter will focus on clinical documentation.

7.1 Clinical Documentation in the EHR

Clinical documentation, also known as **clinical inputs**, contains data related to the patient's clinical status that is entered into the patient's EHR or paper record. Data entered into an EHR can be classified as either structured or unstructured.

Structured data is stored in a specific, organized fashion within a database. Examples of structured data include date of birth, sex, race, lab results, and International Classification of Diseases (ICD) codes. **Unstructured data** is information that is stored in a free-form format that does not adhere to a pre-defined or organized model within a database. Examples of unstructured data include primarily the narrative portions of the EHR such as progress notes, test interpretations, and operative reports. Data will be explored more in depth in Chapter 10.

Manual Data Collection

Data collection for the EHR occurs through a combination of manual and automated methods. **Manual data collection** of demographic and insurance information is often initiated by a staff member upon initial patient contact with a healthcare facility. The data is typically obtained from a preprinted form the patient has completed or during an in-person interview; however, at times, the information is collected over the telephone. A staff member subsequently enters this information into the EHR system. Some healthcare organizations ask patients to enter their own demographic data through a secure, personal internet link that a staff member sends to the patient to begin developing the EHR.

Automated Data Collection

Automated data collection occurs when the data from the initial patient encounter is automatically copied over to each new patient encounter using an automated data capture. Automated data collection is the preferred method of data capture because it requires less personnel time which equates to cost savings, avoids repetitive requests of information from patients, and may allow for more consistent data capture due to the elimination of data entry errors. The era of patients entering EHR data highlights the importance of frontline review for errors and duplication of data. The success of patient-initiated entry of demographic data relies on a healthcare facility's structured auditing and correction procedures to reconcile data errors and/or duplications. As EHR technology has evolved, more data collection has been automated, and healthcare professionals have had to enter less information manually.

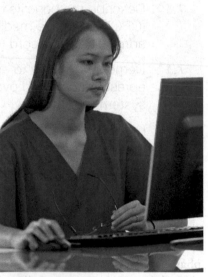

Healthcare workers manually enter demographic and insurance information into the EHR. On subsequent visits, this information is automatically copied over to the next patient encounter.

7.2 Clinical Documentation Cycle

Our discussion of clinical documentation is grouped by the type of provider, including inpatient, outpatient, and long-term care providers. While many of the documentation types and requirements are similar across provider types, there are unique aspects of documentation that are recorded to meet the needs of and care for patients in these different care settings.

We begin our discussion of clinical documentation with the **clinical documentation cycle**, which applies to all provider and care settings (see Figure 7.1). A clinician's initial

Figure 7.1   Clinical Documentation Cycle

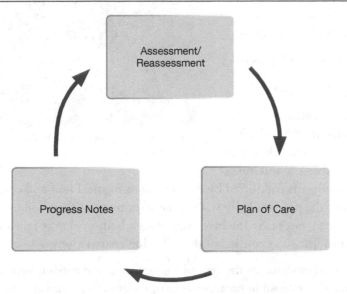

encounter with a patient results in the clinician's evaluation of the patient and development of a plan of care. The plan of care establishes patient health goals and the steps that need to be taken by the patient and the clinician to achieve these goals. At each subsequent interaction, the clinician records progress notes to document the patient's progress toward the established goals. Periodic reassessments or reevaluations of the patient are conducted, and the care plan goals are adjusted in response to changes in the patient's condition. This cycle of assessment, care plan, progress note, and reassessment is the clinical documentation cycle.

7.3 Inpatient Clinical Documentation

While many of the documentation types and requirements are similar across provider types, there are unique aspects of documentation that are recorded to meet the needs and care of patients in inpatient, outpatient, and long-term care settings.

History and Physical Examination

A **history and physical examination (H&P)** is a part of all inpatient encounters with healthcare providers and is a valuable tool for the healthcare provider in the identification of diagnoses. It is also the first step in developing a plan of care. The H&P consists of two main elements: a subjective element and an objective element.

Subjective Element

The **history** is the subjective element of the H&P because it is obtained from the patient or a family member as well as from previous medical records. A **subjective element** is based on personal reporting and opinions and may be biased or difficult to measure. The history begins with the **chief complaint**, which is the patient's stated reason for seeking health services. The chief complaint is then followed by one or more of the following components:

- History of present illness
- Past medical issues

- Allergies

- Medications currently prescribed to the patient

- Family and social histories

Objective Element

The **physical examination** is the **objective element** of the H&P. Objective information is based on facts and not subject to interpreta-

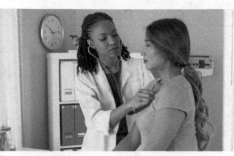

The physical examination is the objective portion of the H&P.

tion. This procedure is conducted by the nursing or medical staff and consists of an investigation of the patient's body systems, an assessment of their condition, and the creation of a treatment plan. The inventory of each body system is called the **review of systems (ROS)**. The ROS consists of the following system assessments:

1. General (documents the general appearance of the patient, such as, "A 66-year-old Asian woman in no acute distress. Patient is alert and able to discuss medical history.")

2. Vital signs (includes the patient's blood pressure, pulse, respiratory rate, pulse oximetry, and body temperature)

3. Head, ears, eyes, nose, and throat (HEENT)

4. Respiratory

5. Cardiovascular

6. Abdominal

7. Gastrointestinal

8. Genitourinary

9. Musculoskeletal

10. Neurologic

Once the healthcare provider has reviewed the history of the patient, physically examined the patient, and evaluated all recent laboratory and diagnostic test results, the provider assesses the patient's diagnoses and decides on a **treatment plan** to remedy the patient's condition.

Depending on the preference of the healthcare provider, the provider may type the H&P directly into the EHR or dictate a report and have a transcriptionist type and upload the report into the patient's EHR.

Tutorial 7.1   EHRNAVIGAT⊕R

Viewing a History and Physical Report

Go to the online course to launch Tutorial 7.1. As an occupational therapist, practice reviewing a patient's history and physical report using the EHR Navigator.

Electronic Health Record Templates

Many of the clinical inputs to an EHR system are accomplished using a **template**, which is a preformatted file that provides prompts to obtain specific, consistent information. For healthcare providers, the use of a template does the following:

- Indicates required fields that must be completed during the documentation process
- Ensures consistent data-gathering techniques among users
- Allows for efficient data entry using structured input options such as drop-down menus and check boxes
- Provides immediate data population of the EHR system
- Avoids the added expense of hiring a transcriptionist to document patient information
- Facilitates easy access to data because of its consistent format, thus avoiding time-consuming searches
- Enables faster and more precise reporting and analysis of data because of its format and consistent elements

Clearly, EHR templates offer several advantages. However, their use should never hinder thorough documentation by a healthcare provider. For any selections not available in drop-down menus, a provider will need to input patient information to ensure accuracy and completeness of the patient record.

Certain patient diagnoses or conditions may dictate the creation of specialized templates that offer information fields tailored to specific documentation needs. Specialized healthcare providers may also need specialized templates. For example, a detailed eye examination template like the one shown in Figure 7.2 would be a useful tool for an ophthalmologist. Depending on the policies of a healthcare organization, staff members may conduct special assessments to determine these special needs.

Care Plan

A **care plan**, also known as a *treatment plan* or *plan of care*, is a patient's road map to better health and is developed and executed by the entire clinical team in conjunction with the patient. Patients express their desired health outcomes at the time of clinical

Figure 7.2 Eye Examination Template

Choose an item. **Visual Acuity OD**	Choose an item. **Visual Acuity OS**
Choose an item. **Pinhole OD**	Choose an item. **Pinhole OS**
Yes ☐No ☐Afferent Pupillary Defect OD	**Yes ☐No ☐Afferent Pupillary Defect OS**
Yes ☐No ☐Dilated OD	**Yes ☐No ☐Dilated OS**
☐ **IOP OD**	☐ **IOP OS**
☐ **CVF OD**	☐ **CVF OS**
Yes ☐No ☐Lid OD WNL	**Yes ☐No ☐Lid OS WNL**
Choose an item. **Lid OD**	Choose an item. **Lid OS**
Yes ☐No ☐Conjunctiva/Sclera OD WNL?	**Yes ☐No ☐Conjunctiva/Sclera OS WNL?**
Choose an item. **Conjunctiva/Sclera OD**	Choose an item. **Conjunctiva/Sclera OS**

CHECKPOINT 7.1

1. Provide two reasons why automated data collection is the preferred method of data capture.

_____

_____

_____

2. Define history and physical examination and identify the two main elements of an H&P.

_____

_____

_____

assessment by medical, nursing, and allied health professionals. The clinicians set realistic, attainable goals for the patient in the form of a care plan and proceed to carry out the care and treatment that will lead to achievement of these goals. A care plan might include physical therapy treatments, the amount of assistance that a patient needs to ambulate or eat, or pain management medications and treatment. Care plans are updated following each clinical assessment, and progress notes are documented to reflect the progress or lack of patient progress toward the care plan goals. See Figure 7.3 for an overview of a patient's care plan in the EHR Navigator.

Nursing Documentation

In an inpatient environment, such as an acute care hospital, rehabilitation hospital, or psychiatric hospital, nurses spend a considerable amount of their shifts documenting the care and treatment of the patients under their responsibility. There are many patient assessments that nurses conduct and document upon admission and throughout a patient's stay. Nurses conduct an admission assessment shortly after the patient's arrival to the hospital room. The admission assessment is similar to the H&P but is completed from a nursing perspective. Major areas on the nursing admission assessment typically include general admission data, patient history, physical assessments of all major body systems, and spiritual, cultural, and social histories and perspectives. Table 7.1 provides more detail of the major assessment areas.

Chapter 8 discusses the Nursing Admission Assessment and additional nursing documentation requirements for inpatient, outpatient, and skilled nursing facilities.

Figure 7.3   Care Plan

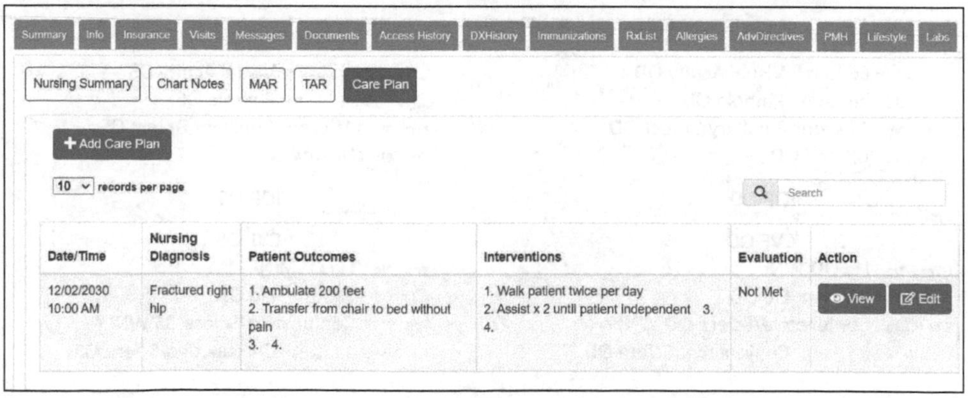

Date/Time	Nursing Diagnosis	Patient Outcomes	Interventions	Evaluation	Action
12/02/2030 10:00 AM	Fractured right hip	1. Ambulate 200 feet 2. Transfer from chair to bed without pain 3. 4.	1. Walk patient twice per day 2. Assist x 2 until patient independent 3. 4.	Not Met	View Edit

Table 7.1 Nursing Admission Assessment

Major Assessment Area	Data Items Included
General Admission Data	• Patient demographics (name, address, date of birth, marital status, etc.) • Admission source (where the patient was admitted from, e.g., home, nursing home, or emergency room) • Reason for admission • Vital signs (temperature, pulse, and blood pressure) • Height and weight • Communication needs (hard of hearing, needs interpreter, etc.) • Advance directives (living will, durable power of attorney for health care, and code status) • Patient belongings (what the patient brought to the hospital, including clothes, glasses, cell phone, and money) • Physicians (including the admitting physician, attending physician, consulting physician, and primary care physician)
Patient History	• Allergies • Medications • Diagnoses • Past diagnoses • Past surgical procedures
Physical Assessments	• Pain assessment • Neurologic assessment • Fall risk assessment • Cardiac assessment • Respiratory assessment • Gastrointestinal assessment • Nutrition assessment • Genitourinary assessment • Skin assessment • Musculoskeletal assessment • Peripheral vascular assessment
Spiritual/Cultural/Social Assessments	• Spiritual needs • Cultural needs • Social situation (lives alone, with spouse, with children, etc.) • Discharge plans (where patient wants to live after discharge)

Progress Notes

Progress notes are the portion of the health record in which healthcare providers of all disciplines document the patient's progress, or lack thereof, in relation to the established goals of the care plan. Healthcare providers may choose to write or transcribe progress notes in any format. For healthcare organizations that have adopted an EHR system, this task can be easily completed using customized templates.

Progress Note Templates

A customized progress note template provides information fields that cater to certain disciplines and specialties. For example, a template for a physical therapy progress note may include checkboxes to indicate whether the patient can bear weight on the right side and on the left side and drop-down menus with options for indicating the patient's range of motion and pain level. A progress note template for a cardiologist may allow healthcare providers to select different causes of syncope (i.e., cardiac, metabolic, or neurologic). Use of a progress note template lessens data entry time and ensures the inclusion of all pertinent data elements.

Tutorial 7.2

EHRNAVIGAT✛R

Entering a Progress Note

Go to the online course to launch Tutorial 7.2. As a nurse, practice entering a progress note into a patient's chart using the EHR Navigator.

Cloned Progress Notes

One area of concern related to EHR progress notes has been the increased use of cloned progress notes. A **cloned progress note** is a note that has been partially or totally copied from an existing progress note. The copied note is then updated by the healthcare provider to include any new information. This shortcut may save time, but it can also result in inaccurate or outdated documentation regarding a patient's health status and progress if the healthcare provider forgets to make the necessary updates to the existing note. Consequently, other healthcare providers may make inappropriate medical decisions based on incorrect patient information, which could have dire consequences for the patient.

Consider This

Dr. Calvin Sebold's progress note for 9/12/2030, 6:20 a.m.:

Patient examined and found in no acute distress. Patient has no complaints at this time. Lab values reviewed and all within normal limits. Continue current plan of treatment.

Nurse Bethany Akin's nurse's note for 9/13/2030, 4:50 a.m.:

Patient complains of nausea and headache. Vital signs: BP 180/101, T 101.8°, P 87, R 12. Resident telephoned and ordered CBC. Abnormal WBC of 9000. Resident telephoned and ordered urine culture. Awaiting results.

Dr. Sebold's progress note for 9/13/2030, 7:10 a.m.:

Patient examined and found in no acute distress. Patient has no complaints at this time. Lab values reviewed and all within normal limits. Continue current plan of treatment.

How does Dr. Sebold's progress note conflict with Nurse Akin's progress note? If you compare Dr. Sebold's progress notes on two different days, you will note that the documentation is identical, indicating the use of a cloned progress note.

Cloned progress notes may also affect the process of coding diagnoses and procedures for reimbursement purposes. Coding classification systems, such as the International Classification of Diseases (ICD) and Current Procedural Terminology (CPT®), require detailed documentation for accurate coding. Coding classification systems will be covered in detail in Chapter 9. Cloned progress notes that do not accurately reflect patient diagnoses and treatment may result in inaccurate code assignment, which in turn could lead to incorrect reimbursement and increased focus and monitoring from pay sources.

The Office of Inspector General (OIG) in the U.S. Department of Health and Human Services is responsible for combating healthcare fraud, waste, and abuse and for working to improve healthcare efficiency. To that end, the OIG routinely audits the billing and coding practices of healthcare organizations. Health record documentation must support code assignment and bills submitted for Medicare and Medicaid reimbursement. The OIG establishes an annual **Work Plan** of areas of healthcare documentation and billing practices to be addressed and audited during the year. The goals of the OIG are to ensure that healthcare organizations maintain accurate coding and billing records and that documentation is accurate and consistent throughout health records.

Consider This

The Emergency Care Research Institute (ECRI) conducted a study looking at the frequency of cloning/copying and pasting in a random sample of 239 EHR notes. The study indicated that 10.8% of notes contained cloned material, and the frequency varied by specialty.

Endocrinology notes were the highest, at 19.5% of notes containing cloned materials, and cardiology was the lowest, at 1.9% containing copied material. Obviously, cloning is a time-saving activity. However, what problems could arise from cloned progress note documentation?

e-Prescribing

Another documentation feature available to users of EHR systems is electronic prescribing, commonly known as **e-prescribing**. This feature allows a physician, nurse practitioner, or physician assistant to electronically transmit medication orders. In an inpatient hospital setting, these medications are transmitted internally to the hospital pharmacy. See Figure 7.4 for an example of an eprescription. The Promoting Interoperability Program that you learned about in Chapter 1 requires hospitals to use e-prescribing functionality with their EHR.

Benefits of e-Prescribing

For healthcare providers, the benefits of e-prescribing include improved prescribing accuracy and efficiency, a decreased potential for medication errors and prescription forgeries, and more accurate and timely billing. e-Prescribing lessens the risk for potential medication errors due to unclear handwriting, illegible faxes, or misinterpreted prescription abbreviations. EHR systems also have the ability to alert a healthcare provider if they prescribe a drug to which the patient is allergic, avoiding a potentially hazardous medication error. Many studies indicate that the use of the e-prescribing

Figure 7.4   Inpatient Eprescription

Add Order

Patient Name:	Date & Time:
Wilkins, Marquita	12/06/2030
	06 : 00 AM

Order: Medication

Drug Name: Plavix   Dose: 75

Drug Form: Tablet   Dose Unit: ☐ g ☐ kg ☐ L ☐ meq ☑ mg ☐ mL

Route of Administration: Oral

Frequency: ☐ BID ☑ QD ☐ QID ☐ QOD ☐ TID ☐ Q4h ☐ Q6h ☐ Q8h ☐ PRN ☐ Other: Other Frequency

Route of Administration: Oral

Frequency: ☐ BID ☑ QD ☐ QID ☐ QOD ☐ TID ☐ Q4h ☐ Q6h ☐ Q8h ☐ PRN ☐ Other: Other Frequency

Date & Time:

Start: 12/06/2030   10 : 00 AM

End: 12/10/2030   06 : 00 PM

Ordering physician: Holzer, Gregory

Order Type: Telephone   ☑ RBV* Required

Cancel   Sign and Save

feature of EHR systems has reduced medication errors by 12%–15%, which translates to 17.4 million medication errors averted per year. e-Prescribing also benefits patients in terms of improved accuracy in medication administration, more effective and efficient communication between patients and prescribers, and timely notifications for refills. Overall, e-prescribing improves patient care quality.

The e-prescribing component of an EHR includes an alert function that notifies the prescribing healthcare provider of drug-to-drug interactions, drug-to-food interactions, and the patient's

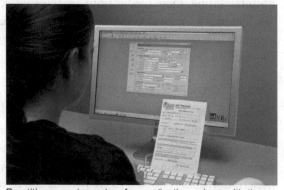

Practitioners enter orders for medications along with the patient's pharmacy location into the patient's EHR, and the prescription is automatically transferred to the pharmacy.

allergies to medications. These alerts are grouped into a hierarchy of potential risk and seriousness of the interactions or allergies, and healthcare prescribers may override less serious interactions or allergies and continue to prescribe the medication. For example, if there is only one medication that will be effective in treating a life-threatening illness and the potential drug-to-drug interaction may result in a minor drop in blood pressure, the physician may determine that the need for the medication is worth the minor blood pressure decrease.

Challenges of e-Prescribing

Although e-prescribing affords many benefits to both patients and healthcare providers, there are also some challenges associated with the use of this technology. When EHRs were first implemented, the major challenge of fully implementing e-prescribing involved the dispensing of controlled substances. A **controlled substance** is a drug (primarily a narcotic) declared by US federal or state law to be illegal for sale or use by the general public unless

dispensed per a healthcare provider's prescription. The basis for determining whether a drug is a controlled substance is the drug's potential for addiction, abuse, or harm.

Although US federal and state laws governing the distribution of controlled substances were in place prior to 1970, in that year the drug counterculture of the 1960s led the US government to enact stronger legislation regarding the manufacture and distribution of narcotics, stimulants, depressants, hallucino-

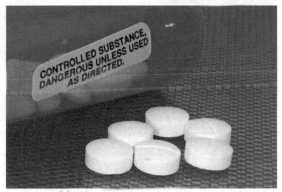

As e-prescribing for controlled substances was approved by each state, EHR systems had to be updated to include those medications and include the appropriate controls.

gens, anabolic steroids, and chemicals used in the illicit production of controlled substances. This legislation, known as the **Controlled Substances Act of 1970**, placed tight controls on the pharmaceutical and healthcare industries and outlined five schedules of controlled substances based on their potential for harm. This legislation established additional procedures for healthcare providers writing prescriptions for controlled substances. These procedures required that prescribers use hard-copy or printed prescriptions when ordering Schedule II controlled substances. Consequently, the use of eprescriptions for these substances had to be approved by individual US state boards of pharmacy before this technology could be implemented. In August 2015, Vermont became the final state to permit e-prescribing for all medications, including all controlled substances.

Even though the legal barrier regarding controlled substances has been eliminated, using e-prescribing to order controlled substances is still a challenge because many EHR systems have not upgraded software to handle the e-prescribing of controlled substances. In addition, many providers are uncomfortable using e-prescribing for many of the frequently abused painkillers, such as oxycodone, hydrocodone, and morphine, fearing that breaches in the security of the EHR may allow for fraudulent prescriptions.

Another challenge associated with e-prescribing is the lack of interoperability between healthcare facility EHR software and some pharmacy software. An eprescription is not useful to a patient if they are unable to fill it at the pharmacy. If a pharmacy's software does not communicate with the healthcare facility's EHR, a traditional handwritten prescription must be used.

Consider This

Prescriptions that have been handwritten by physicians or other prescribers pose a number of potentially serious problems. The combination of handwriting style and the use of abbreviations can lead to difficulty in reading and filling the prescription accurately. This can result in mistaken drug names, dosages, and strengths. Another issue with handwritten prescriptions is that they can be easily altered by drug seekers. In light of these issues, how does the use of e-prescribing decrease the potential for medication errors and prescription forgeries?

CHECKP+INT 7.2

1. List three benefits of e-prescribing.

_____

_____

_____

2. What legal barrier previously prevented e-prescribing from being fully implemented?

_____

_____

_____

Managing Orders

As you learned in Chapter 3, computerized provider order entry (CPOE) is a functionality present in all EHR systems. CPOE is also shorthand for the order itself. Providers, typically physicians, physician assistants, and nurse practitioners, use the CPOE function to order medications, diagnostic tests, procedures, and treatments for the care and treatment of their patients. Other clinicians, such as pharmacists, physical therapists, occupational therapists, respiratory therapists, and speech pathologists may also be able to initiate CPOEs depending on state laws regarding their scope of practice. Provider orders are also needed for consultations, resuscitation, transfers, and discharges. While the primary purpose of CPOE is to facilitate patient care, another important purpose of CPOE is the automatic generation of charges that are used in the billing process. When a CPOE is entered into the EHR, a charge for the medication, diagnostic test, and so on is automatically generated and transmitted to the organization's billing system, where it will be processed and transmitted on a claim to the appropriate payer (i.e., Medicare, Medicaid, or a commercial insurance payer). The billing and claims management processes are covered in Chapter 10.

In the design and maintenance of EHR software, providers and clinicians should be involved in the design of order screens and templates to ensure that medications, diagnostic tests, procedures, and treatments can be ordered thoroughly and accurately. For example, a CPOE template for ordering mechanical ventilation for a patient should be designed with physicians whose medical specialty is respiratory in conjunction with respiratory therapists. The template ensures that all the mechanical ventilation settings are included in the order to enable a respiratory therapist to provide high-quality patient care.

The medical staff of an inpatient facility is primarily responsible for the care rendered and should formally review and approve all EHR templates and order screens.

Portable Medical Orders

A portable medical order is a type of medical order that is entered into the EHR and then shared with other providers, either electronically or via paper if a provider does not have access to the patient's EHR. Medical orders regarding life-sustaining treatments are frequently written as a portable order for patients and patients' families to have on hand to share with future providers. There is no national standard for the content to be included in a portable order for life-sustaining treatments, so the content may vary by state and EHR system. Typically, a life-sustaining treatments order will include a patient's directives related to whether they wish to be resuscitated in the event of a cardiac arrest, if they wish to be put on mechanical ventilation, or if they wish to receive comfort care only. Do Not Resuscitate, or DNR, is a common term used to describe the life-sustaining treatments order. It is extremely important for a DNR order to be followed to ensure that a patient's wishes are honored.

Consider This

Patient Eleanor, who has a portable medical order for life-sustaining treatment, arrived via ambulance at a hospital emergency room in acute heart failure and respiratory distress. Eleanor's daughter shared her mother's portable medical order for life-sustaining treatments with the EMTs, who then shared it with the emergency room physician. The emergency room physician and staff were made aware of Eleanor's wishes and acted accordingly.

Eleanor's portable medical order for life-sustaining treatments indicated that she did not wish to be resuscitated in the event of a cardiac arrest. When Eleanor subsequently suffered a cardiac arrest in the emergency room, the emergency room physician and staff honored her wishes and did not resuscitate her. If the physician had not been made aware of Eleanor's portable medical order, what would have been the likely outcome?

Electronic Medication Administration Record

Documentation of medications administered to patients by nurses and other qualified healthcare providers is found in the medication administration record (MAR). When the MAR is in electronic format, it is referred to as the **electronic medication administration record (eMAR)**. The eMAR benefits the patient and increases efficiency for the care team. The use of the eMAR instead of paper records has been connected to a 45% reduction in medication errors, resulting in high quality of care for patients and better efficiency for the healthcare staff. Nursing staff spend less time on documentation when they record the information in the eMAR, and providers can quickly and easily see what medication was administered and when without needing to track down a paper MAR. More information regarding the eMAR can be found in Chapter 14.

Flowsheets

A **flowsheet** is a type of documentation tool used to record patient-related values over time. A flowsheet displays a patient's progress regarding anything that a provider needs to monitor such as weight, fluid input, lab values, and blood glucose levels. Common flowsheets found in EHR documentation include:

- Vital Signs Flowsheet: Documents and charts blood pressure, pulse, and respirations at a frequency ordered by a provider

- Blood Sugar Values Flowsheet: Documents the blood glucose values of diabetic patients before and after meals and more frequently, as ordered, to determine the necessity for insulin injections or medications

- Intake and Output Flowsheet: Documents the amount of fluid that a patient receives orally and intravenously as well as the amount of urine produced by the patient within a 24-hour period

Specialty flowsheets can be designed to track anything that a provider wants to monitor.

Therapy Documentation

Clinicians providing therapy care and treatment also follow the clinical documentation cycle that was discussed earlier in this chapter. When developing a plan of care, a physical therapist would ask a patient what their goals are and then discuss if the patient's desires are realistic and attainable. There are many types of therapy provided to patients, but the four major types are physical, occupational, speech, and respiratory. The therapists in each of these specialty areas address different aspects of rehabilitation, and their documentation reflects these differences. Therapists focus on a patient's ability to perform their **activities of daily living (ADLs)**, which include all the fundamental skills that an individual needs to be able to perform so they can independently care for themselves. These fundamental skills include eating, bathing, dressing, and toileting as well as mobility.

Physical Therapy Documentation

The goal of physical therapy is to improve a patient's mobility and to alleviate the pain that is associated with the patient's movement. The physical therapist's assessment of a patient includes documentation of the patient's ability to walk, how far they can walk, whether they need assistance with walking, and any pain experienced when walking as well as their ability to raise their arms, bend over, transfer from a chair to a bed, and so on. The physical therapist's contribution to the care plan reflects goals to improve a patient's mobility and will likely include the use of adaptive devices such as a walker or cane. The physical therapist documents a progress note on a daily basis or more often as warranted to record the patient's progress or lack of progress toward their care plan goals. The patient is reassessed, and the care plan is adjusted as needed. All care and treatment must be documented in the EHR because it serves as a legal document for the provider. If care or treatment is not documented, it is not considered to have occurred.

Occupational Therapy Documentation

While physical therapy addresses the gross movement and mobility of the patient, the purpose of occupational therapy is to address the fine motor skills of the patient, such as buttoning clothes, picking up eating utensils, and using pen and paper. Occupational therapists use the clinical documentation cycle to record the care and treatment they provide.

Speech Therapy Documentation

Speech therapists, also known as *speech-language pathologists*, treat patients for conditions involving language, communication, voice, and swallowing. In an inpatient setting, speech-language pathologists are generally consulted to evaluate a patient's ability to swallow food and liquids to determine the best type of diet for them. For example, a patient with significant swallowing problems may need a pureed diet to prevent them from aspirating food into their lungs. The speech therapist establishes a plan of care that will slowly advance a patient's diet as their swallowing disorder permits. Again, speech therapists use the clinical documentation cycle to record their care and treatment.

Respiratory Therapy Documentation

Respiratory therapists follow the clinical documentation cycle in the treatment of patients with respiratory disorders. Respiratory disorders may be short term, for example, pneumonia that benefits from bronchodilator therapy, or long term, such as black lung disease that requires lifelong oxygen therapy. In an inpatient setting, respiratory therapists assume a critical role when treating patients who are on a ventilator (historically known as an *iron lung*). Mechanical ventilation requires the use of flowsheets to document ventilator settings and the patient's progress toward weaning from the ventilator.

7.4 Outpatient Clinical Documentation

There are many similarities between inpatient and outpatient documentation; however, there are several differences that are driven by the needs of the patients and providers in the different settings. In inpatient settings, documentation occurs over several days, whereas in an outpatient setting the encounter may last for only 15–30 minutes.

History and Physical Examination

As discussed previously, the H&P is a valuable tool for the healthcare provider in the identification of diagnoses and is the first step in developing a plan of care. The same is true for outpatient settings such as physician's offices and outpatient clinics. The outpatient H&P consists of the subjective and objective elements; however, depending on the reason for the patient's visit, the physician may conduct a complete ROS or a selective ROS that focuses on the body systems involved with the patient's chief complaint(s). For example, a high school student whose chief complaint is that they wish to participate in sports will likely need a complete ROS to ensure their health status is appropriate for participation in the sport. However, a 10-year-old whose chief complaint is throat pain will likely receive only a general examination along with a check of vital signs and a review of the HEENT system.

In an outpatient setting, such as a physician's office, there are several H&P templates that are available for use. These templates include fields to record the annual history and the physical examination for patients who are well and asymptomatic. In addition, pediatric physician's offices may have H&P templates that are specific to the age of the child at the time of the examination and to the systems reviewed at that age.

Electronic Chart Note Templates

In an outpatient setting, the progress notes or chart notes are often templates based on the patient's chief complaint or the reason for the visit. In the EHR Navigator, you will find many examples of templates specific to a chief complaint that you might see in a live EHR system of a physician's practice. These include:

- Abdominal Pain Chart Note
- Auto Accident Follow-up Chart Note
- Breast Cancer Chart Note
- CHF Chart Note
- Constipation Chart Note
- Headache Chart Note
- Knee Pain Chart Note
- Pediatric Otitis Media Chart Note
- UTI Chart Note

In addition to progress note and chart note templates, there is an opportunity to document a free text chart note. This chart note is important to have in every EHR system as templates are typically used only for the most frequent types of encounters. For example, a free text chart note would be documented when a patient reports vague symptoms such as fever, shortness of breath, and lethargy. The diagnosis is not readily apparent, so the provider would document findings in a free text note.

Electronic Superbill

The electronic superbill, also called an *encounter form*, is an itemized form that allows charges to be captured from a patient visit. Instead of an automatic charge capture process used in inpatient settings, outpatient settings typically use an electronic superbill in which the provider enters the reason for the visit and the time and level of service that the provider rendered. Testing that is performed in the physician's office, such as rapid strep tests or tympanometry, is also entered on the electronic superbill.

Outpatient Eprescription

The e-prescribing process in the outpatient setting is the same as the e-prescribing process in the inpatient setting. The only two notable differences between e-prescribing in the inpatient and outpatient settings are:

1. Eprescriptions are transmitted to various community pharmacies in the outpatient setting rather than to the hospital's pharmacy in an inpatient setting.

2. Prescription refills are more prevalent in the outpatient setting as providers are treating patients for chronic conditions that require long-term medications.

The e-prescribing component of the EHR in the outpatient setting also includes an alert function that notifies the prescribing healthcare provider of drug-to-drug interactions, drug-to-food interactions, and the patient's allergies to medications.

Tutorial 7.3 **EHR**NAVIGAT♦R

Modifying a Patient's ePrescription

Go to the online course to launch Tutorial 7.3. As a physician, practice modifying a patient's eprescription using the EHR Navigator.

Tutorial 7.4 **EHR**NAVIGAT♦R

Overriding a Drug Allergy Notification

Go to the online course to launch Tutorial 7.4. As a physician assistant, practice adding an eprescription and overriding a drug allergy notification using the EHR Navigator.

Tutorial 7.5 **EHR**NAVIGAT♦R

Reporting an Immunization

Go to the online course to launch Tutorial 7.5. As a medical assistant, practice reporting an immunization using the EHR Navigator.

7.5 Skilled Nursing and Rehab Clinical Documentation

Clinical documentation in a skilled nursing and rehab setting follows most of the same requirements as an inpatient setting such as a hospital. The most notable documentation difference in a skilled nursing and rehab setting is the Minimum Data Set (MDS), which is used to assess patients, also known as *residents*, and drive reimbursement to the skilled nursing facility.

Minimum Data Set

The MDS is part of the federally mandated process for clinical assessment of all residents in Medicare- and Medicaid-certified nursing homes. This process provides a comprehensive assessment of each resident's functional capabilities and helps nursing home staff identify health problems. A care plan is derived from the MDS to specify the care needs of the patient, or resident. See Figure 7.5 for an excerpt from the MDS in EHR Navigator.

Figure 7.5 Excerpt from Minimum Data Set

Resident: Esparza, Miguel   Identifier: 1772506   Date: 12-02-2030

MINIMUM DATA SET (MDS) - Version 3.0
RESIDENT ASSESSMENT AND CARE SCREENING
Nursing Home Comprehensive (NC) Item Set

MDS Quick Navigation Section Tabs

A. Identification Information   B. Hearing, Speech, and Vision   C. Cognitive Patterns   D. Mood   E. Behavior   F. Preferences for Customary Routine and Activities   G. Functional Status   GG. Functional Abilities and Goals

H. Bladder and Bowel   I. Active Diagnoses   J. Health Conditions   K. Swallowing/Nutritional Status   L. Oral/Dental Status   M. Skin Conditions   N. Medications   O. Special Treatments, Procedures, and Programs

P. Restraints and Alarms   Q. Participation in Assessment and Goal Setting   V. Care Area Assessment (CAA) Summary   X. Correction Request   Z. Assessment Administration

Section A	Identification Information

A0050. Type of Record

Enter Code ☐

1. Add new record -> Continue to A0100, Facility Provider Numbers
2. Modify existing record -> Continue to A0100, Facility Provider Numbers
3. Inactivate existing record -> Skip to X0150, Type of Provider

A0100. Facility Provider Numbers

A. National Provider Identification (NPI):

B. CMS Certification Number (CCN):

C. State Provider Number:

A0200. Type of Provider

Enter Code ☐

Type of Provider
1. Nursing Home (SNF/NF)
2. Swing Bed

A0310. Type of Assessment

Enter Code ☐

A. Federal OBRA Reason for Assessment
01. Admission assessment (required by day 14)
02. Quarterly review assessment
03. Annual assessment
04. Significant change in status assessment
05. Significant correction to prior comprehensive assessment
06. Significant correction to prior quarterly assessment
99. None of the above

Enter Code ☐

B. PPS Assessment
PPS Scheduled Assessments for a Medicare Part A Stay
01. 5-day scheduled assessment
02. 14-day scheduled assessment
03. 30-day scheduled assessment
04. 60-day scheduled assessment
05. 90-day scheduled assessment
PPS Unscheduled Assessments for a Medicare Part A Stay
07. Unscheduled assessment used for PPS (OMRA, significant or clinical change, or significant correction assessment)
Not PPS Assessment
99. None of the above

Chapter Summary

Clinical documentation and reporting are at the core of the EHR system, making this system an interactive repository of timely, valuable, and possibly lifesaving data.

Data collection for the EHR occurs through a combination of manual and automated methods. Automated data collection is the preferred method of data capture because it requires less personnel time, avoids repetitive requests of information from patients, and allows for more consistent data. Patient demographic data is usually entered manually at the patient's first encounter with the healthcare organization and is automated at subsequent visits.

The clinical documentation cycle consists of recording a provider's initial evaluation of a patient, establishing and documenting a care plan, documenting the patient's progress toward care plan goals and closing the documentation cycle by recording a reassessment of the patient's condition.

History and physical examination results, progress notes, assessments, consultations, care plans and operative reports are examples of documents that may be manually or electronically added to the EHR. An area of concern related to EHR progress notes has been the increased use of cloned progress notes. Healthcare providers must ensure that their documentation is accurate at all times.

Diagnostic tests such as laboratory results are ideally transferred directly from the laboratory computer to the EHR. e-Prescribing has greatly benefited patients and providers, with improved accuracy in medication administration and efficiency related to communication and refills.

A portable medical order is a type of medical order that is entered into the EHR and then shared with other providers, either electronically or via paper if a provider does not have access to the patient's EHR. Medical orders regarding life-sustaining treatments are frequently written as a portable order.

Electronic medication administration records (eMAR), flowsheets, therapy documentation and the Minimum Data Set (MDS) are other types of clinical documentation.

Without the capability for exchange of clinical data inputs and outputs, the EHR system would function merely as a static, electronic file folder. From filling eprescriptions to the emergency review of laboratory results, the electronic exchange of clinical information has proven to be invaluable to patients and their caregivers.

Review and Assessment

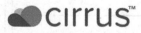

The following Review and Assessment activities are also available online in the Cirrus online course. Your instructor may ask you to complete these activities online. Cirrus also provides access to flash cards, a crossword puzzle, and practice quizzes to help strengthen your understanding of the chapter content.

Acronyms/Initialisms

Study the following acronyms discussed in this chapter. Go to the online course for flash cards of the acronyms and other chapter key terms.

CPOE: computerized provider order entry

CPT®: Current Procedural Terminology

eMAR: electronic medication administration record

H&P: history and physical examination

HEENT: head, ears, eyes, nose, and throat

ICD: International Classification of Diseases

OIG: Office of Inspector General

ONC: Office of the National Coordinator for Health Information Technology

ROS: review of systems

Check Your Understanding

To check your understanding of this chapter's key concepts, answer the following questions.

1. The documentation cycle includes which of the following steps, in the correct order?

   a. assessment, plan of care, progress notes, and reassessment

   b. history and physical examination and progress notes

   c. history and physical examination, plan of care, and eprescriptions

   d. plan of care, progress notes, and assessment/reassessment

2. Which document contains the results of the examination of a patient's body systems?

   a. operative report

   b. radiology report

   c. laboratory report

   d. history and physical examination (H&P)

3. Which of the following statements concerning e-prescribing are *true*?

   a. e-Prescribing is the electronic generation and transmission of prescriptions.

   b. e-Prescribing increases the efficiency of healthcare practices.

   c. e-Prescribing assists prescribers by telling them which medication they should order for each diagnosis.

   d. Both *a* and *b* are true.

4. The abbreviation ROS means a

   a. review of systems on the history and physical examination.

   b. record of steroid use in e-prescribing.

   c. report of substance abuse.

   d. review of syndromic surveillance.

5. Which of the following would probably *not* be documented in a patient's care plan?

    a. goal for ambulation

    b. pain management medications

    c. target hemoglobin value

    d. family history of breast cancer

6. True/False: The e-prescribing feature of an EHR system is an optional meaningful use function.

7. True/False: A template is a preformatted file that provides prompts to obtain specific, consistent information.

8. True/False: If a physician's office does *not* interface with a laboratory's computer, there is no way to incorporate laboratory results into the EHR system.

9. True/False: A physician who copies and pastes documentation from one progress note to another is creating cloned notes.

10. True/False: Per US law, Schedule II controlled substances *cannot* be ordered via e-prescribing.

Go on the Record

To build on your understanding of the topics in this chapter, complete the following short-answer activities.

1. Explain why a healthcare provider might use cloned progress notes.

2. Describe the benefits of e-prescribing.

3. List three body systems examined during an H&P.

4. Describe the two elements of an H&P.

5. Explain how Northstar Medical Center can prove that its EHR system meets the core requirements of meaningful use.

Navigate the Field

To gain practice in handling challenging situations in the workplace, consider the following real-world scenarios and identify how you would respond to each.

1. You are the health information manager at a local hospital. A physician on the medical staff does not understand how to add H&P notes to a patient's EHR. He explains that he "always used to handwrite the H&P." You explain to the physician that he can no longer handwrite his H&P notes, and you give him two options of how he can add his H&P notes to the EHR. Describe these two options.

2. You are a laboratory manager at a local hospital. Your laboratory systems can interface with the hospital's EHR system to automatically provide test results. However, there are times when this process does not function properly and results have to be entered manually. As the laboratory manager, you want to develop a procedure for doing this. What steps might you include in

this procedure? Write a one-page procedure for manually entering laboratory results into the hospital's EHR system when the laboratory computer cannot automatically transfer the laboratory results to the hospital's EHR system.

Think Critically

Continue to think critically about challenging concepts and complete the following activities.

1. As the quality manager at a local hospital, you are conducting an audit of physician progress notes to ensure that the progress notes accurately reflect the condition of the patient and are not simply cloned notes depicting inaccuracies.

   Patient Scenario #1: Progress note of 10/4/2030, 07:45: Infectious disease note: No fevers/chills. Tolerating antibiotics without difficulty. Lungs clear. Abdomen soft with positive bowel sounds. PICC without phlebitis. Vanc trough value of 10/2/2030 is 14.0.

   Which of the following progress notes is accurately written according to Patient Scenario #1 if the patient's status is completely the same as it was on 10/4/2030?

   _____ a. Progress note of 10/5/2030, 10.00: Infectious disease note: No changes from progress note of 10/4/2030, 07:45.

   _____ b. Progress note of 10/5/2030, 16:00: Infectious disease note: No fevers/chills. Tolerating antibiotics without difficulty. Lungs clear. Abdomen soft with positive bowel sounds. PICC without phlebitis. Vanc trough value of 10/2/2030 is 14.0.

   _____ c. Progress note of 10/5/2030, 14:00: Infectious disease note: Temp of 101.8°F today. Tolerating antibiotics without difficulty. Lungs clear. Abdomen soft with positive bowel sounds. PICC without phlebitis. Vanc trough value of 10/2/2030 is 14.0.

   Patient Scenario #2: Progress note of 04/12/2030, 08:10: Pulmonary note: Patient doing well on trach collar. Afebrile. Chest clear. No edema. Chronic respiratory failure. Change trach to #6 and start capping speech to evaluate for swallowing.

   Which of the following progress notes is accurately written according to Patient Scenario #2 if the patient's status is completely the same as it was on 04/12/2030, except the patient now has a fever of 101.4°F?

   _____ a. Progress note of 04/13/2030, 14:15: Pulmonary note: Patient doing well on trach collar. Fever of 101.4°F. Chest rales heard. No edema. Chronic respiratory failure. Change trach to #6 and start capping speech to evaluate for swallowing.

   _____ b. Progress note of 04/13/2030, 14:10: Pulmonary note: Patient doing well on trach collar. Afebrile. Chest clear. No edema. Chronic respiratory failure. Change trach to #6 and start capping speech to evaluate for swallowing.

   _____ c. Progress note of 04/13/2030, 11:10: Pulmonary note: Patient doing well on trach collar. Temp of 101.4°F. Chest clear. No edema. Chronic respiratory failure. Change trach to #6 and start capping speech to evaluate for swallowing.

2. Perform an internet search to determine the laboratory results that must be reported to your state public health agency. Select another state and perform an internet search to determine the laboratory results that must be reported to that state's public health agency. How do the required test results compare? What tests are in common? Which are different? Why do you think some required test results vary from state to state? Why are some tests similar?

Make Your Case

Consider the scenario and then complete the following project.

You are a nurse at a medical office committed to community outreach and education. Your office uses e-prescribing software and wants to conduct a meeting for patients and guests to explain this technology. Develop a presentation for the meeting that explains the functions and benefits of using e-prescribing.

Explore the Technology

EHRNAVIGAT☰R *Complete the EHR Navigator practice assessments that align to each tutorial and the assessments that accompany Chapter 7 located in the online course.*

Chapter 8 Electronic Health Records for Nursing

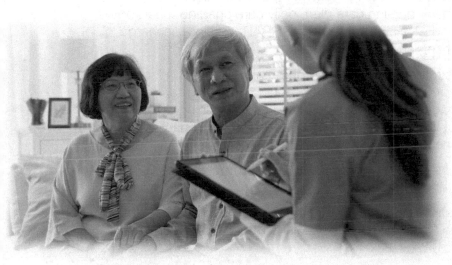

Field Notes

"In my position as the Clinical Quality Improvement
Officer for a large suburban hospital, one of the statistics
I have most enjoyed reporting to our medical staff and
administration is the significant decrease in medication
errors that we've enjoyed since the implementation of the
hospital-wide EHR."

– Michele Lamping, MBA, BSN, C-EFM, NE-BC

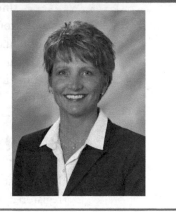

Learning Objectives

8.1 Discuss the vital role that nursing staff play in the provision and documentation of patient care in inpatient and outpatient settings.

8.2 Explain the flow of EHR documentation completed by nurses in an inpatient setting.

8.3 Demonstrate nursing EHR documentation in an inpatient hospital setting, including admission orders, nursing admission assessment, infection control assessment, fall risk assessment, skin assessment, pain assessment, pressure injury risk assessment, nursing care plan, daily care charting, chart notes, eMAR and eTAR, I&O flowsheets, SBAR, nursing discharge assessment, and transfer form.

8.4 Demonstrate nursing EHR documentation in an inpatient skilled nursing and rehabilitation setting including a long-term care nursing admission assessment, delirium screening, Minimum Data Set (MDS), and long-term care nursing discharge assessment.

8.5 Explain the flow of EHR documentation completed by nurses in an outpatient setting.

8.6 Demonstrate nursing EHR documentation in an outpatient setting, including SOAP notes and specialized templates such as a pediatric physical exam.

Communication is a key component in the provision of quality health care. Healthcare providers must communicate important patient information in a timely, accurate manner, and this communication is largely accomplished via the electronic health record (EHR). Nursing staff play a vital role in the provision and documentation of patient care.

In this chapter, you will learn about the different types of nurses and how nurses document patient care in inpatient facilities, long-term care facilities, and outpatient facilities.

8.1 Nursing Staff

Nursing staff includes certified nursing assistants, licensed practical nurses, and registered nurses. These different titles denote different educational levels, certification, and licensures as well as the roles and responsibilities in the care of patients. Each of these different nurses can work in various healthcare settings, such as hospitals, long-term care facilities, physician's offices, and other outpatient settings. Although roles and responsibilities vary among the different categories of nursing staff, the primary responsibility of all nursing staff is advocacy for the patients in their care by attempting to meet their healthcare needs in a safe, comfortable environment. It is the responsibility of the nursing staff to carry out the orders prescribed by physicians, physician assistants, and nurse practitioners. **Scope of practice** refers to the allowable procedures and functions that healthcare professionals may perform according to their state licensures. Nurses are ranked according to their level of education and licensure, with certified nursing assistants at the lower end and registered nurses at the higher end of that hierarchy.

Certified Nursing Assistants

Certified nursing assistants (CNAs) work in a variety of healthcare settings, including hospitals, long-term care facilities, home health care, rehabilitation hospitals, and psychiatric facilities, with most CNAs working in long-term care. CNAs provide a significant amount of direct patient care by taking vital signs, checking blood glucose levels, and assisting patients with their activities of daily living (ADLs). ADLs include eating, bathing, toileting, dressing, and moving (e.g., turning in bed, transferring from bed to chair, and walking), and CNAs respond to these requests and needs of their patients.

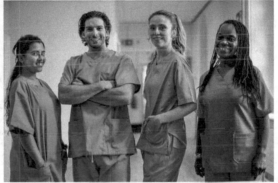

The requirements for CNAs, also known as **STNAs (state-tested nursing assistants)**, **SRNAs (state-registered nursing assistants)**, **GNAs (geriatric nursing assistants)**, and **LNAs (licensed nursing assistants)**, vary by state. Most states require CNAs to take a state-approved program and pass a certification exam. Periodic recertification is usually a requirement as well.

Nurses have the responsibility of caring for patients in a variety of healthcare settings, such as hospitals, long-term care facilities, and physician's offices.

Licensed Practical Nurses

Licensed practical nurses (LPNs), also known as **licensed vocational nurses (LVNs)** in California and Texas, have a high school diploma, attended an LPN program of 9–18 months, and passed a state licensure exam. LPNs perform basic nursing functions such as taking blood pressure readings and other vital signs, catheter care, and wound care. Some states include administering medications to long-term care residents in the scope of practice of LPNs. LPNs work under the supervision of an RN or a physician.

Registered Nurses

Registered nurses (RNs) are typically assigned a group of patients in a healthcare setting and are responsible for the overall assessment, care planning, and treatment of those patients. The RN assumes a leadership role in assessment, care, and treatment by supervising LPNs and CNAs caring for their patients. RNs hold an associate or bachelor's degree from an approved nursing school and must pass state board exams.

8.2 Nursing in Inpatient Settings

In an inpatient setting, the nursing staff begin patient care and documentation upon the admission of the patient and continue care and documentation throughout the stay and discharge of the patient. Since the nursing staff spend the most time of any group of healthcare providers caring for the patient, they are placed in the main role of documenting patient data for use by other healthcare providers.

The inpatient setting section of this chapter outlines and allows you to practice the basic documentation required by nursing staff in most inpatient settings. One of the challenges for all healthcare providers is to keep a caring, responsive approach with the patient while using an EHR system. Standing or sitting in front of a computer while asking the patient questions without maintaining eye contact and without warm, caring conversation is not the type of nursing care that will promote healing and positive patient outcomes or opinions. As you study this chapter, envision yourself interacting with a patient while asking your patient questions, conducting assessments, and providing care. Become familiar enough with the documentation you need to enter into the EHR so that you can focus on having a caring conversation with your patient that solicits most, if not all, the information you need for your documentation. Practicing your interaction with patients and technology as you study and become familiar with EHR documentation requirements will help you become the caring, healing nurse you want to be.

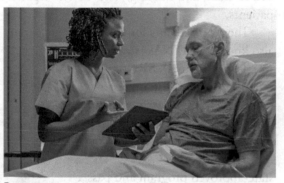

Documenting patient care in an EHR while maintaining compassion and warmth is a skill you will need to develop throughout your nursing career.

Admission Orders and Transfer

To enable nursing staff to begin their care of an inpatient upon admission, there must be admission orders in place. **Admission orders** include, at a minimum, instructions for the patient's diet; medications; activities; diagnostic testing, including laboratory tests and radiology tests; and monitoring orders.

An admission order template contains these categories with space for the physician to add specific orders. In addition, many hospitals have specific admission order templates developed for common diagnoses such as myocardial infarction, congestive heart failure, and acute mental status change to assist the medical staff with following best-practice protocols that have been developed by physician specialists. Admission orders may be generated in several different ways, including **transfer orders** from the emergency department (ED), transfer orders from another inpatient hospital, or physician admission orders for an elective admission. Patients transferred from a long-term care facility or other outpatient facility (e.g., a surgical center) are typically triaged in the ED rather than being directly admitted to a hospital unit. Admission orders for these patients will be generated by the ED. Regardless of the source of the admission orders, the admitting physician must approve them. This is typically accomplished with a review of the orders via a telephone call from the admitting nurse to the admitting physician. These admission orders are then considered valid and in effect via the facility's telephone order policy and must be signed by the admitting physician within a time period specified by facility policy.

Once admission orders have been documented and signed by the admitting physician, the orders populate the EHR in the appropriate sections and notify hospital staff of action needed to be taken. For example, medications will populate the medication administration record (MAR) and the fill list for the pharmacy staff, radiology tests will populate the radiology technician's schedule of tests to be performed, and so on.

Tutorial 8.1

EHRNAVIGATOR

Starting a Patient's Admissions Orders

Go to your online course to launch Tutorial 8.1. As a nurse, add admissions orders to a patient's chart for a preoperative patient.

Tutorial 8.2

EHRNAVIGATOR

Completing a Patient's Admissions Orders

Go to your online course to launch Tutorial 8.2. As a nurse, continue to add the admissions orders to a patient's chart for a preoperative patient.

CHECKPOINT 8.1

1. Define *scope of practice*.

_____

_____

_____

_____

2. Admission orders include all of the following *except*

a. labs.

b. transfer.

c. diet.

d. medications.

8.3 Assessments Conducted by Nurses

An important duty of all healthcare providers is accurate, timely assessment of the patients under their care. **Assessment** includes evaluations of subjective and objective information, resulting in patient risk values, diagnoses, and conditions, depending on the focus of the assessment. The first assessment done by nurses is the admission assessment. In addition to the admission assessment, there are several assessments that are completed throughout a patient's stay, as their condition warrants. Hospital policies and procedures will govern the completion of these assessments. Assessments that may be completed throughout the stay of the patient include the following:

- Infection control
- Fall risk assessment
- Pain assessment
- Skin assessment
- Pressure injury risk assessment

We will cover the purpose and documentation requirements for each assessment.

Nursing Admission Assessment

Upon admission, the nursing staff must conduct an **admission assessment** of the patient. The completion of this assessment is typically assigned to the admitting nurse, who has been assigned the responsibility of welcoming the patient to the nursing unit, obtaining admission orders, conducting all admission documentation, and scheduling all the initial care and treatment of the patient. Admission assessments are very detailed and cover the following:

- Personal, family, and social data
- Vital signs
- Medical history
- Pain assessment
- Fall risk assessment
- Review of all body systems
- Advanced directives
- Educational and discharge needs

It is imperative that the admission assessment be complete and accurate as it establishes the condition of the patient upon admission. This has always been an important responsibility for nursing staff but even more so in recent years as payers, including Medicare, Medicaid, and commercial insurance, do not pay for hospital-acquired complications or comorbidities. For example, the costs associated with the care, treatment, and additional days in the hospital resulting from a pressure sore, urinary tract infection, or fracture that developed or occurred while in the hospital will not be covered or paid for by payers. What happens if the admitting nurse fails to note one of these conditions upon admission? The saying, "If it wasn't documented, it wasn't done," means that the hospital would experience a loss of reimbursement due to the failure of the nurse to appropriately document the existence of the patient's condition upon admission. Figure 8.1 illustrates the nursing admission assessment.

Starting a Nursing Admission Assessment
Go to your online course to launch Tutorial 8.3. As a nurse, begin a Nursing Admission Assessment.

Figure 8.1 Nursing Admission Assessment

Add Chart Note

Title: CAD   Type: Nursing Admission Assessment   Time Entered: 12/02/2030 04 : 30 PM

Patient Info | Vital Signs & History | Assessments | Body System Review | Additional & Advance Directive

Patient: Donaldson, Vance

Accompanied by: Spouse

Language Barriers: Y ☑N
Interpreter Needed: Y ☑N
Admitted to: S-134
Admitting diagnosis: CAS

Mode of Admission: ☑Ambulatory Stretcher Wheelchair Other
Transported with: Oxygen Monitor IV Other
Valuables: ☑None

Dentures/partials: Y ☑N
Hearing Aids: Y ☑N
Prosthesis: Y ☑N
If yes, list:
The patient's preference for learning:

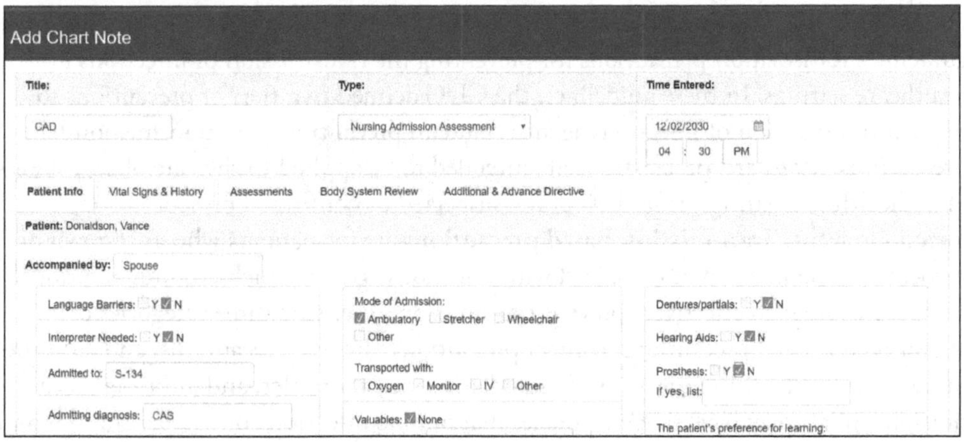

Tutorial 8.4   EHRNAVIGATOR

Entering Health Information in a Nursing Admission Assessment
Go to your online course to launch Tutorial 8.4. As a nurse, continue populating the Nursing Admission Assessment by entering the patient's vital signs, allergies, and health problems.

Tutorial 8.5   EHRNAVIGATOR

Entering Pain and Body Systems Review Information in a Nursing Admission Assessment
Go to your online course to launch Tutorial 8.5. As a nurse, enter the patient's pain assessment information and the results of the body systems review on the Nursing Admission Assessment.

Tutorial 8.6   EHRNAVIGATOR

Completing a Nursing Admission Assessment
Go to your online course to launch Tutorial 8.6. As a nurse, complete the review of systems for the patient and sign and save the Nursing Admission Assessment.

Infection Control Assessment

Many patients, especially those transferred from another inpatient facility, have infections that warrant isolation to a particular room and special precautions that need to be followed by staff and visitors. By the mid-1970s, **healthcare-associated infections (HAIs)** were recognized as a major threat connected to medical care. Efforts to prevent and control HAIs have led to profound changes in the ways that those infections are perceived and managed in the United States and abroad. Programs that focused on preventing and controlling HAIs were rare in US hospitals in the early 1970s but are now present in virtually every hospital in the nation and in many hospitals abroad.

In 2007, the Centers for Disease Control and Prevention (CDC) published specific guidelines for isolation precautions for preventing the transmission of infections in healthcare settings. In these guidelines, the CDC defined two tiers of precautions to prevent transmission of infectious agents: standard precautions and transmission-based precautions. **Standard precautions** are intended to be applied to the care of *all* patients in *all* healthcare settings, regardless of the suspected or confirmed presence of an infectious agent. **Transmission-based precautions** are for patients who are known or suspected to be infected or colonized with infectious agents, which requires additional control measures to effectively prevent transmission. There are three categories of transmission-based precautions: contact precautions, droplet precautions, and airborne precautions. In addition to the use of standard, contact, droplet, and airborne precautions, hospitals may have specific policies that outline infection control precautions and procedures that must be used as well. For example, a hospital policy may state that patients who are infected with methicillin-resistant *Staphylococcus aureus* (MRSA) may reside together in a semiprivate room, but staff and visitors must wear appropriate protective items, including gown and gloves. The protective clothing is meant to protect both the staff or visitor and the patient.

The need to accurately document the infection status of a patient is important because this documentation is used not only by nursing floor staff and visitors but also by every healthcare provider encountering the patient, such as radiology staff conducting diagnostic testing or operating room staff conducting procedures.

Upon admission and throughout the stay of the patient, the nursing staff are responsible for documenting the infection status of the patient. This documentation should include, at a minimum, the following:

- Infection status of the patient (a patient has an active infection, does not have an active infection, or does not have an active infection but is a carrier—someone who does not have active symptoms of an infection but has specific infectious bacteria living in the nose or on the skin)

- Type of organism (e.g., MRSA or vancomycin-resistant enterococci)

- Source of the infection (e.g., sputum or blood)

- Type of isolation precautions to be used by staff and visitors (e.g., standard, contact, droplet, or airborne)

An infection control assessment is illustrated in Figure 8.2.

EXPAND YOUR LEARNING 📶

For more detailed information regarding universal precautions, visit the CDC website at https://EHR3.ParadigmEducation.com/CDC.

Tutorial 8.7 | **EHR**NAVIGAT✛R

Entering an Infection Control Form

Go to your online course to launch Tutorial 8.7. As a nurse, complete, sign, and save an Infection Control form.

Fall Risk Assessment

Falls occur more often with advancing age and are a major threat to older adults' quality of life, often causing a decline in self-care ability and participation in physical

Figure 8.2   Infection Control Assessment

| | | | 10 : 30 | AM |

Active Infection:

☑ Yes

☐ No

☐ Carrier

Isolation precautions:

Choose multiple

☑ Standard

☐ Contact

☐ Droplet

☐ Airborne

☐ Other

Organism:

Choose multiple

☐ MRSA

☐ VRE

☑ Influenza

☐ TB

Source:

Choose multiple

☐ Abscess

☐ Blood

☐ Wound

☐ Sputum

and social activities. Each year, approximately 30%–40% of people aged 65 years and older who live in the community (as opposed to an inpatient care setting) fall. Roughly half of all falls result in an injury, of which 10% are serious, and injury rates increase with age.

Risk factors have been identified that indicate that a patient may have an increased likelihood of falling. These risk factors include the following:

- Age-related changes
- Cognitive deficits
- Gait, strength, or balance deficits
- Sensory deficits
- Chronic conditions
- Acute illnesses
- Behaviors and choices
- Medications
- Footwear
- Assistive devices
- Home and neighborhood features
- Alcohol and drug use
- Support from caregivers

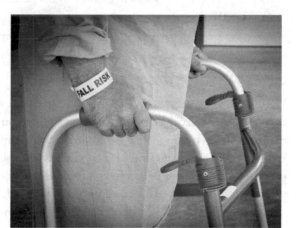

Patients at risk of a fall should wear a special fall risk bracelet and have their risk calculated in the EHR.

Clinical assessments by a healthcare provider combined with individualized treatment of identified risk factors have been found to reduce the rate of falls. Therefore, it is important for patients to be screened upon admission for risk of falls so appropriate care and treatment may be provided. It is also important to periodically reassess fall risk throughout a patient's stay and upon a significant change in condition, medications, or other fall risk factors.

EXPAND YOUR LEARNING

According to the CDC, the direct medical costs for falls total nearly $50 billion annually, and the average hospital cost for a fall injury is more than $30,000. Go to https://EHR3 .ParadigmEducation .com/STEADI to learn more about fall risks and the CDC's program aimed at reducing the incidence of falls.

Figure 8.3   Fall Risk Assessment

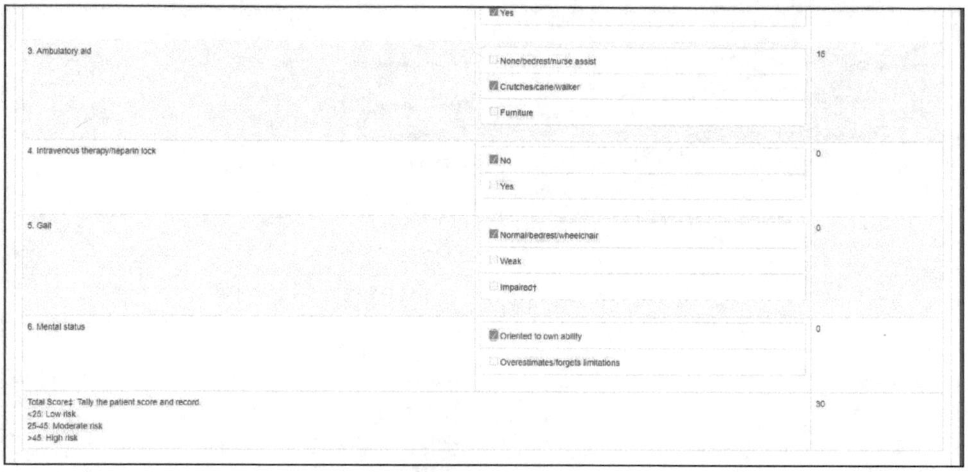

	☑ Yes	
3. Ambulatory aid	☐ None/bedrest/nurse assist	15
	☑ Crutches/cane/walker	
	☐ Furniture	
4. Intravenous therapy/heparin lock	☑ No	0
	☐ Yes	
5. Gait	☑ Normal/bedrest/wheelchair	0
	☐ Weak	
	☐ Impaired	
6. Mental status	☑ Oriented to own ability	0
	☐ Overestimates/forgets limitations	
Total Scores: Tally the patient score and record. <25: Low risk. 25–45: Moderate risk >45: High risk		30

ON THE JOB

The nurse must interview the patient and their family or caregivers for a complete and accurate fall risk assessment.

A **fall risk assessment** includes scoring the presence or absence of fall risk factors, resulting in a cumulative score that indicates the degree to which a patient is at risk for falling. For example, a patient who has a history of falling, has secondary diagnoses, has an IV, is weak and uses a walker, and forgets to ask staff for assistance with ambulation would have a high fall risk score, resulting in fall risk prevention protocols. Figure 8.3 illustrates a fall risk assessment.

Tutorial 8.8   EHRNAVIGAT✛R

Completing a Fall Risk Assessment
Go to your online course to launch Tutorial 8.8. As a nurse, complete a Fall Risk Assessment.

Skin Assessment

Upon admission of a patient, a comprehensive **skin assessment** must be performed. The skin assessment may be a part of a nursing admission assessment tool or a separate assessment process. The rationale for completing a comprehensive skin assessment is twofold. First, any and all skin injuries and conditions (e.g., skin tears, bruises, scabs, rashes, or pressure injuries) must be carefully identified and documented to ensure that all injuries and conditions are known and appropriately treated. Additionally, skin injuries and conditions that are not identified upon admission may be attributed to the care or lack of care by the provider. As discussed, failing to record injuries and conditions upon admission could result in a reduction in reimbursement from the insurance payer. Failure to identify serious conditions might also result in a lawsuit against the provider and/or actions taken by accrediting or government agencies if a serious pattern of skin conditions, such as hospital-acquired pressure injuries, were found to be a consistent problem at the facility.

A comprehensive skin assessment begins with a head-to-toe assessment of all skin surfaces, including the patient's scalp and nails. As each skin injury and condition is identified, a description of the skin must be documented. This description may include skin color, temperature, turgor, moisture status, integrity, and size/measurements,

Figure 8.4   Sample Skin Assessment Illustration

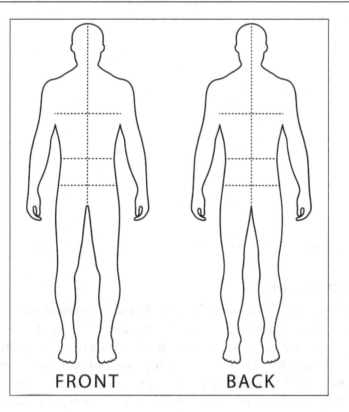

if applicable. If a current or healed pressure injury is identified, the length, width, depth, and stage of the ulcer must be documented. A body image is typically used to document the location of the skin injuries and conditions, such as in Figure 8.4.

Locations of skin conditions and injuries are noted on the body image with sequential numbers or letters. Corresponding descriptions of each identified site are documented, as shown in Figure 8.5.

Figure 8.5   Skin Assessment

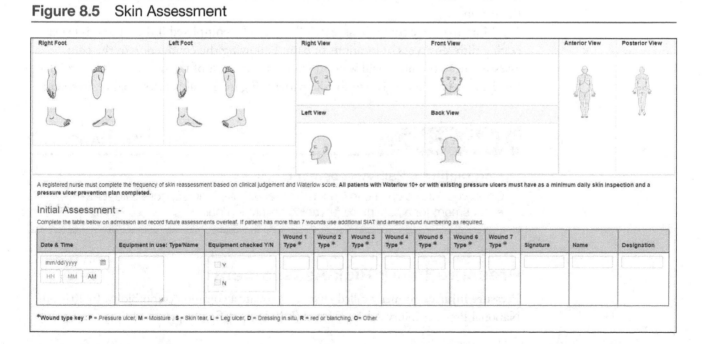

Figure 8.6   Pain Assessment

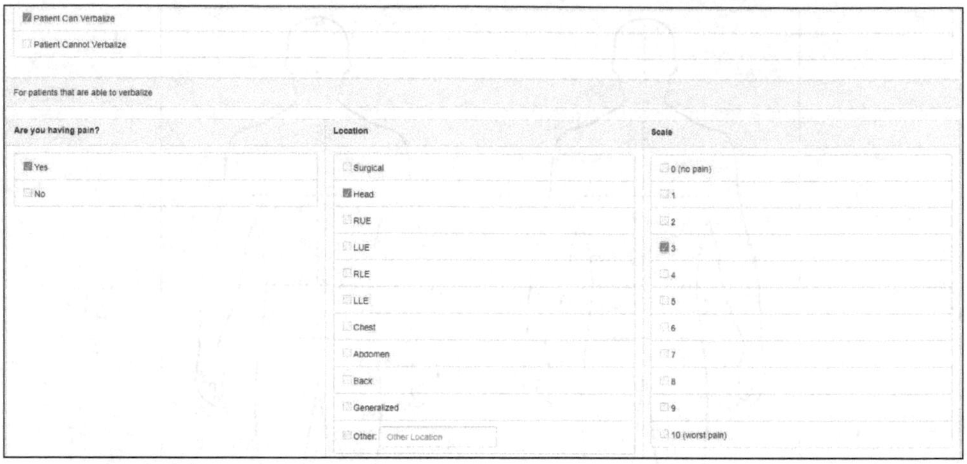

☑ Patient Can Verbalize		
☐ Patient Cannot Verbalize		

For patients that are able to verbalize

Are you having pain?	Location	Scale
☑ Yes	☐ Surgical	☐ 0 (no pain)
☐ No	☑ Head	☐ 1
	☐ RUE	☐ 2
	☐ LUE	☑ 3
	☐ RLE	☐ 4
	☐ LLE	☐ 5
	☐ Chest	☐ 6
	☐ Abdomen	☐ 7
	☐ Back	☐ 8
	☐ Generalized	☐ 9
	☐ Other: Other Location	☐ 10 (worst pain)

ON THE JOB

During a fall risk assessment, a patient may not clearly verbalize whether they need help, so the nurse must pay close attention to the patient's body language and expression for signs that help is needed.

Pain Assessment

Controlling a patient's pain is a major focus for all healthcare providers, especially the nursing staff, who work to make patients as comfortable as possible during their treatment and healing processes. Pain is either acute or chronic. Acute pain can be described as pain that lasts for a short period of time, such as hours, days, or weeks, and is caused by an injury, infection, or inflammation. Acute pain may occur following a procedure or be associated with a brief disease process or condition, such as a migraine headache or pinched nerve. Chronic pain can be described as pain that may be continual and lasts for a long period, such as months or years.

Whether the pain is acute or chronic, the first step in assisting patients with the management of their pain is to assess the pain. The **pain assessment** includes the type of pain, acute or chronic; the location of the pain; the intensity of the pain; and what, if anything, helps to relieve the pain. The nurse will want to assess the patient's pain in a caring, empathetic manner, focusing on the patient rather than on an EHR computer screen, demonstrating that the nurse is interested in the care, healing, and comfort of the patient.

More than one pain assessment will need to be completed if the patient is experiencing different types or locations of pain. Following the conduction of the pain assessment(s), the nurse will want to work with the rest of the healthcare team to plan for the best pain management for the patient. Figure 8.6 illustrates a pain assessment.

Tutorial 8.9   EHRNAVIGAT⊕R

Completing a Pain Assessment

Go to your online course to launch Tutorial 8.9. As a nurse, complete a Pain Assessment for a patient experiencing severe leg pain.

Pressure Injury Risk Assessment

Pressure injuries, formerly called *pressure ulcers*, are a common comorbidity. In 2016, the National Pressure Injury Advisory Panel (NPIAP) redefined a pressure injury as follows:

A pressure injury is localized damage to the skin and underlying soft tissue usually over a bony prominence or related to a medical or other device. The injury can present as intact skin or an open ulcer and may be painful. The injury occurs as a result of intense and/or prolonged pressure or pressure in combination with shear. The tolerance of soft tissue for pressure and shear may also be affected by microclimate, nutrition, perfusion, co-morbidities and condition of the soft tissue.

Pressure injuries are classified by a staging system that was also defined by the NPIAP. The stages are listed below along with their descriptions. For further information or resources, visit the NPIAP website at https://EHR3.ParadigmEducation.com/NPIAP.

- Stage 1 pressure injury: nonblanchable erythema of intact skin

- Stage 2 pressure injury: partial-thickness skin loss with exposed dermis

- Stage 3 pressure injury: full-thickness skin loss

- Stage 4 pressure injury: full-thickness skin and tissue loss

- Unstageable pressure injury: obscured full-thickness skin and tissue loss

- Deep tissue pressure injury: persistent nonblanchable deep red, maroon, or purple discoloration

Many risk factors have been identified with the development of pressure injuries. These risk factors include advanced age, poor nutritional status, poor circulation, incontinence, low body weight, and physical or cognitive impairment. It is important for an inpatient facility such as a hospital or nursing home to identify a patient's risk for pressure injury development so appropriate treatment and procedures can be undertaken to prevent pressure injury development. There are several assessment templates that are widely used in the United States, including the Braden Scale, Norton Scale, and Waterlow Scale. All of these templates assess the patient's pressure injury risk score by assigning numerical values to risk factors, resulting in a total patient score that summarizes the patient's risk of developing a pressure injury. Figure 8.7 shows a pressure injury risk assessment.

Figure 8.7   Pressure Injury Risk Assessment

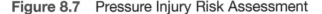

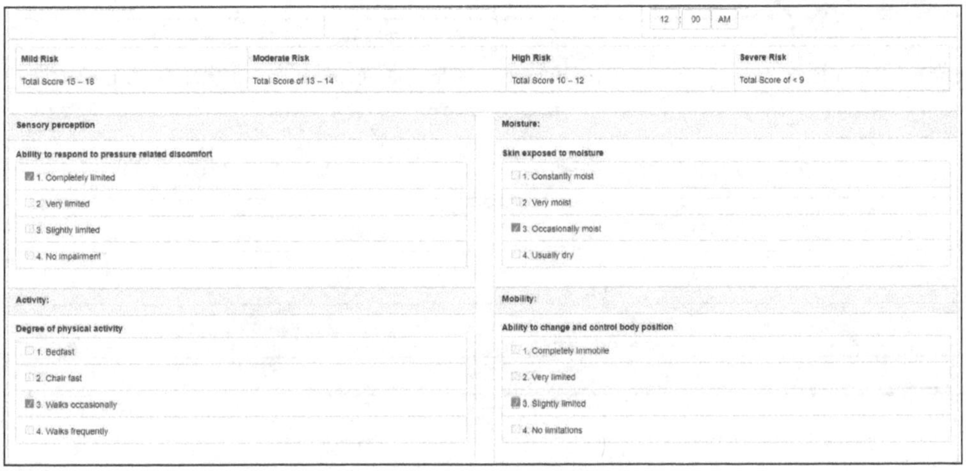

			12 : 00 AM
Mild Risk	**Moderate Risk**	**High Risk**	**Severe Risk**
Total Score 15 – 18	Total Score of 13 – 14	Total Score 10 – 12	Total Score of < 9

Sensory perception	**Moisture:**
Ability to respond to pressure related discomfort	Skin exposed to moisture
☑ 1. Completely limited	☐ 1. Constantly moist
☐ 2. Very limited	☐ 2. Very moist
☐ 3. Slightly limited	☑ 3. Occasionally moist
☐ 4. No impairment	☐ 4. Usually dry

Activity:	**Mobility:**
Degree of physical activity	Ability to change and control body position
☐ 1. Bedfast	☐ 1. Completely immobile
☐ 2. Chair fast	☐ 2. Very limited
☑ 3. Walks occasionally	☑ 3. Slightly limited
☐ 4. Walks frequently	☐ 4. No limitations

Why is it so important for a facility to assess a patient's risk of developing a pressure injury? First and foremost, pressure injuries affect patient comfort and healing by causing pain and often infection. Second, pressure injuries can be difficult to heal due to a patient's medical conditions, such as poor circulation, incontinence, limited mobility, and poor nutritional status. Many times, surgical interventions such as debridement or skin flaps are required. These procedures take an additional toll on already compromised patients, resulting in more pain, longer hospital stays, and increased cost of care. In addition, pressure injuries may contribute, in general, to worse patient prognosis and/or increased risk of death.

Prevention strategies need to be undertaken by nursing and allied health staff to reduce the risk of pressure injury development. The strategies implemented will depend on the level of risk identified on the pressure injury risk assessment. Common prevention procedures include the use of specialty beds such as low–air loss mattresses, frequent turning of patients in bed from right side to left side to back, nutritional supplements, and heel protectors.

A patient's risk for developing a pressure injury should be assessed upon admission, reassessed as a patient's condition changes, and documented accordingly within the EHR.

Wound Assessment

Once a wound has been identified, it must be treated and the treatment documented. This is accomplished through frequent wound assessments that document the size and appearance of the wound. An example of a wound assessment is found in Figure 8.8.

Tutorial 8.10   **EHR**NAVIGAT◆R

Completing a Wound Assessment

Go to your online course to launch Tutorial 8.10. As a nurse, complete a Wound Assessment for a patient with a postoperative wound.

CHECKP◆INT 8.2

1. Explain why it is important for a facility to assess a patient's risk for developing a pressure injury.

2. What four items are documented on a pain assessment?

Figure 8.8 Wound Assessment

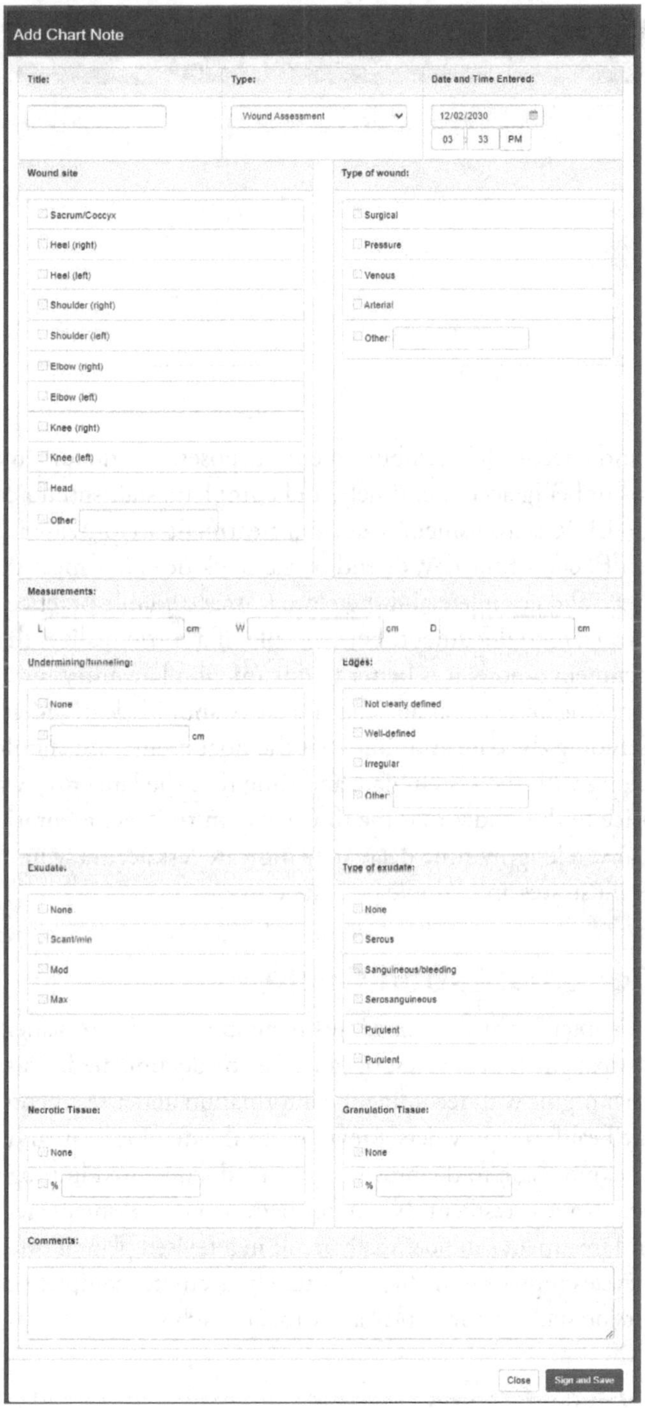
Add Chart Note

Title:
Type: Wound Assessment
Date and Time Entered: 12/02/2030 03 : 33 PM

Wound site
- Sacrum/Coccyx
- Heel (right)
- Heel (left)
- Shoulder (right)
- Shoulder (left)
- Elbow (right)
- Elbow (left)
- Knee (right)
- Knee (left)
- Head
- Other

Type of wound:
- Surgical
- Pressure
- Venous
- Arterial
- Other

Measurements:
L cm W cm D cm

Undermining/tunneling:
- None
- cm

Edges:
- Not clearly defined
- Well-defined
- Irregular
- Other

Exudate:
- None
- Scant/min
- Mod
- Max

Type of exudate:
- None
- Serous
- Sanguineous/bleeding
- Serosanguineous
- Purulent
- Purulent

Necrotic Tissue:
- None
- %

Granulation Tissue:
- None
- %

Comments:

Close Sign and Save

8.4 Daily Charting

Nursing staff must document the patient care rendered in the EHR. The documentation must be accurate, timely, and complete, as the EHR is a main communication tool in the provision of high-quality care. The EHR also serves as a legal document for

Figure 8.9   Late Entry in Documentation

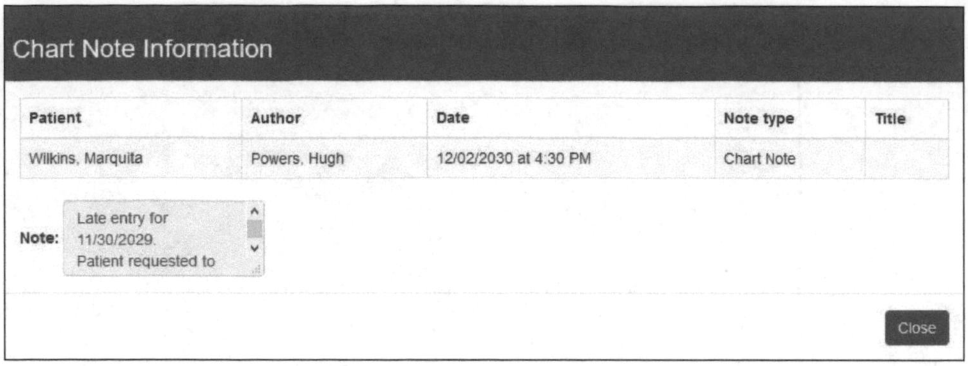

Chart Note Information					
Patient	**Author**	**Date**		**Note type**	**Title**
Wilkins, Marquita	Powers, Hugh	12/02/2030 at 4:30 PM		Chart Note	

Note: Late entry for 11/30/2029. Patient requested to

Close

the institution and a record for reimbursement purposes. For documentation to meet the requirements of being accurate, timely, and complete, staff should continually document in the EHR as assessment, care, and treatment are provided. Waiting until the end of the shift, end of the day, or end of the week does not meet the definition of accurate, timely, and complete and therefore is unacceptable practice. Having said that, it is never too late to document. For example, if a nurse realizes that they have neglected to document a note, it is better to document a late entry into the EHR as opposed to not having an entry at all. The late entry should clearly identify that it is a late entry by including the date and time that the documentation should have been entered. This, along with the system date and time that the late entry was documented, will serve as notice to the reader that the time delay in the documentation should be considered, because a lengthy time delay may indicate less accuracy in the documentation. Figure 8.9 illustrates an example of a late entry.

Clinical Documentation Cycle

As discussed in Chapter 7, when care and treatment are provided to patients (both inpatients and outpatients), the process of care must be documented. This documentation follows a cycle that begins with recording the information and assessments reviewed and conducted by the healthcare providers, progresses to the development and documentation of the plan of care, moves on to the provision of care documented in progress notes, and finally cycles back to a reassessment. New information and assessments regarding the results of care and treatment can potentially result in a revised plan of care. The clinical documentation cycle emphasizes the need for timely, accurate, complete EHR documentation by the nursing staff, as nurses play a key role in each step.

Nursing Plan of Care

The **nursing plan of care** is a working communication tool for nurses to share nursing diagnoses, desired patient outcomes related to the diagnoses, the interventions that the nursing staff will perform or direct, and evaluation indicating if the outcome was achieved (i.e., met or not met). Nursing diagnoses are related to but different from medical diagnoses. As defined by NANDA International (formerly the North American Nursing Diagnosis Association), a "medical diagnosis is a concept that defines a disease process or injury," and nursing diagnoses are "human responses to potential or actual health problems." The following are examples of medical diagnoses and related nursing diagnoses.

Figure 8.10 Plan of Care

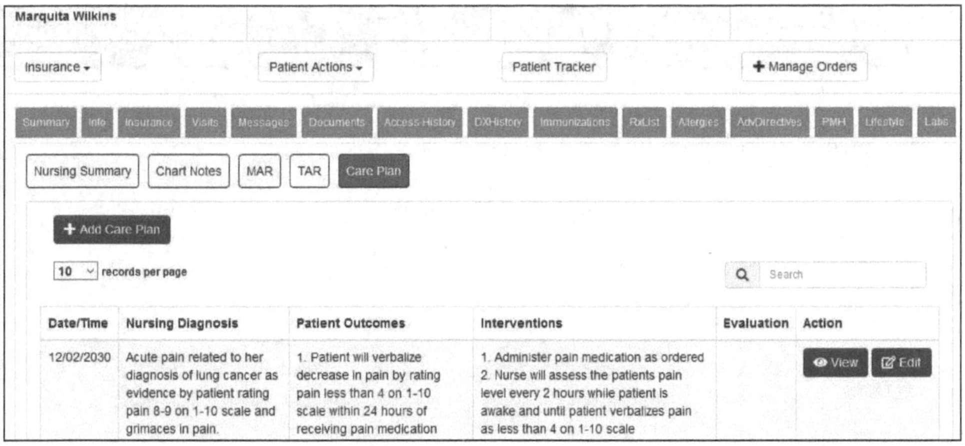

Example 1: A patient who has a *medical diagnosis* of malignant neoplasm of the lung might have the following *nursing diagnoses* that relate to the medical diagnosis:

- Difficulty breathing

- Acute chest pain

- Anxiety related to the change in health status

Example 2: A patient who has a *medical diagnosis* of cerebrovascular accident might have the following *nursing diagnoses* that relate to the medical diagnosis:

- Difficulty swallowing

- Difficulty speaking

- Anxiety related to an inability to communicate

In many facilities, the nursing plan of care is not a part of the organization's legal, permanent EHR record, just as it was not previously a part of the legal, permanent paper record. In fact, the nursing plan of care, when included in the paper record, was written in pencil, erased, and updated from shift to shift. Sometimes a portion of the care plan may be written on a white board in the patient's room. Whether the nursing plan of care is a part of the organization's legal health record is defined in organizational policy. Figure 8.10 illustrates an electronic nursing plan of care.

Daily Nursing Notes

There are two types of nursing notes that are a part of the legal record and that may be documented daily according to organizational policies and procedures. One type of nursing note, the nursing daily care assessment, is a summary of the patient's status, the care rendered, and the patient's response to care and treatment for a specific time, such as a 12-hour shift. Depending on facility policy, nursing notes that include the patient's status along with the care and treatment provided may be documented in the EHR every shift or once a day. A nursing daily care assessment is in template format to ensure that all necessary documentation is included. A sample nursing daily care assessment is found in Figure 8.11.

Figure 8.11 Nursing Daily Care Assessment

Chart Note Information

Patient	Author	Date	Note type	Title
Wilkins, Marquita	Powers, Hugh	12/02/2030 at 4:30 PM	Nursing Daily Care Assessment	

Date	Time	Patient
12/02/2030		Wilkins, Marquita

Patient Status

☑ Asleep

☐ In bed

☑ In chair

☐ In bathroom

Patient Requests

☐ Pt requests met

☐ Other:

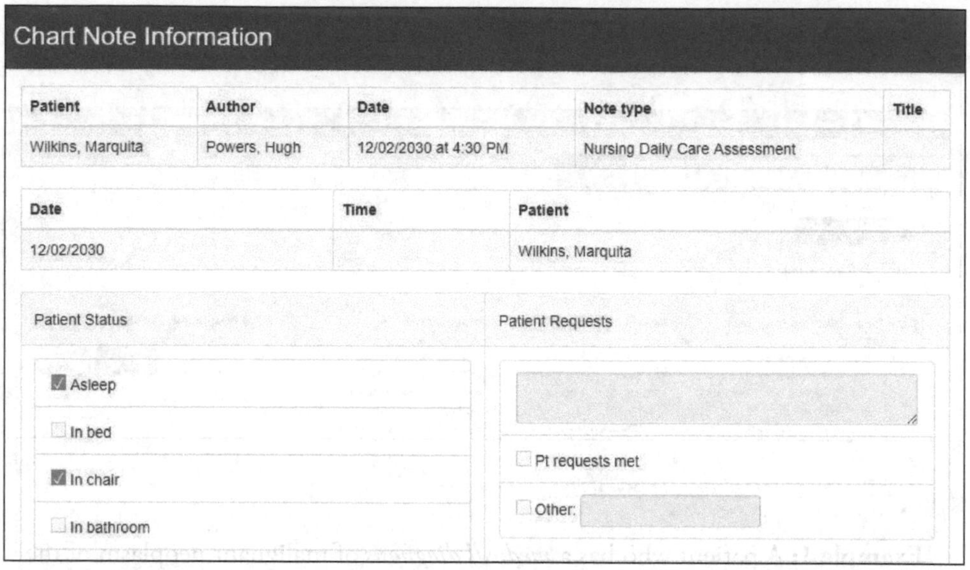

Figure 8.12 Episodic Nursing Note

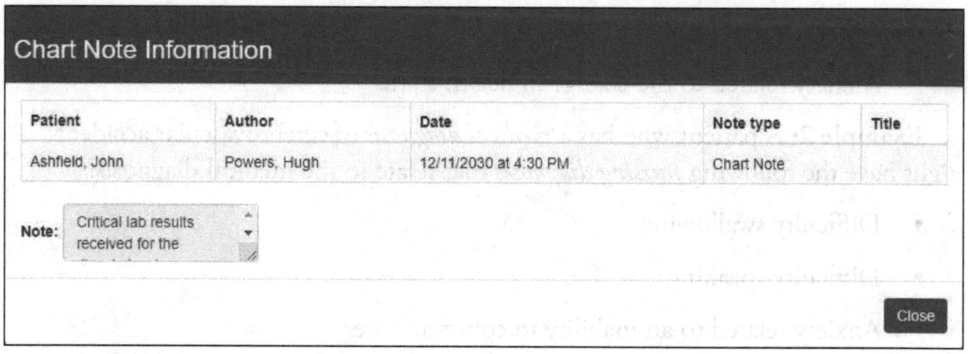

Chart Note Information

Patient	Author	Date	Note type	Title
Ashfield, John	Powers, Hugh	12/11/2030 at 4:30 PM	Chart Note	

Note: Critical lab results received for the

Close

A second type of daily nursing note is a free text episodic chart note. Episodic nursing notes are completed when something significant or unusual occurs—for example, the patient falls, there is a critical lab test result, or the patient successfully weans from the ventilator. Figure 8.12 shows an episodic nursing note.

Tutorial 8.11 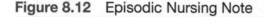 EHRNAVIGATOR

Completing a Nursing Daily Care Assessment

Go to your online course to launch Tutorial 8.11. As a nurse, enter the patient's status and requests in a Nursing Daily Care Assessment.

Tutorial 8.12 EHRNAVIGATOR

Adding a Chart Note

Go to your online course to launch Tutorial 8.12. As a nurse, add a free text chart note to a patient's visit.

8.5 Electronic Documentation of Medications and Treatments

Documentation of medications administered to patients by nurses and other qualified healthcare staff is found in the medication administration record (MAR). When the MAR is in electronic format, it is referred to as the **electronic medication administration record (eMAR)**.

Electronic Medication Administration Record

Once a medication has been ordered and signed, the order must be acknowledged by the nurse before the medication becomes active and is ready to be administered. When the nurse is administering the medication, he or she must scan the medication and scan the patient's wristband. The eMAR documents the date and time of the administration of the medication. If a medication is not administered as ordered—for example, due to patient refusal or when it is contraindicated due to the patient's condition, such as insulin being held due to a low blood glucose level or hypertension medication being held due to a low blood pressure reading—the nurse must document the reason for the non-administration. If a scanner is unavailable, the barcode numbers must be manually entered.

Negative patient outcomes may occur when medications are not correctly administered at the ordered times. The eMAR alerts nurses of overdue medications.

Figure 8.13 is an example of an eMAR screen displaying medications that need to be administered to the patient.

Bar-Coded Medication Administration

Bar-coded medication administration (BCMA) was first implemented in 1999 in US veterans hospitals and helped to reduce medication errors by requiring medications to have identifying barcodes that would be scanned before patient administration, thereby reducing the risk that the wrong medication would be administered to the patient. When coupling BCMA with the eMAR functionality of the EHR, medication errors are

Figure 8.13   eMAR—Medications to Be Administered

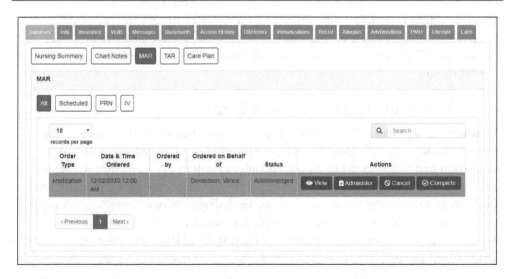

Figure 8.14   eMAR—Barcode Scanning

Administer Medication

Administer ▾

Scan the patient's bracelet

☐ Scanner broken

☑ Scanner not available

Bracelet barcode

23892390

Scan the Medication

☐ Scanner broken

☑ Scanner not available

Medication barcode

128912890

Close   Administer

further reduced. Scanning the barcode on the patient's wristband along with the bar-coded medication verifies the administration of the correct medication to the appropriate patient as ordered. The administering nurse must document when a barcode scanner is not working or not available. Figure 8.14 is an example of a bar-coding screen.

There is a standard for safe medication administration that is known as the *seven "rights" of medication*

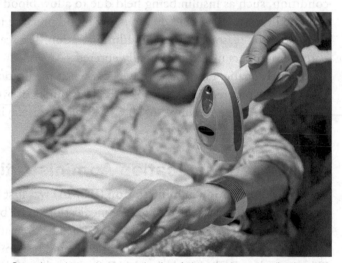

Scanning a barcode on a patient's wristband reduces medication errors by ensuring the correct medication is being administered to the correct patient.

administration; they include right patient, right medication, right dose, right route, right time, right reason, and right documentation (see Figure 8.15). Nurses and healthcare professionals are aware of this standard as the best practice for medication administration. The EHR supports the successful achievement of proper medication administration.

Reduction in Adverse Drug Events

An **adverse drug event (ADE)** occurs when a patient is negatively affected upon the administration of a medication. An ADE may result in a minor condition such as indigestion or a rash or could be serious enough to result in a patient's death. The ADE may occur with a drug-to-drug interaction, a drug-to-food interaction, a patient allergy to the drug, or a negative reaction due to the patient's diagnoses or condition. With paper medical records, pharmacists were responsible for manually reviewing medications ordered for inpatients to identify potential ADEs. With EHRs, potential drug interactions are identified immediately by the software. Physicians or nurses receive an electronic alert

Figure 8.15   Seven "Rights" of Medication Administration

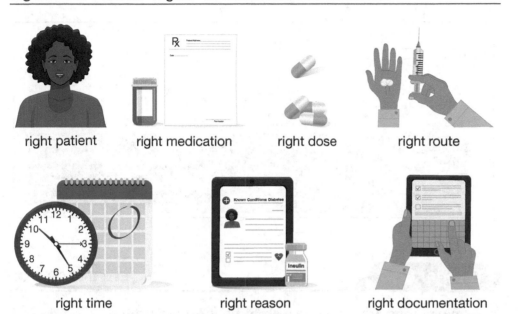

right patient   right medication   right dose   right route

right time   right reason   right documentation

when attempting to enter a medication order that might interact with another drug or is contraindicated due to the patient's allergies, diagnoses, or conditions. This improvement alone has resulted in significantly increasing patient safety by reducing ADEs.

Electronic Treatment Administration Record

The **electronic treatment administration record (eTAR)** documents patient treatments that are not medications and functions the same way as the eMAR. A treatment must be ordered and the order acknowledged before it becomes active. Some examples of common inpatient treatments include the following:

- Therapy (e.g., physical, occupational, speech, or respiratory)

- Intake and output (I&O)

- Low–air loss bed

- Wound care treatments

As treatments are rendered, caregivers must document completion of the treatments in the eTAR. When treatments are not performed as ordered—for example, when the patient refuses or the treatment is contraindicative to the patient's condition—the caregiver must document the reason why the treatment was not rendered. Figure 8.16 illustrates a typical eTAR screen.

Tutorial 8.13   **EHR**NAVIGAT✛R

Administering Medication in a Medication Administration Record

Go to your online course to launch Tutorial 8.13. As a nurse, you will add a medication order, acknowledge the order, administer a medication, and record the administration in the eMAR.

Figure 8.16   eTAR

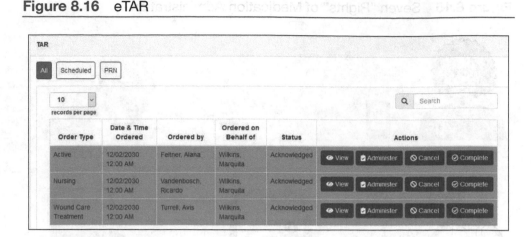

Tutorial 8.14   **EHR**NAVIGAT⊕R

Administering Treatment in a Treatment Administration Record

Go to your online course to launch Tutorial 8.14. As a nurse, you will add a treatment order, acknowledge the order, administer a treatment, and record the administration in the eTAR.

8.6 Intake and Output Flowsheet

A flowsheet is a document that allows the tracking of patient health data over a period of time, such as patient intake and output and vital signs. **Intake and output (I&O) monitoring** of fluids is very important in assessing and controlling patient hydration and fluid balance. Close monitoring of I&O is imperative for patients with conditions such as congestive heart failure, kidney disease, and malnutrition and for many postoperative patients. Fluids that are measured as **intake** include fluids taken by mouth, feeding tubes, and intravenous catheters. **Output** is fluid that is measured from the kidneys, the gastrointestinal tract, drainage tubes, and wounds. Physicians frequently order the monitoring of a patient's I&O; however, I&O monitoring does not require a physician's order. Nurses have the responsibility to identify when I&O monitoring is indicated and to initiate this monitoring and documentation in the EHR. Nursing assistants frequently document patients' I&O as they collect food trays and refill water pitchers as well as empty catheters and assist patients to the restroom. Nurses bear the ultimate responsibility for overseeing the nursing assistants and documentation to ensure accurate recording of fluid I&O. Documentation of the I&Os on a flowsheet helps the nurse see fluctuations in intake or output at a glance. Refer to Figure 8.17 for an example of an I&O flowsheet.

Figure 8.17   Intake and Output Flowsheet

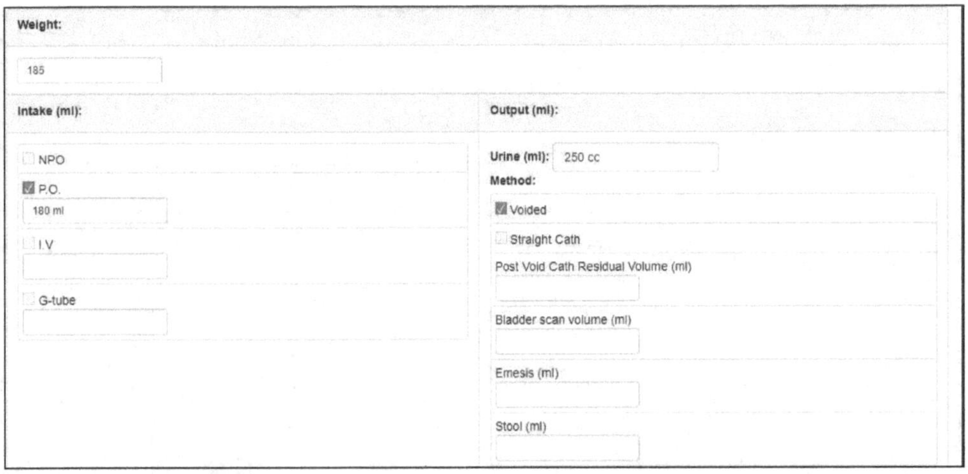

Weight:

185

Intake (ml):

☐ NPO

☑ P.O.

180 ml

☐ I.V

☐ G-tube

Output (ml):

Urine (ml):   250 cc

Method:

☑ Voided

☐ Straight Cath

Post Void Cath Residual Volume (ml)

Bladder scan volume (ml)

Emesis (ml)

Stool (ml)

Tutorial 8.15

EHRNAVIGAT✛R

Completing an Intake/Output Flowsheet

Go to your online course to launch Tutorial 8.15. As a nurse, enter the patients intake and output values in the intake/output flowsheet.

8.7 Vital Signs Flowsheet

Monitoring vital signs is very important in assisting healthcare providers identify whether a patient is stable and recovering or getting worse. The vital signs that are monitored include body temperature, pulse, respirations, blood pressure and pulse oximetry. Vital signs are typically ordered to be monitored frequently, sometimes every 15 minutes if a patient is very ill. Figure 8.18 is an example of a Vital Signs Flowsheet with vitals taken every 4 hours. A visual representation of a patient's vital signs, in the form of a graph, can be viewed to quickly identify a patient's status, as shown in Figure 8.19.

Figure 8.18   Vital Signs Flowsheet

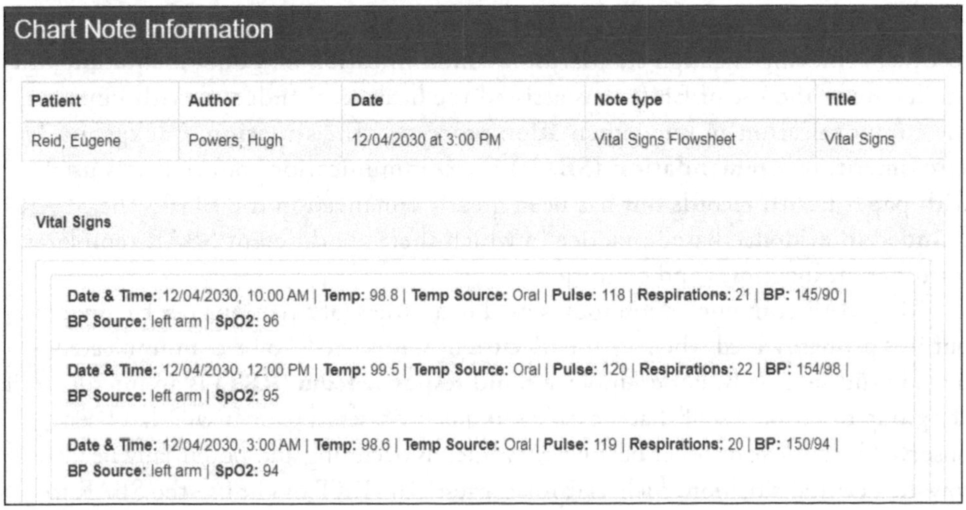

Chart Note Information

Patient	Author	Date	Note type	Title
Reid, Eugene	Powers, Hugh	12/04/2030 at 3:00 PM	Vital Signs Flowsheet	Vital Signs

Vital Signs

> **Date & Time:** 12/04/2030, 10:00 AM | **Temp:** 98.8 | **Temp Source:** Oral | **Pulse:** 118 | **Respirations:** 21 | **BP:** 145/90 |
> **BP Source:** left arm | **SpO2:** 96

> **Date & Time:** 12/04/2030, 12:00 PM | **Temp:** 99.5 | **Temp Source:** Oral | **Pulse:** 120 | **Respirations:** 22 | **BP:** 154/98 |
> **BP Source:** left arm | **SpO2:** 95

> **Date & Time:** 12/04/2030, 3:00 AM | **Temp:** 98.6 | **Temp Source:** Oral | **Pulse:** 119 | **Respirations:** 20 | **BP:** 150/94 |
> **BP Source:** left arm | **SpO2:** 94

Figure 8.19   Vital Signs Graph

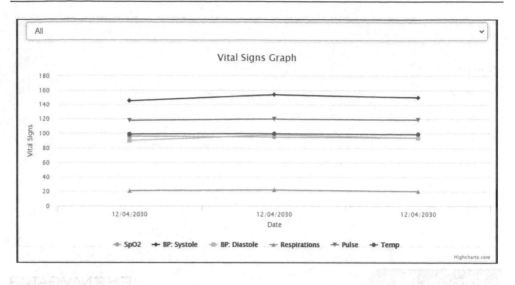

Tutorial 8.16   EHRNAVIGAT✛R

Recording a Patient's Vital Signs

Go to your online course to launch Tutorial 8.16. As a nurse, record two sets of a patient's vital signs.

8.8 Situation, Background, Assessment, Recommendation

Treating hospital inpatients is a complicated process involving hundreds of clinical and support staff with the common goal of positive patient outcomes. As previously discussed, to accomplish positive patient outcomes, timely, accurate, and complete communication is imperative. This is achieved via thorough health record documentation and clinicians dedicated to this goal. With paper medical records, achieving the high standards of communication and documentation was challenging. The use of EHRs has assisted the healthcare industry with improving the communication and documentation processes. The **situation**, **background**, **assessment**, **recommendation (SBAR)** is a communication tool that was used with paper health records but has been greatly enhanced in the EHR. The SBAR is founded in evidence-based practice in which there are different SBAR templates for different diagnoses and conditions.

The SBAR communication tool is used in a variety of situations per facility policy, but it is primarily used when a patient's current status needs to be communicated quickly and succinctly. For example, a **rapid response team (RRT)** is an interdisciplinary group of hospital staff that are called to quickly assess a patient who has been observed by a nurse or other healthcare worker as declining and potentially headed toward a critical situation, such as cardiac arrest. The RRT might use the SBAR to quickly receive the patient's current status. Since the goal of the RRT is to identify the cause(s) of the patient's decline and intervene with care that will prevent a patient's further decline, time is of the essence, and the SBAR facilitates rapid communication and intervention.

Communication is enhanced with the use of SBARs during nursing shift handoffs as it replaces what was previously solely an oral handoff. During an oral handoff, important information regarding the patient's status may not be relayed, or there might be too much information to be remembered. The SBAR provides an avenue of communication that is more thorough and may be referenced during the following shifts. The Joint Commission has identified inadequate handoff communication as a common problem that can result in minor to severe harm to patients. Similar to the SBAR, the Joint Commission has developed a handoff communication tool that it refers to as a Targeted Solutions Tool. Another communication tool mentioned by the Joint Commission is the I-PASS, which stands for *illness severity, patient summary, action list, situation awareness and contingency plans, and synthesis by receiver.* Whatever tool a facility implements, it is important that accurate handoff communication is recognized as a critical process in the attainment of high-quality patient care. Figure 8.20 illustrates a sample SBAR.

Figure 8.20 Sample SBAR

Chart Note Information				
Patient	Author	Date	Note type	Title
Wilkins, Marquita	Powers, Hugh	12/02/2030 at 4.30 PM	SBAR	

S

Situation:

This is [Candace Alejo, RN], I'm calling from unit: [4North]. I am calling about patient:

The problem I am calling about is: [shortness of breath]. I have just assessed the patient.

The patient's code status is:	Vital signs are:	I am concerned about the:
☐ DNRCC	**Blood pressure** 220/100	☐ blood pressure because it is less than 90 or 30mmHg below usual
☐ DNRCC-Arrest	**Pulse** 96	☐ pulse because it is over 125 or less than 45
☑ Full Code	**Respiration** 22	☐ respiration because it is less than 10 or over 30
	Temperature 98.5	☐ temperature because it is less than 96 or over 104
	O2 sat 88	☑ O2 Sat because it is <90% despite oxygen
		☑ Other: High BP

Continues

Figure 8.20   Sample SBAR—*Continued*

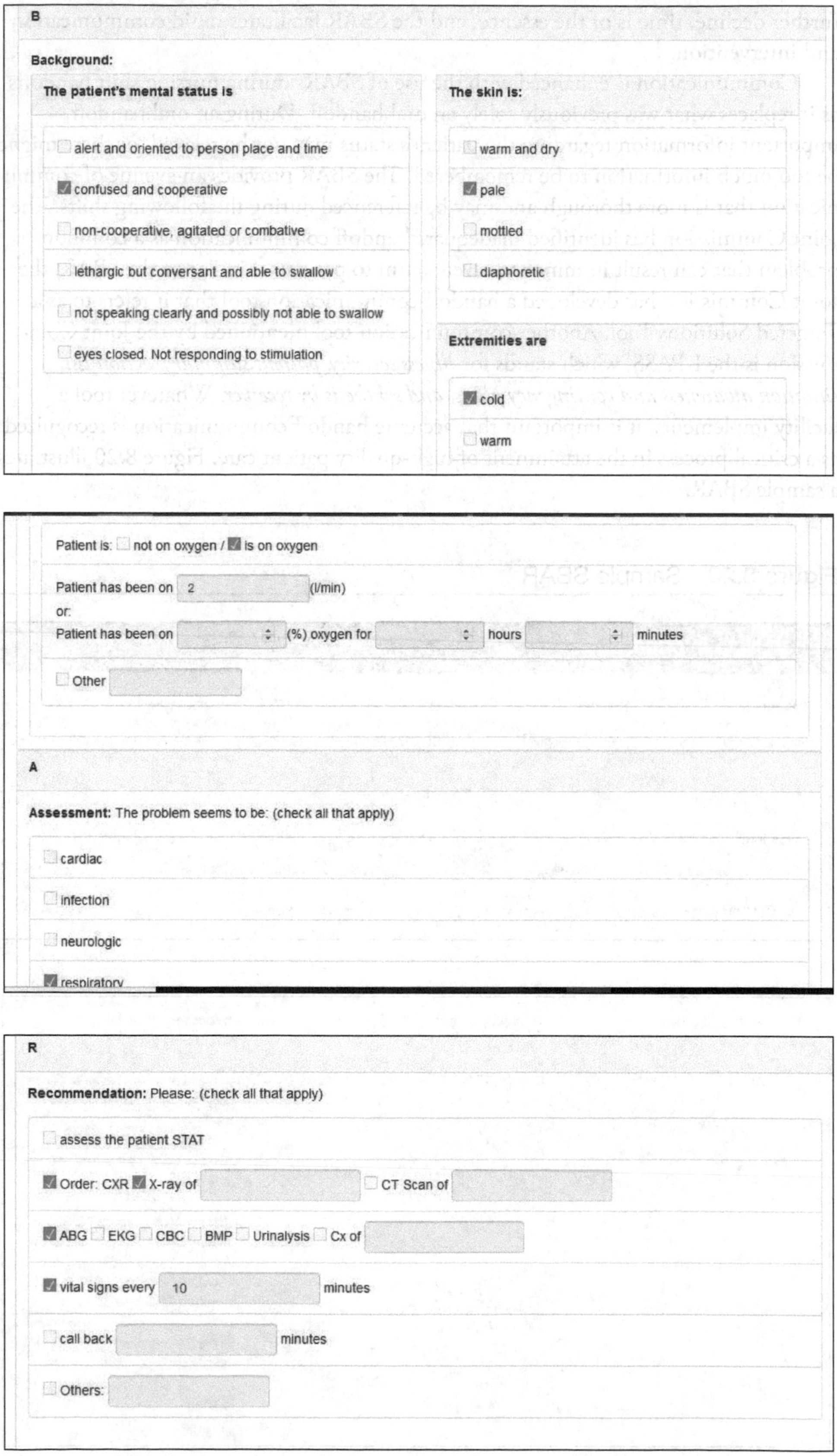

B

Background:

The patient's mental status is	The skin is:
☐ alert and oriented to person place and time	☐ warm and dry
☑ confused and cooperative	☑ pale
☐ non-cooperative, agitated or combative	☐ mottled
☐ lethargic but conversant and able to swallow	☐ diaphoretic
☐ not speaking clearly and possibly not able to swallow	**Extremities are**
☐ eyes closed. Not responding to stimulation	☑ cold
	☐ warm

Patient is: ☐ not on oxygen / ☑ is on oxygen

Patient has been on 2 (l/min)

or:

Patient has been on ___ (%) oxygen for ___ hours ___ minutes

☐ Other ___

A

Assessment: The problem seems to be: (check all that apply)

☐ cardiac

☐ infection

☐ neurologic

☑ respiratory

R

Recommendation: Please: (check all that apply)

☐ assess the patient STAT

☑ Order: CXR ☑ X-ray of ___ ☐ CT Scan of ___

☑ ABG ☐ EKG ☐ CBC ☐ BMP ☐ Urinalysis ☐ Cx of ___

☑ vital signs every 10 minutes

☐ call back ___ minutes

☐ Others: ___

Tutorial 8.17   **EHR**NAVIGAT✛R

Completing the SBAR

Go to the online course to launch Tutorial 8.17. As a nurse, complete the SBAR for a patient with an elevated temperature.

CHECKP✛INT 8.3

1. Why are flowsheets used in healthcare documentation?

2. What are the seven "rights" of medication administration?

8.9 Nursing Discharge Documentation

When patients are discharged from an inpatient hospital stay, they typically require follow-up care post-discharge. Follow-up care may be provided at their home via home healthcare services, at a skilled nursing and rehab facility, or at a physician's or surgeon's office. Depending on the type of follow-up care needed, some documentation of the patient's status at the time of discharge will be needed by the healthcare providers for continuity of care. In other words, for high-quality care to continue for the patient, the next group of caregivers will need to know the patient's diagnoses, procedures performed, test results, medications, and orders for continued care. Ideally, the healthcare providers who are providing the post-discharge care have direct access to the patient's EHR to obtain information about the patient's status; however, direct access or universal interoperability is still a goal of many healthcare providers and EHR systems. When direct access is not available, copies of portions of the patient's EHR—along with documented summaries such as a physician discharge summary, nursing discharge assessment, and transfer forms—need to be provided to the organizations assuming responsibility for the patient's post-discharge care.

Nursing Discharge Assessment

A **nursing discharge assessment** is completed upon the discharge of a patient from an inpatient facility to document the patient's condition and status at the time of discharge. This document should be provided to the patient's primary care physician as well as any healthcare providers that will be following up with the patient post-discharge. Facility policy defines the type and amount of information on the nursing discharge

Figure 8.21 Nursing Discharge Assessment

Chart Note Information

Patient	Author	Date	Note type	Title
Wilkins, Marquita	Powers, Hugh	12/02/2030 at 4:30 PM	Nursing Discharge Assessment	

Date & Time	Patient
12/02/2030 12:00 PM	Wilkins, Marquita

Discharge Disposition	Advanced Directives	Discharge Diagnosis(es)
☐ Home, self-care ☑ Home with home health	Does the patient have an Advanced Directive? ☑ Yes	Traumatic open fracture, femur

assessment template and should ensure that a clear picture of the patient's condition and care needs at the time of discharge are documented. Figure 8.21 illustrates a nursing discharge assessment.

Transfer Form

Upon discharge from a hospital, when patients are being transferred to another facility or level of care, a transfer form should be completed to provide continuity of care. The **transfer form** is similar to a nursing discharge assessment in that it indicates the status and condition of the patient upon discharge, such as prognosis, advance directives in place, follow-up appointments scheduled, and diagnoses. The major difference between a nursing discharge assessment and a transfer form is the individual responsible for completion. The nursing discharge assessment is completed by a nurse. The transfer form must be signed by a physician or physician extender as it contains orders to be carried out by the receiving organization. For example, a long-term care facility accepting the patient will need orders for medications, therapy, and testing to be able to initiate care and treatment. The patient will then be assessed by nurses, physicians, and therapists who may advise changes to the treatment orders. Similarly, a patient who is transferred home with home health services will require a transfer form for the home agency to initiate treatment. The only discharged patients who would not have a transfer form completed are those who are transferred to home without home health services and those who expire in the hospital. Figure 8.22 illustrates a transfer form.

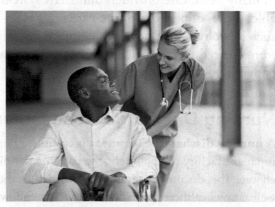

When patients transfer from one facility (e.g., a hospital) to another (e.g., a long-term care facility) nurses must fill out a transfer form.

Figure 8.22   Transfer Form

Title:	Type:	Time Entered:
Transfer to LTCi	Transfer Form ▾	12/04/2030 📅
		04 : 15 PM

Patient	Date and Time of Transfer:
Patient Name: Donaldson, Vance	12/04/2030 📅 04 : 15 PM
Patient DOB:1988-05-15T00:00:00.000Z	
	Transfer From: Northstar Medical Center
Emergency Contact Information	Transfer To: Northstar Skilled Nursing and Rehab ▾
Emergency Contact Name: Sara Donaldson	Advance Directives:
Emergency Contact Relationship: Spouse	
Emergency Contact Phone Number: 513-999-1252	
	Attending Physician: Select Physician ▾
	Surgeon: Select Surgeon ▾

8.10 Nursing Documentation in Skilled Nursing and Rehabilitation Settings

A **skilled nursing facility** is an inpatient setting with the staff and equipment available to provide skilled nursing care and, in most cases, skilled rehabilitative (physical, occupational, speech, and respiratory) services. A skilled nursing facility may also provide other related health services, such as renal dialysis. The term *skilled care* is a Medicare-defined term that describes care and treatment that can be provided only by qualified healthcare professionals such as physicians, nurses, and physical, occupa-tional, speech, and respiratory therapists. To be admitted to a skilled nursing and rehabilitation facility, a patient must need skilled nursing care and/or rehabilitation services on a daily basis, and the patient must have a qualifying stay in an acute care hospital before admission to the skilled nursing and rehabilitation facility. A **qualifying stay** is a hospital stay of at least 3 days during the 30 days before admission to the skilled nursing facility.

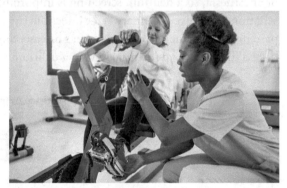

Patients in a skilled nursing facility may receive occupational therapy.

Similar to a hospital, in a skilled nursing and rehabilitation setting, the nursing staff begin patient care and documentation upon the admission of the patient and continue care and documentation throughout the stay and discharge of the patient. One significant difference in the nursing admission documentation in a skilled nursing and rehabilitation facility, as opposed to an acute care hospital, is that nurses receive a significant amount of hospital documentation to review regarding the patient's prior hospital stay. It is important for the admission nurse to review all available documenta-tion upon admission of the patient to ensure that all of the patient's needs are planned for. Even more so in a skilled nursing facility versus a hospital, the nursing staff spend the most time of any group of healthcare providers caring for the patient. Physicians do not visit skilled nursing facility patients daily, which puts more responsibility on the nursing staff to identify changes in healthcare conditions. Again, they are placed in the main role of documenting patient data for use by other healthcare providers.

Long-Term Care Nursing Admission Assessment

The nursing admission assessment for a patient in a long-term care facility is similar to that for a hospital patient, with a few differences:

- The term **resident** is used rather than *patient*, indicating a facility that is homelike and (usually) requires a longer length of stay.

- The reason for admission to a long-term care facility that provides two levels of care, skilled care and long-term care, should be specified on the admission assessment. As we have discussed, **skilled care** refers to skilled nursing or rehabilitation services that are provided by licensed health professionals such as nurses and physical therapists and are ordered by a doctor. **Long-term care** refers to that which is more custodial in nature, such as treatment of chronic conditions and assistance with ADLs that are primarily provided by patient care assistants with oversight by nursing and an attending physician.

Figure 8.23 illustrates a long-term care Nursing Admission Assessment.

Delirium Screening

The identification and assessment of delirium in residents of long-term care facilities is important because elderly individuals are at high risk for experiencing delirium. The elderly experience longer cognitive recovery times when exposed to even small amounts of anesthesia, so a delirium screening is important to conduct post-procedure when sedation is involved. Urinary tract infections are another common cause of delirium in patients with dementia or Alzheimer's disease. Since many long-term care residents have a diagnosis of dementia, having a delirium screening protocol in place is necessary

Figure 8.23 Long-Term Care Nursing Admission Assessment

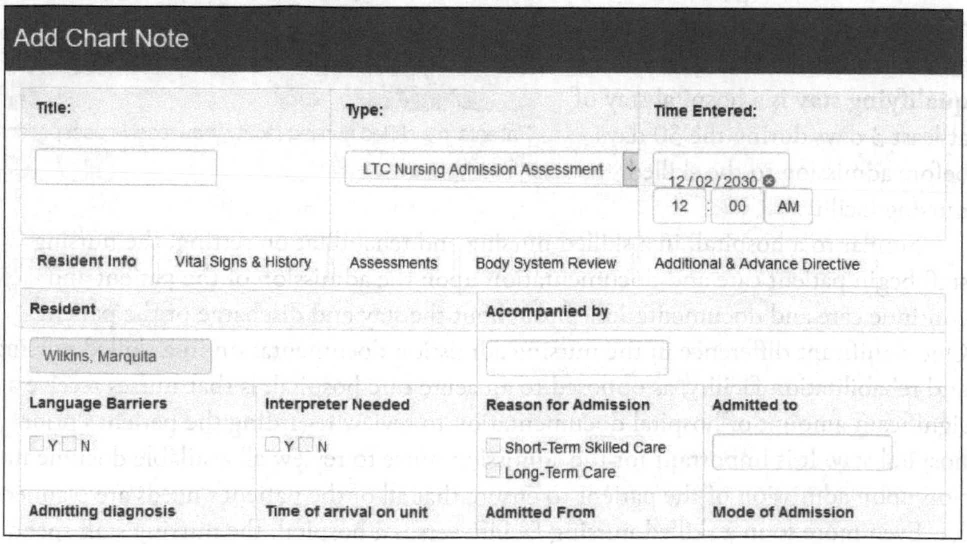

Figure 8.24   Delirium Screening

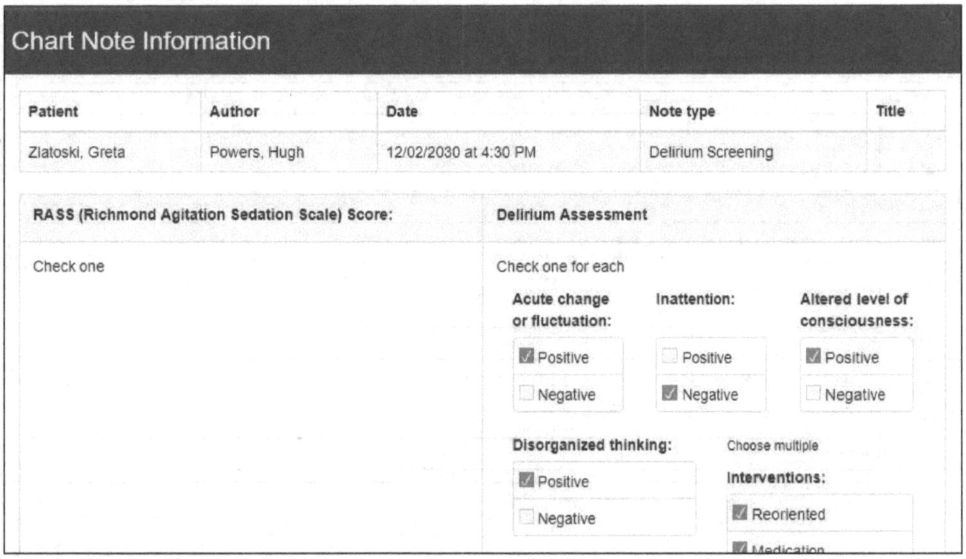

Chart Note Information				
Patient	**Author**	**Date**	**Note type**	**Title**
Zlatoski, Greta	Powers, Hugh	12/02/2030 at 4:30 PM	Delirium Screening	

RASS (Richmond Agitation Sedation Scale) Score:

Check one

Delirium Assessment

Check one for each

Acute change or fluctuation:	Inattention:	Altered level of consciousness:
☑ Positive	☐ Positive	☑ Positive
☐ Negative	☑ Negative	☐ Negative

Disorganized thinking: Choose multiple

☑ Positive   **Interventions:**

☐ Negative   ☑ Reoriented

☑ Medication

to identify patients with delirium. There are many standardized tools that have been developed by different organizations and healthcare providers, including the Richmond Agitation and Sedation Scale (RASS). The RASS assesses for acute changes or fluctuations in consciousness, attention, and thinking. The RASS also includes the identification of interventions that are used to improve the patient's agitation and delirium. Figure 8.24 illustrates a typical delirium screening tool.

Minimum Data Set

The MDS is a standardized, primary screening and assessment tool of health status for all residents of Medicare- and Medicaid-certified nursing homes. The MDS was implemented in 1988 and has gone through several revisions, with the MDS 3.0 version in effect at this time. The MDS provides a way for clinicians to assess a resident's functional capabilities and identify health problems. Comprehensive MDS assessments must be completed upon admission to the nursing facility, periodically throughout the patient's stay, and upon discharge. The MDS is required to be completed by an RN along with input from therapists and other allied health professionals. The RN responsible for MDS completion is usually a specifically trained MDS nurse or coordinator because the MDS is a long and complicated assessment.

MDS information is transmitted electronically by nursing homes to the national MDS database at the Centers for Medicare & Medicaid Services (CMS) and serves as a basis for reimbursement for Medicare and Medicaid residents. The MDS has considerable ramifications involving reimbursement and state and federal health inspections, also known as *surveys*. The accurate completion of MDS assessments results in accurate reimbursement to the skilled nursing facility. Inaccurate completion of MDS assessments may result in lower reimbursement than deserved or reimbursement that is too high, which might open the facility to claims of fraud or abuse. Nursing facilities experience annual federal or state health inspections/surveys to ensure that regulations governing the care and treatment of nursing facility residents are being followed. Publicly available survey results for each nursing facility list the regulations that are

EXPAND YOUR LEARNING

An interactive website at https://EHR3 .ParadigmEducation .com/NursingHomes lists US nursing facilities, deficiencies, and fines. A CMS website, Nursing Home Compare (https://EHR3 .ParadigmEducation.com/ NursingHomeCompare), is available to the public to compare nursing homes on a five-star quality rating system that includes health inspection data, staffing ratios, and quality measure information.

Adult children helping their parents search for and select a nursing facility increasingly use websites such as Nursing Home Compare. Since much of the quality measurement information comes from the completion of the MDS, you can see why it is imperative that the MDS is accurate.

Figure 8.25 MDS Form

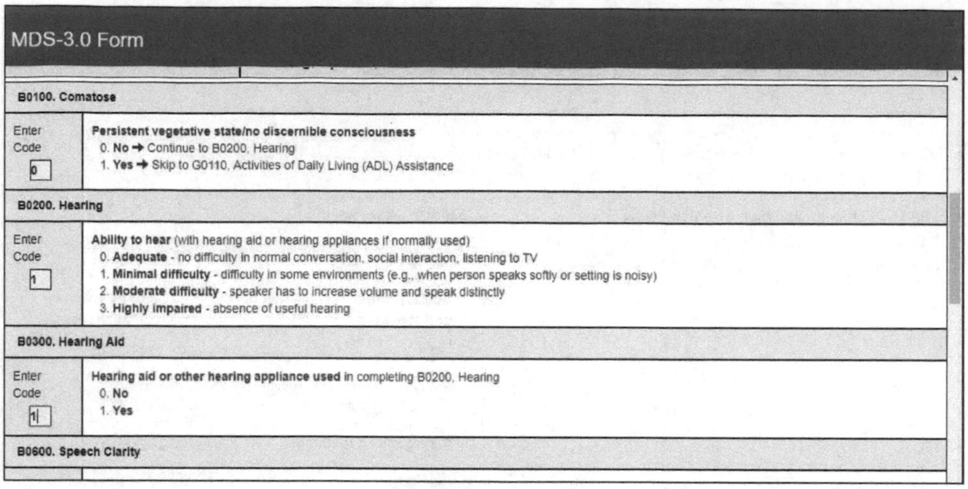

MDS-3.0 Form

B0100. Comatose

Enter Code	Persistent vegetative state/no discernible consciousness
0	0. No → Continue to B0200, Hearing
	1. Yes → Skip to G0110, Activities of Daily Living (ADL) Assistance

B0200. Hearing

Enter Code	Ability to hear (with hearing aid or hearing appliances if normally used)
1	0. Adequate - no difficulty in normal conversation, social interaction, listening to TV
	1. Minimal difficulty - difficulty in some environments (e.g., when person speaks softly or setting is noisy)
	2. Moderate difficulty - speaker has to increase volume and speak distinctly
	3. Highly impaired - absence of useful hearing

B0300. Hearing Aid

Enter Code	Hearing aid or other hearing appliance used in completing B0200, Hearing
1	0. No
	1. Yes

B0600. Speech Clarity

not being followed, also known as **deficiencies**. Fines may be assigned to the facility depending on the seriousness of the deficiencies. Fines can be significant—one of the highest fines ever imposed exceeded $1.5 million.

For more information and resources regarding the MDS, visit the CMS website at https://EHR3.ParadigmEducation.com/CMS.

Figure 8.25 illustrates an MDS form.

Long-Term Care Nursing Discharge Assessment

Just as a nursing discharge assessment is completed upon the discharge of a hospital patient, a nursing discharge assessment should be completed upon the discharge of a long-term care resident. Residents from a long-term care facility are usually discharged to home with home health services, to an acute care hospital for inpatient acute care, or to another long-term care facility, perhaps to be geographically closer to family or friends or to receive specialized services, such as dialysis or Alzheimer's care, that their current facility does not offer. The **long-term care nursing discharge assessment** is very similar to the nursing discharge assessment from the hospital, with the choices of discharge disposition being the only notable difference. As a transfer form is completed for patient transfers from the acute care hospital to other healthcare providers, a transfer form is also completed for patient transfers from the long-term care facility to another healthcare provider. A nurse is responsible for the completion of a long-term care nursing discharge assessment that must be done in an accurate, complete, and timely fashion to facilitate high-quality continued care. Figure 8.26 shows a long-term care nursing discharge assessment.

Tutorial 8.18   **EHR**NAVIGATOR

Starting a Nursing Discharge Assessment
Go to your online course to launch Tutorial 8.18. As a nurse, start a Nursing Discharge Assessment.

Figure 8.26   Long-Term Care Nursing Discharge Assessment

Date	Time	Resident
12/02/2030	12 : 00 AM	Gupta, Amala

Discharge Disposition	Advanced Directives	Discharge Diagnosis(es)
☐ Home, self-care	**Does the resident have an Advanced Directive?** ☑ Yes ☐ No	CAD
☑ Home with home health		**Procedures Performed**
☐ Hospital, acute care		
☐ Hospital, long-term acute care	**Copy attached?** ☑ Yes ☐ No	☐ Refer to property list for detail of belongings accompanying resident
☐ Skilled nursing facility		**Last PO Intake**
☐ Inpatient rehab facility		
☐ Hospice		10:30 AM
☐ Expired		

Tutorial 8.19

EHRNAVIGAT✚R

Completing a Nursing Discharge Assessment

Go to your online course to launch Tutorial 8.19. As a nurse, complete the Nursing Discharge Assessment.

CHECKP✚INT 8.4

1. The MDS is documented in which healthcare setting(s)?

_____

_____

2. What is the purpose of a nursing discharge assessment?

_____

_____

8.11 Nursing in Outpatient Settings

Nurses provide care in a number of outpatient settings, including physician offices, clinics, ambulatory surgery centers, dialysis centers, and mental health facilities. While the basic requirements that health record documentation be accurate, timely, and thorough hold true just as they do in inpatient settings, the types of documentation that nurses complete in outpatient settings have some significant differences from nursing documentation in inpatient settings.

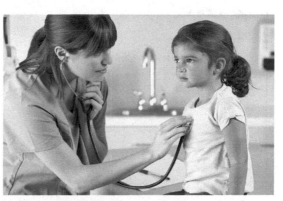

Nurses in a physician's office take vital signs and perform other care before the doctor visits the patients.

In outpatient settings, the time that nurses spend with their patients is much shorter than in inpatient settings. For example, a nurse might see a patient for only five minutes in a physician's office or for several hours in an ambulatory surgical center or dialysis center, as opposed to 12 hours per day for several days in an inpatient setting such as a hospital or nursing facility. This requires a nurse to be efficient in their assessment and treatment skills and to document immediately upon assessment and treatment.

Consider This

Consider a nurse in an ambulatory surgery center who treats 15 patients in a day. What would happen if the nurse waited until the end of the day to document assessment and treatment notes for all 15 patients? Undoubtedly, there would be at least some errors in documentation and perhaps confusion among patients.

SOAP Note

The most common nursing documentation in an outpatient setting is in the form of a nursing note such as a SOAP note. The **SOAP note** is a popular form of nursing note as it contains the subjective, objective, assessment, and plan components all in one note.

- **Subjective:** the information expressed by the patient, such as how they are feeling, when the symptoms started, and what eases symptoms

- **Objective:** factual data such as physical exam results, lab, and diagnostic test results

- **Assessment:** the diagnosis or suspected diagnosis that is made based on the subjective and objective data

- **Plan:** the plan of care and treatment for the diagnosis of the patient such as medications, diagnostic tests, and follow-up appointments

Figure 8.27 illustrates a SOAP note.

Figure 8.27   SOAP Note

CC
Abdominal pain
S
Patient reports sharp pains in upper abdomen. Also reports frequent diarrhea.
O
Examination reveals slightly enlarged pancreas and slight icterus.
A
Acute pancreatitis
P
Patient instructed to be admitted to Northstar Medical Center for IV fluids and treatment.

| Tutorial 8.20 | **EHR**NAVIGAT⊕R |

Entering a SOAP Note

Go to your online course to launch Tutorial 8.20. As a nurse, add a SOAP note to the patient's visit.

Figure 8.28   Pediatric Physical Exam

Diet	Illnesses	Stools
No concerns	strep	1/day

Meds/Vitamins	Accidents	Sleep patterns
multivitamin	No concerns	12 hrs

Exposure to tobacco smoke	Growth development
none	Hops on one foot Counts 4 pennies Copies a square Catches, throws a ball Plays with several children Recognizes 3-4 colors Knows opposites Knows name, address, phone number

Objective

General	Head	Eyes	Ears
well-nourished and developed No abuse/neglect evident	☑ no lesions	PERRLA conjunctivae	Canals clear TMs normal

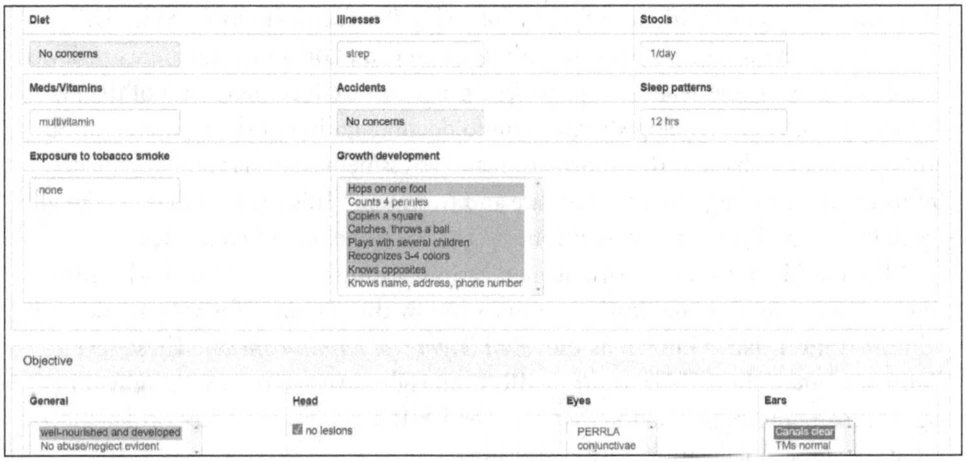

Specialized Templates

A physical examination focused on the type of patient or body system is also a common outpatient documentation completed by nurses. One example is a pediatric physical exam that might be completed in a physician's office or ambulatory surgical center. Just as any physical exam, this is completed to document the condition of the patient at the time of the visit. Figure 8.28 shows a completed Pediatric Physical Exam template.

Chapter Summary

Nursing staff play a vital role in the provision and documentation of patient care. CNAs, LPNs, and RNs make up the nursing staff, and each plays a role and has different responsibilities in the care and treatment of patients and documentation.

As each member of the nursing staff performs their duties and documentation in the EHR, one of the challenges is to keep a caring, responsive approach with the patient. Standing or sitting in front of a computer asking the patient questions without maintaining eye contact and without warm, caring conversation is not the type of nursing care that will promote healing and positive patient outcomes or opinions. It is important for nurses to become familiar enough with the documentation they are entering in the EHR to be able to conduct a conversation with the patient, allowing them to be the caring, healing nurses they wish to be.

Nursing documentation in an inpatient setting includes admission orders and nursing admission assessments as well as other special assessments, MARs, and discharge assessments. Nursing admission assessments are very detailed and include a patient's personal, family, and social information along with their medical history. Objective findings by the examining nurse are also included in the admission assessment, such as pain and fall risk assessments, a review of all body systems, advanced directives, and educational and discharge needs. Assessments that may be completed throughout the stay of the patient include infection control, fall risk, pressure injury risk, pain, and skin assessments.

Nurses document on a daily basis in an inpatient setting and at the time of visit or treatment in an outpatient setting by following the documentation cycle. The documentation cycle begins with recording the information and assessments reviewed and conducted by the healthcare providers; progresses to documentation of the plan of care that has been developed; moves on to documentation of the provision of care; and finally circles back to the information and assessment step that documents new information regarding the results of care and treatment. This last step may potentially result in a revised plan of care—and the cycle of documentation continues.

The eMAR documents patient medication administration. When administering and documenting medications, nurses follow the standard for safe medication administration that is known as the *seven "rights" of administration*. These seven rights include right patient, right medication, right dose, right route, right time, right reason, and right documentation. The EHR supports the successful achievement of proper medication administration.

The eTAR documents patient treatments that are not medications. As with medications, when treatments are not performed as ordered—such as when the patient refuses or the treatment is contraindicative to the patient's condition—the nurse must document the reason the treatment was not rendered.

Monitoring of fluid I&Os is very important in assessing and controlling patient hydration and fluid balance, which is needed by patients with certain conditions. Documentation of the I&Os is made on a flowsheet to provide identification of fluctuations in intake or output at a glance.

The SBAR is a communication tool that is used by nurses and other healthcare providers in a variety of situations, such as shift changeover reporting and RRT communication.

Upon the discharge of a patient from an inpatient facility, a discharge assessment is completed to document the patient's condition and status at the time of discharge. When patients are being transferred to another inpatient facility, such as a skilled nursing facility, a transfer form is also completed.

In a skilled nursing facility, individuals are known as residents. Admission orders and admission nursing assessments are a part of nursing documentation requirements in a skilled nursing facility, similar to hospital documentation. A significant difference in nursing documentation in a skilled nursing facility is the MDS. The MDS provides a thorough assessment of the residents at scheduled intervals, which is used for planning care and treatment as well as reporting and reimbursement purposes.

Nursing documentation in an outpatient setting is more abbreviated than that in an inpatient setting, as the patient is seen for a much shorter period. The SOAP note is one of the most widely used documentation templates in the outpatient setting.

No matter the setting, inpatient or outpatient, nursing staff play a vital role in the provision and documentation of patient care.

Review and Assessment

The following Review and Assessment activities are also available online in the Cirrus online course. Your instructor may ask you to complete these activities online. Cirrus also provides access to flash cards, a crossword puzzle, and practice quizzes to help strengthen your understanding of the chapter content.

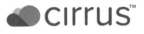

Acronyms/Initialisms

Study the following acronyms discussed in this chapter. Go to the online course for flash cards of the acronyms and other chapter key terms.

ADE: adverse drug event

BCMA: bar-coded medication administration

eMAR: electronic medication administration record

eTAR: electronic treatment administration record

HAI: healthcare-associated infection

I&O: intake and output

MDS: minimum data set

SBAR: situation, background, assessment, recommendation

SOAP: subjective, objective, assessment, plan

Check Your Understanding

To check your understanding of this chapter's key concepts, answer the following questions.

1. Nurses play a vital role in

   a. maintenance of health information.

   b. communication of patient information.

   c. documentation of patient care.

   d. submitting health information for claims.

2. Nursing staff includes all the following *except*

   a. CNAs.

   b. CSTs.

   c. LPNs.

   d. RNs.

3. Assessment includes all the following *except*

   a. subjective information.

   b. diagnoses and conditions.

   c. risk values.

   d. plan of care.

4. Which of the following is an outpatient setting where a nurse would provide care?

   a. ambulatory surgery unit

   b. surgery unit

   c. coronary care unit

   d. rehabilitation unit

5. Which of the following lists the correct order of the documentation cycle?

   a. plan of care, physician orders, provision of care, and information and assessment

   b. physician orders, provision of care, information and assessment, and plan of care

   c. information and assessment, plan of care, physician orders, and provision of care

   d. provision of care, information and assessment, plan of care, and physician orders

6. True/False: Admission orders include instructions for the patient's diet, medications, activities, diagnostic testing, and monitoring orders.

7. True/False: A qualifying stay for admission to a skilled nursing and rehabilitation facility consists of a hospital stay of at least 5 days during the 30 days before admission.

8. True/False: The term *patient* is used in a long-term care setting, indicating that a facility is homelike.

9. True/False: The CDC defined two tiers of precautions to prevent transmission of infectious agents, including standard and transmission-based precautions.

10. True/False: A fall risk assessment includes only scoring the absence of fall risk factors.

Go on the Record

To build on your understanding of the topics in this chapter, complete the following short-answer activities.

1. List the components and describe the purpose of the inpatient admission assessment conducted by nurses.

2. Discuss the risk factors included in the fall risk assessment and how it impacts a patient's care.

3. Pressure injuries are classified by a staging system. Describe the stages of pressure injuries.

4. There are four components of the documentation cycle. Describe each cycle component and discuss how each component impacts patient care.

5. Describe the eMAR process.

Navigate the Field

To gain practice in handling challenging situations in the workplace, consider the following real-world scenarios and identify how you would respond to each.

1. As the nurse manager in the medical/surgical unit at Northstar Medical Center, you have determined that you need to educate your nursing staff on the prevention strategies for patients that are at a risk of developing pressure ulcers. What are the strategies that you would discuss with your nursing staff?

2. You are a nurse at Northstar Physicians and a new RN has joined your nursing team. You need to explain the importance of the SOAP note to the new nurse. Describe each component of the SOAP note.

Think Critically

Continue to think critically about challenging concepts and complete the following activities.

1. As a nurse on the medical/surgical unit at Northstar Medical Center, you typically complete two types of nursing notes during your shift. Describe the similarities and differences as well as the importance of the daily nursing notes.

2. You have received an order for your patient to receive medication. You will use the eMAR to administer the medication order. Describe the standard for safe medication administration that is known as the seven "rights" of medication administration.

Make Your Case

Consider the scenario and then complete the following project.

You are a nurse at Northstar Skilled Nursing and Rehab Center. As the MDS nurse, you are responsible for collecting the data used to assess the resident's functional capabilities and to identify health problems. You have been asked to develop an MDS training plan for a nurse who will be joining the MDS Department. Develop a presentation that explains the required components of the MDS documentation.

Explore the Technology

Complete the EHR Navigator practice assessments that align to each tutorial and the assessments that accompany Chapter 8 in your online course.

EHRNAVIGAT✛R

Chapter 9 Diagnostic and Procedural Coding

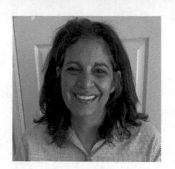

Field Notes

"The EHR completely streamlined the coding process for the healthcare enterprise I work for that has 150 hospitals located around the country. Prior to the implementation of the EHR, paper medical records needed to be scanned every three days for all inpatients to give the corporate coders up-to-date documentation for concurrent coding. This was very time consuming and required coders to decipher handwriting from scanned documents. With the EHR, coders are able to access medical records from all 150 hospitals immediately upon entry by the providers."

– Jody Pruss, Health Information Technician

9.1 Define *nomenclature* and identify its role in the electronic health record (EHR).

9.2 Define *classification systems* and identify specific classification systems used for coding for each healthcare delivery system.

9.3 Discuss the purposes of diagnostic and procedural coding.

9.4 Discuss the classification systems used to code diagnoses and procedures, including the *International Classification of Diseases*, Current Procedural Terminology, Healthcare Common Procedure Coding System, Current Dental Terminology, and the *Diagnostic and Statistical Manual of Mental Disorders*, Fifth Edition.

9.5 Discuss how EHRs affect coding processes.

9.6 Define and describe *computer-assisted coding*.

9.7 Define and discuss important coding concepts, such as *concurrent coding* and *present on admission*.

9.8 Discuss external and internal coding auditing.

9.9 Demonstrate coding processes utilizing EHR software.

W hether in an inpatient healthcare setting such as a hospital, nursing home, or long-term acute care hospital, or an outpatient setting such as an ambulatory surgical center or a behavioral health clinic, there are individuals tasked with assigning and validating diagnostic and procedural codes to represent the patient's diseases or conditions and the treatment rendered. These individuals are known as **clinical coders**, medical coders, or coders, and they are responsible for assigning accurate codes based on health record documentation and coding guidelines. These codes are then used for reimbursement, research, decision making, public health reporting, quality improvement, resource utilization, and healthcare policy and payment.

The practice of accurately coding diagnoses and procedures is a complicated process but can be facilitated by the use of electronic health records (EHRs). The adoption of an EHR system allows coders in every healthcare setting to easily access patient health data as well as billing and reimbursement systems. This improved access, along with the increased legibility of documentation, results in a more streamlined approach to coding and billing. However, EHRs can be of assistance in the reimbursement

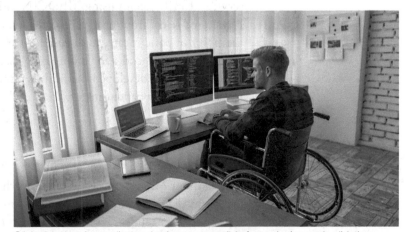

Clinical coders (or medical coders) are responsible for assigning and validating accurate codes based on health record documentation.

process only if clinical and support staff members are properly trained in complete and accurate documentation.

9.1 Nomenclature Systems

Nomenclatures and *classification systems* are two terms frequently—but incorrectly—used interchangeably. **Nomenclature** refers to a common system of naming things. When used in a discussion of EHRs, *nomenclature* refers to a system of common clinical and medical terms, with codes to represent diseases, procedures, symptoms, and medications. SNOMED CT (Systematized Nomenclature of Medicine Clinical Terms) is a federally sanctioned nomenclature to be used with EHRs. Another common nomenclature system is MEDCIN. The term *nomenclature* is used interchangeably with *terminology*.

EXPAND YOUR LEARNING 📶

To learn more about SNOMED CT and its applications with EHR systems, go to https://EHR3 .ParadigmEducation .com/SNOMED to view an informational video.

SNOMED CT

SNOMED CT is a standardized vocabulary of clinical terminology used by healthcare providers for clinical documentation and reporting, and it is considered the most comprehensive healthcare terminology in the world.

Federal and private developers of EHR systems can purchase a license to incorporate SNOMED CT in their systems. SNOMED CT was recommended and adopted as a federal Consolidated Health Informatics standard. However, even with the federal adoption of SNOMED CT as a standard, EHR systems have not consistently implemented SNOMED CT. For example, some facilities use the nomenclature system MEDCIN in their EHR systems.

MEDCIN

MEDCIN, which is a naming system primarily used in physicians' offices, was developed by Medicomp Systems, Inc., and is derived from the US Centers for Medicare & Medicaid Services (CMS) guidelines for evaluation and management coding/charges. Because MEDCIN's vocabulary has been mapped to the evaluation and management Current Procedural Terminology (CPT®) codes that physicians use for billing their services, EHR systems using MEDCIN assist with the coding and billing processes. Physicians select from nearly 300,000 standard clinical data elements in MEDCIN, at the point of patient care, to document treatment rendered. These data elements are mapped to CPT® codes for billing purposes. In addition to the standard vocabulary, MEDCIN has a developed medical terminology interface that facilitates interoperability as it relates to patient information exchange.

9.2 Classification Systems

A **classification system**, as used in health care, is a standardized coding method that organizes diagnoses and procedures into related groups to facilitate reimbursement, reporting, and clinical research. The two most widely used classification systems are the **International Classification of Diseases (ICD)** and **Current Procedural Terminology (CPT®)**. Hospitals, medical offices, long-term care facilities, ambulatory care centers, and many other healthcare institutions use ICD and CPT®.

Other classification systems include the *Diagnostic and Statistical Manual of Mental Disorders*, **Fifth Edition (DSM-5)**, used to classify psychiatric disorders; the **Healthcare Common Procedure Coding System (HCPCS)**, used to code ancillary services and procedures; and **Current Dental Terminology (CDT®)**, used to code dental procedures.

Under the Health Insurance Portability and Accountability Act of 1996 (HIPAA), the US government adopted specific code sets for diagnoses and procedures required of healthcare facilities for all billing transactions. These specific code sets include ICD for diagnosis coding in all settings and hospital inpatient procedure coding, CPT® for physician services and procedures, CDT for dental claims, HCPCS for ancillary services and procedures, and National Drug Codes for drugs.

Purposes of Diagnostic and Procedural Coding

The use of standardized classification systems such as ICD and CPT® has a direct impact on health care, because the data is used for the following purposes:

- Reimbursement—enabling healthcare facilities and providers to bill for services and treatment rendered

- Research—helping researchers with studies and clinical trials

- Decision making—supporting healthcare systems with operational and strategic planning

- Public health—assisting the Centers for Disease Control and Prevention (CDC) and other public health programs to monitor contagious diseases and other health risks

- Quality improvement—aiding healthcare providers with clinical, safety, financial, and operational quality improvement activities

- Resource utilization—supporting administrative and financial healthcare executives with tracking and monitoring the use of resources

- Healthcare policy and payment—assisting government and private agencies with establishing and updating healthcare policies and payment systems

International Classification of Diseases Coding

The history of the ICD (shown in Figure 9.1) can be traced back to the eighteenth century, during which a classification system was developed in England and implemented for the statistical study of infant mortality rates. Although the classification system was rudimentary, it served its purpose at the time and accurately estimated an appalling trend: England's 36% child mortality rate before the age of six years. William Farr (1807–1883), one of the first medical statisticians, worked with the General Register Office in England and became interested in disease and mortality statistics. Farr used the classification system to categorize diseases by anatomic site and to monitor mortality rates.

Bertillon and the *International List of Causes of Death*

In 1891, the International Statistical Institute in Chicago commissioned Jacques Bertillon, chief of statistical services of the city of Paris, to create a classification system based on Farr's work. This new classification system, presented to the institute in 1893,

Figure 9.1 ICD Timeline

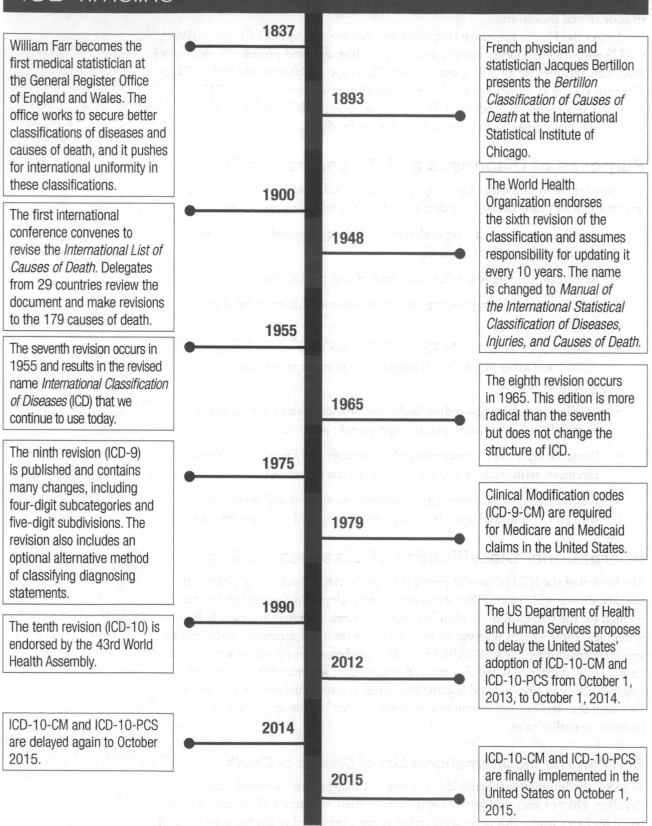

ICD Timeline

1837
William Farr becomes the first medical statistician at the General Register Office of England and Wales. The office works to secure better classifications of diseases and causes of death, and it pushes for international uniformity in these classifications.

1893
French physician and statistician Jacques Bertillon presents the *Bertillon Classification of Causes of Death* at the International Statistical Institute of Chicago.

1900
The first international conference convenes to revise the *International List of Causes of Death*. Delegates from 29 countries review the document and make revisions to the 179 causes of death.

1948
The World Health Organization endorses the sixth revision of the classification and assumes responsibility for updating it every 10 years. The name is changed to *Manual of the International Statistical Classification of Diseases, Injuries, and Causes of Death*.

1955
The seventh revision occurs in 1955 and results in the revised name *International Classification of Diseases* (ICD) that we continue to use today.

1965
The eighth revision occurs in 1965. This edition is more radical than the seventh but does not change the structure of ICD.

1975
The ninth revision (ICD-9) is published and contains many changes, including four-digit subcategories and five-digit subdivisions. The revision also includes an optional alternative method of classifying diagnosing statements.

1979
Clinical Modification codes (ICD-9-CM) are required for Medicare and Medicaid claims in the United States.

1990
The tenth revision (ICD-10) is endorsed by the 43rd World Health Assembly.

2012
The US Department of Health and Human Services proposes to delay the United States' adoption of ICD-10-CM and ICD-10-PCS from October 1, 2013, to October 1, 2014.

2014
ICD-10-CM and ICD-10-PCS are delayed again to October 2015.

2015
ICD-10-CM and ICD-10-PCS are finally implemented in the United States on October 1, 2015.

became known as the *Bertillon Classification of Causes of Death* and was referenced as such until its first revision in 1900, when it was renamed the *International List of Causes of Death*. Twenty-six countries, including the United States, began to use and revise the *International List of Causes of Death*.

Emergence of the ICD

The *International List of Causes of Death* continued to evolve through several revisions until 1948, when the First World Health Assembly of the World Health Organization (WHO) endorsed the sixth revision of the classification system and renamed it the *Manual of the International Statistical Classification of Diseases, Injuries, and Causes of Death*. This sixth revision marked the beginning of a new era in international vital and health statistics. Governments began to establish national committees on vital and health statistics, correlate statistical activities within their countries, and coordinate statistical activities with other countries and the WHO.

The seventh revision occurred in 1955 and resulted in the revised name *International Classification of Diseases* (ICD), a title still used today. The eighth revision (ICD-8) was released in 1965, and the ninth revision (ICD-9) was published in 1975.

ICD-9

By 1977, the US National Center for Health Statistics convened a steering committee to provide expertise and advice in the development of a clinical modification of ICD-9 to be used solely by the United States. This clinical modification would make it more applicable to the diseases experienced by US patients and would include the level of detail requested by the country's researchers and statisticians. The US version was titled *ICD-9, Clinical Modification* (ICD-9-CM).

There have been annual updates to the 1977 version of ICD-9-CM to include new codes, delete codes, and modify existing codes. The Coordination and Maintenance Committee of the ICD-9-CM is responsible for maintaining the classification system and is composed of four cooperating parties: the American Hospital Association (AHA), the CMS, the American Health Information Management Association (AHIMA), and the National Center for Health Statistics. In addition to developing new and revised ICD-9-CM codes, the committee also provides coding guidance for ICD-9-CM and publishes clarifications of coding issues in *Coding Clinic*, published by the AHA. The clarifications of coding questions and issues that are published in *Coding Clinic* are considered official interpretations of and guidance on coding issues and must be followed for accurate coding.

ICD-10

None of the revisions to ICD-9 and ICD-9-CM were extensive until the tenth revision (ICD-10) was adopted by the World Health Assembly in 1990. ICD-10 is vastly different from ICD-9. There were approximately 13,000 codes in ICD-9. Now there are approximately 68,000 codes in ICD-10 to allow for more specific coding and reporting of diagnoses and procedures. The format of the ICD-10 codes is also much different from that of ICD-9. The codes in ICD-9 are primarily numeric (000.1–999.99), with combination alphanumeric codes being limited to three sections, namely, the Morphology of Neoplasms (M codes), External Causes of Injury and Poisoning (E codes), and Factors Influencing Health Status and Contact with Health Services (V codes). All of the ICD-10 codes are alphanumeric (A00–T98, V01–Y98, and Z00–Z99). On October 1, 2015, the United States formally adopted a version of ICD-10 known as the *International Classification of Diseases, Tenth Revision, Clinical Modification* (ICD-10-CM) to classify diseases and conditions in all healthcare settings.

In conjunction with the adoption of ICD-10-CM, the United States also adopted a new system for classifying inpatient medical procedures and treatments. This new classification is called the *International Classification of Diseases, Tenth Revision, Procedural Coding System* (ICD-10-PCS). ICD-10 was originally scheduled for implementation in the United States in 2013. Both the AHA and the American Medical Association (AMA) requested a delay to allow healthcare providers and organizations time to fully prepare and test systems to ensure a smooth transition from ICD-9 to ICD-10. The implementation was then set for 2014 and again delayed to 2015. ICD-10-CM and ICD-10-PCS were finally implemented in 2015.

EXPAND YOUR LEARNING

The WHO was created by the United Nations in 1948 and is responsible for providing leadership on global health matters, shaping the health research agenda, setting norms and standards, articulating evidence-based policy options, providing technical support to countries, and monitoring and assessing global health trends. The WHO also provides training tools for projects such as ICD-11. To identify these tools, conduct a search of the organization's website at https://EHR3.ParadigmEducation.com/Classifications.

ICD-11

ICD-11 has been developed and approved by the WHO. Globally, countries may implement ICD-11 in January 2022 or any time thereafter. ICD-11 will likely be implemented in the United States between 2025 and 2030, depending on whether the United States makes clinical modifications to ICD-11 as were made with ICD-10. It is important to note that ICD-11 is an alphanumeric classification system used only to code diagnoses. The WHO does not develop a procedural coding system. The ICD-10-PCS will remain in use in the United States with code updates occurring annually. ICD-11 is the first version of the ICD classification system that has been designed for use in EHR systems. It is expected to make the implementation of ICD-11 less costly and less labor intensive. Continuing toward the goal of being able to code diagnoses with greater specificity, ICD-11 contains 55,000 diagnosis codes compared with 14,400 in ICD-10. It is anticipated that the CMS will implement a clinical modification of ICD-11 to increase the number of codes and provide for greater specificity, therefore, enhancing data use. For example, the WHO version of ICD-10 contained 14,400 diagnosis codes, and the ICD-10-CM had 69,000 codes. Tables 9.1 and 9.2 show comparisons of ICD-9, ICD-10, and ICD-11 codes.

Table 9.1   Example Diagnosis Codes

Diagnosis	ICD-9-CM Code	ICD-10-CM Code	ICD-11 Code
Diabetes mellitus, Type 2	250.00	E11.9	5A11
Fracture of neck of femur (fractured hip)	820.00	S72.019A	ABO.1 plus additional anatomy code

Table 9.2   Example Procedure Codes

Procedure	ICD-9-CM Code(s)	ICD-10-PCS Code
Percutaneous transluminal coronary angioplasty (PTCA)	00.66, 36.07, 00.47, 00.41 (all four codes required)	0272342
Appendectomy	47.01	0DTJ4ZZ

CPT® Coding

CPT® is the classification system that describes medical, surgical, and diagnostic services, and it is used to report the procedures and services rendered to patients, including all surgical, radiologic, and anesthetic procedures, as well as other diagnostic screenings, such as laboratory and pathology studies. The sites for these services include hospitals, nursing homes, ambulatory centers, medical offices, and other patient care facilities. CPT® codes are used to report procedures and services when billing both private and public insurance companies.

CPT® is published by the AMA and is updated every January. The AMA is also responsible for the creation and maintenance of CPT® codes. A CPT® editorial panel meets three times per year to discuss issues associated with new and emerging technologies as well as difficulties encountered with procedures and services and their relation to CPT® codes. The panel is composed of 17 members. Eleven are nominated by the AMA, and the remaining six individuals are nominated by entities such as private insurance companies or professional healthcare organizations.

Individuals who use CPT® codes must stay current and always use the most recent manual to bill for services. There are more than 8,000 CPT® codes ranging from 00100 through 99607. In addition, two-digit modifiers may be added to certain CPT® codes to clarify or modify the description of the procedure.

Healthcare Common Procedure Coding System

CPT® codes are part of the Healthcare Common Procedure Coding System (HCPCS). HCPCS—pronounced "hick picks"—is divided into Levels I and II. Level I of HCPCS is composed of CPT® codes and is used to bill physician services and procedures. Level II of HCPCS is commonly referred to as *National Codes* and is primarily used to bill for products, supplies, and services not included in the CPT® codes, such as ambulance services, durable medical equipment, prosthetics, orthotics, and supplies. HCPCS codes are published annually by the CMS.

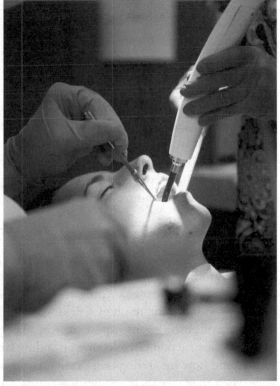

Current Dental Terminology Coding

The code set on dental procedures and nomenclatures that is used in the United States is Current Dental Terminology (CDT). CDT is published and annually updated by the American Dental Association (ADA). CDT is a set of dental procedural codes used to report all dental services, with the exception of some oral surgery procedures.

Current Dental Terminology (CDT) is used to code dental services.

Dentists use ICD codes to report diagnoses and CDT codes to report the dental procedures and services. The CDT codes are also used with ICD codes for billing purposes.

DSM-5 Coding

DSM-5 refers to the *Diagnostic and Statistical Manual of Mental Disorders,* Fifth Edition. DSM-5, published by the American Psychiatric Association (APA), is a manual that contains codes for every known behavioral health condition. The manual is designed to coincide with ICD, but the two coding systems are not identical. ICD diagnosis codes are used for billing purposes, but they are not detailed enough for researchers, clinicians, policy makers, health insurance companies, pharmaceutical companies, and psychiatric drug regulatory agencies. DSM codes are not included as approved codes in the HIPAA transaction and code set standards for electronic data interchange for billing purposes. Mental health providers rely on the DSM as a supportive diagnostic tool. To submit claims for reimbursement purposes, DSM codes are crosswalked to ICD codes. **Crosswalking** is the act of translating a code in one code set to a code in another code set.

CHECKPOINT 9.1

1. List three purposes of diagnostic and procedural coding.

   a. _____

   b. _____

   c. _____

2. What was the implementation date of ICD-10 in the United States?

   _____

3. In what year is ICD-11 expected to be implemented in the United States?

   _____

9.3 Code Assignment

Traditionally, coders have used hard- or soft-cover coding manuals to assign ICD, CPT®, and DSM-5 diagnostic and procedure codes. Depending on the classification system, coders have used as many as two books at a time, such as when coding with ICD-10-CM/PCS. For those healthcare organizations with a low volume of health records to code, the use of coding manuals may be effective. However, with high volumes of health records to code, using several cumbersome manuals slows down the coding process.

Using Encoders versus Print Coding Manuals

To remedy the difficult process of coding from many different print manuals, clinical encoders/groupers were adopted by these high-volume facilities in the 1990s. A **clinical encoder** is a software program that helps coding professionals navigate coding pathways with the end result of assigning codes. It is important to note that many coding certification exams require the test taker to code from coding books. Therefore, classroom instruction often focuses on coding from manuals to ensure that students understand how the coding classification systems work and how to apply that knowledge when they take their certification exams. Coders must understand how to assign codes using both encoder software and printed coding manuals.

Diagnosis-Related Groups

A **diagnosis-related group (DRG)** is a patient classification system that groups hospital inpatients of similar age, sex, diagnoses, and treatments. Each DRG is associated with a specific dollar amount that the hospital expects to be reimbursed for in relation to the treatment provided. The first DRG system, the Medicare **inpatient prospective payment system (IPPS)**, was implemented in 1983 to reimburse acute care hospitals for the treatment of Medicare patients. Since then, many other payers, such as Medicaid and commercial payers, have adopted the Medicare DRG system for the reimbursement of inpatient care for their insured members. The purpose of a DRG system is to relatively equalize payments to hospitals for providing the same care to patients with the same clinical characteristics. Prior to the implementation of the Medicare DRG system, acute care hospitals were reimbursed for whatever they charged Medicare or other payers. Take a look at a simplified example of pre-DRG and post-DRG payments for two patient scenarios in the following Consider This box.

Medicare and Medicaid patients may be grouped together using a diagnosis-related group classification system for coding purposes.

Consider This

Patient A

Final principal diagnosis: acute respiratory failure

Principal procedure: mechanical ventilation, more than 96 hours

Patient B

Final principal diagnosis: acute myocardial infarction

Principal procedure: coronary artery bypass

Hospital Name	Patient A Reimbursement Before Medicare DRG ($)	Patient A Reimbursement After Medicare DRG ($)	Patient B Reimbursement Before Medicare DRG ($)	Patient B Reimbursement After Medicare DRG ($)
City Hospital	63,588	47,184	24,160	33,238
Tender Care Hospital	52,140	47,184	44,321	33,238
Bayview Hospital	38,690	47,184	45,870	33,238
Grace Hospital	47,545	47,184	63,923	33,238

Analyze the table above. Why do reimbursement rates for Patients A and B vary among hospitals in the time before the Medicare DRG implementation? Why are the reimbursement rates the same for Patients A and B among the hospitals under the Medicare DRG system? Under the Medicare DRG system, why is the reimbursement for Patient A not the same as Patient B?

Consider This

Through the Medicare inpatient prospective payment system (IPPS), the US government spends more than $130 billion every year in payments to acute care hospitals for inpatient care. Because the IPPS depends on diagnostic and procedural coding to calculate the payments to acute care hospitals, what would happen if coding staff incorrectly coded charts 10% of the time?

9.4 Coding and the Electronic Health Record

The use of an EHR system has a positive impact on the coding of health records. It facilitates efficient concurrent and final coding processes, greater accuracy in code assignments, and improved access to health records.

The Coding Process

Healthcare facilities initiate the billing process for patient visits after each visit or admission. The healthcare facility prepares the claims to be sent to the insurance carrier, and upon submission, payments are made to the healthcare facility. A **medical coder**, a career option in the health information management field, plays a key role in the billing process by coding diagnoses and procedures in preparation for billing claims.

Medical coding is the process of assigning and validating standardized alphanumeric identifiers to the diagnoses and procedures documented in a health record. A **diagnosis** is a statement or conclusion that describes a patient's illness, disease, or health problem. A **medical procedure** is an activity performed on an individual to improve health, treat disease or injury, or identify a diagnosis. Healthcare professionals must document diagnoses and procedures in the health record, and the medical coders use that information to assign the appropriate codes for billing and research purposes.

But not all healthcare professionals record diagnoses and procedures in a uniform way. For example, two physicians might describe the same condition in different terms, as shown in Figure 9.2. Assigning standardized alphanumeric codes to this medical data makes it easier to interpret immediately, share, compare, classify, and manipulate the data for reimbursement, research, and planning.

Coded data is used by healthcare providers to seek reimbursement from the government, private insurance companies, and other third-party payers. A **third-party payer** is an entity other than the patient that is financially responsible for payment of the medical bill. Patients who pay for the entire visit themselves are referred to as **self-pay patients**. Third-party payers are so named because there are typically three parties involved in the care of the patient:

- Party 1: the patient
- Party 2: the healthcare provider
- Party 3: the entity, other than the patient, that pays the medical bill

Figure 9.2 Comparison of Medical Notes

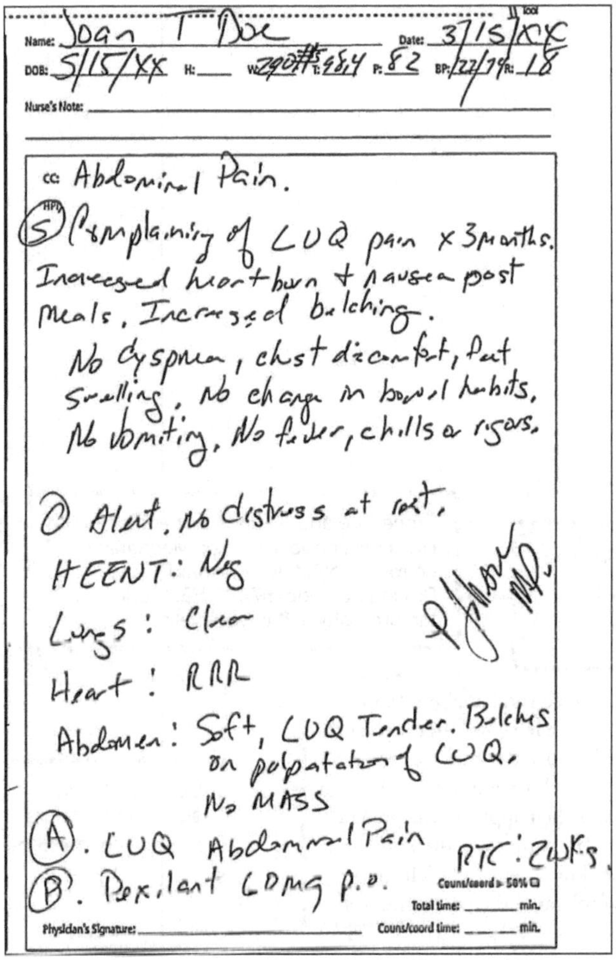
Name: Joan T Doe Date: 3/15/XX
DOB: 5/15/XX Ht: ___ Wt: 180# T: 98.4 P: 82 BP: 122/74 R: 18
Nurse's Note:

CC: Abdominal Pain.
HPI
(S) Complaining of LUQ pain x 3 months. Increased heartburn + nausea post meals, Increased belching.
No dyspnea, chest discomfort, feet swelling, no change in bowel habits, No vomiting, No fever, chills or rigors.

(O) Alert, no distress at rest,
HEENT: Neg
Lungs: Clear
Heart: RRR
Abdomen: Soft, LUQ Tender. Belches on palpatation of LUQ. No MASS

(A). LUQ Abdominal Pain
(P). Dexilant 60mg p.o. RTC: 2wks

Couns/coord > 50% ☐
Total time: ___ min.
Physician's Signature: ___ Couns/coord time: ___ min.

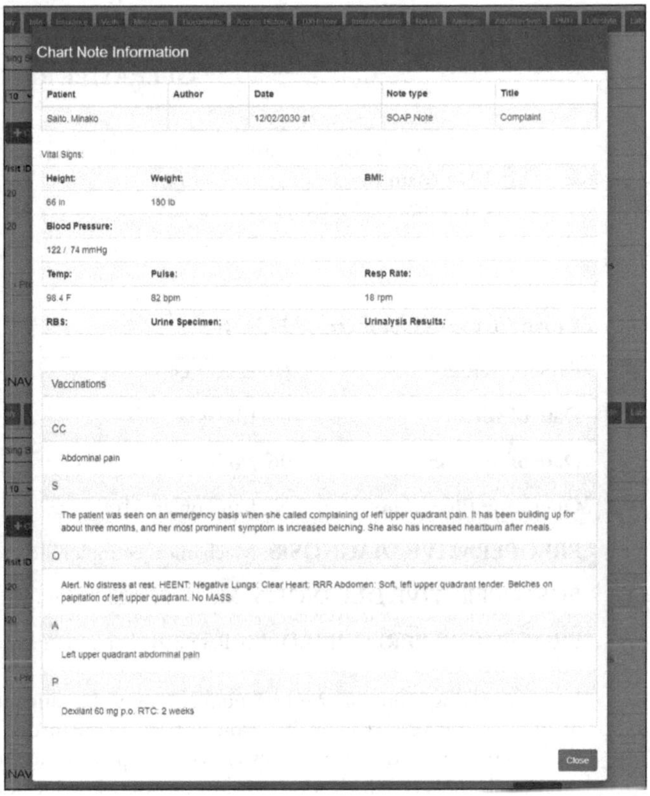
Chart Note Information

Patient	Author	Date	Note type	Title
Saito, Minako		12/02/2030 at	SOAP Note	Complaint

Vital Signs:

Height:	Weight:	BMI:
66 in	180 lb	

Blood Pressure:
122 / 74 mmHg

Temp:	Pulse:	Resp Rate:
98.4 F	82 bpm	18 rpm
RBS:	Urine Specimen:	Urinalysis Results:

Vaccinations

CC

Abdominal pain

S

The patient was seen on an emergency basis when she called complaining of left upper quadrant pain. It has been building up for about three months, and her most prominent symptom is increased belching. She also has increased heartburn after meals.

O

Alert. No distress at rest. HEENT: Negative Lungs: Clear Heart: RRR Abdomen: Soft, left upper quadrant tender. Belches on palpitation of left upper quadrant. No MASS

A

Left upper quadrant abdominal pain

P

Dexilant 60 mg p.o. RTC: 2 weeks

Close

Coded data is also used in public health management to monitor the incidence and prevalence of diseases as well as death rates. To monitor health trends, nations track **morbidity**, which consists of the rates of diseases in a population, and **mortality**, the rate of death in a population—these rates are typically expressed as statistics and percentages. Coded information enables the storage and retrieval of diagnostic information for clinical, epidemiologic, and quality control purposes.

Reporting Codes from the Health Record

The health record and the documentation it contains is the starting point for reporting medical codes. An **operative report** is a form of clinical documentation that contains the details of a particular surgery or procedure performed on a patient. Figure 9.3 illustrates the different parts of an operative report for tarsorrhaphy, a procedure in which the eyelids are partially sewn together to narrow the opening.

The steps in reporting codes from an operative report are generally the following:

1. Read the report and verify that the diagnoses and procedures listed at the top of the report are supported by the documentation of the procedure provided in the body of the report (sometimes called the *operative technique*). If the documentation supports a different procedure or diagnosis

Figure 9.3   Example of an Ophthalmologic Operative

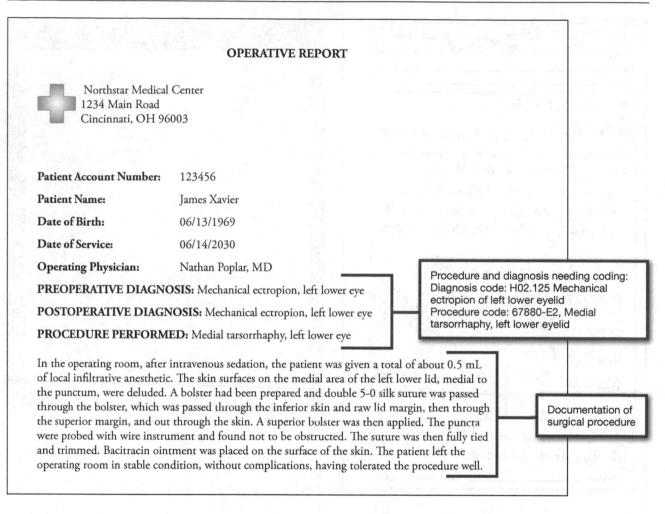

OPERATIVE REPORT

Northstar Medical Center
1234 Main Road
Cincinnati, OH 96003

Patient Account Number: 123456

Patient Name: James Xavier

Date of Birth: 06/13/1969

Date of Service: 06/14/2030

Operating Physician: Nathan Poplar, MD

PREOPERATIVE DIAGNOSIS: Mechanical ectropion, left lower eye

POSTOPERATIVE DIAGNOSIS: Mechanical ectropion, left lower eye

PROCEDURE PERFORMED: Medial tarsorrhaphy, left lower eye

> Procedure and diagnosis needing coding:
> Diagnosis code: H02.125 Mechanical ectropion of left lower eyelid
> Procedure code: 67880-E2, Medial tarsorrhaphy, left lower eyelid

In the operating room, after intravenous sedation, the patient was given a total of about 0.5 mL of local infiltrative anesthetic. The skin surfaces on the medial area of the left lower lid, medial to the punctum, were deluded. A bolster had been prepared and double 5-0 silk suture was passed through the bolster, which was passed through the inferior skin and raw lid margin, then through the superior margin, and out through the skin. A superior bolster was then applied. The puncta were probed with wire instrument and found not to be obstructed. The suture was then fully tied and trimmed. Bacitracin ointment was placed on the surface of the skin. The patient left the operating room in stable condition, without complications, having tolerated the procedure well.

> Documentation of surgical procedure

than that listed by the physician, the coder should review the facility policies and procedures, which typically instruct the coder to query the provider for additional information.

2.   Identify the correct codes for the diagnoses and procedures using resources such as coding manuals and coding software.

3.   Enter the medical codes into the EHR to prepare the account for billing.

Concurrent and Final Coding

Final bills are typically held in a suspended status for three days after patient discharge to allow for final charge entry, documentation, insurance verification, and final coding. Patient accounts not able to be final billed to the insurance company or responsible party because of a lack of final coding, insurance verification, or other data errors are considered **discharged not final billed (DNFB)**. These accounts are flagged as DNFB and are included on a data report produced by the EHR system. This report is monitored daily by health information managers, coders, and other staff members in healthcare organizations. For coders, this report highlights the oldest outstanding accounts and the accounts with the highest unbilled account balances. The EHR system further assists the coder by providing coding **work-list reports**. These reports present the patient accounts for coding in a priority order, beginning with the oldest accounts with the highest balances. For those coders who use physical paper records rather than an EHR system, a major contributor to a DNFB list is the delay in locating the paper record.

For coders, an EHR system can perform **concurrent coding**, which is the task of coding while a patient is still receiving treatment in a hospital. This concurrent coding accelerates the final coding process that is completed upon discharge of the patient, by allowing coders to query healthcare providers for necessary documentation regarding diagnoses and procedures over the course of a particular patient's stay. Consequently, the coder has all the documentation needed upon patient discharge to allow for final coding.

The financial managers of healthcare organizations promote concurrent coding because the process speeds up final billing procedures, thereby reducing the number of unbilled accounts. Even though there are many contributing factors involved in the final billing process, health information management (HIM) departments, and coding staff in particular, are held accountable for the inability of an organization to produce final bills to payers due to a lack of final coding.

Accuracy in Code Assignments

As previously discussed in Chapters 1 and 2, EHRs eliminate the problems of illegible handwriting that exist in most paper health records. Illegible handwriting can result in inaccurate coding when coders miss or miscode diagnoses because they cannot read the healthcare provider's handwriting. The EHR also improves coding through more accurate documentation. Physicians may be prompted to enter more information based on the templates built in the EHR system. EHRs can therefore reduce the number of errors due to incomplete or vague diagnostic or procedural information.

As the coder navigates through the EHR, separate clinical encoder software windows are open for support. As a result, the clinical coder can read and enter the patient's diagnoses and procedures rendered to a patient into the encoder, resulting in the applicable codes. The coder may automatically generate physician queries and highlight or make notations to the EHR that do not change or affect the legality of the health record. A **physician query** is a request, typically from a coder or a case manager, to add documentation to the health record that clarifies a diagnosis or procedure performed (see Figure 9.4). Physician queries may be issued to providers concurrently or retrospectively. AHIMA has published best-practice guidance on the query process in its *Guidelines for Achieving a Compliant Query Practice*. In an EHR, all physician queries are automatically routed to the appropriate physician's message inbox and displayed when the physician logs in to the system.

The use of clinical encoders and physician queries assists coders in establishing the most accurate code assignments. Accurate code assignments, in turn, result in appropriate reimbursement for healthcare organizations. Although organizations must ensure that health record documentation is complete and accurate, its staff members cannot educate or encourage physicians to document simply for the purpose of claiming a higher-paying DRG and, therefore, increased reimbursement. This maneuver is referred to as **upcoding** and is illegal. Unintentional upcoding is considered **abuse**, whereas intentional upcoding is considered **fraud**. Those convicted of fraud or abuse may receive monetary fines or jail time.

Figure 9.4 Example of a Physician Query

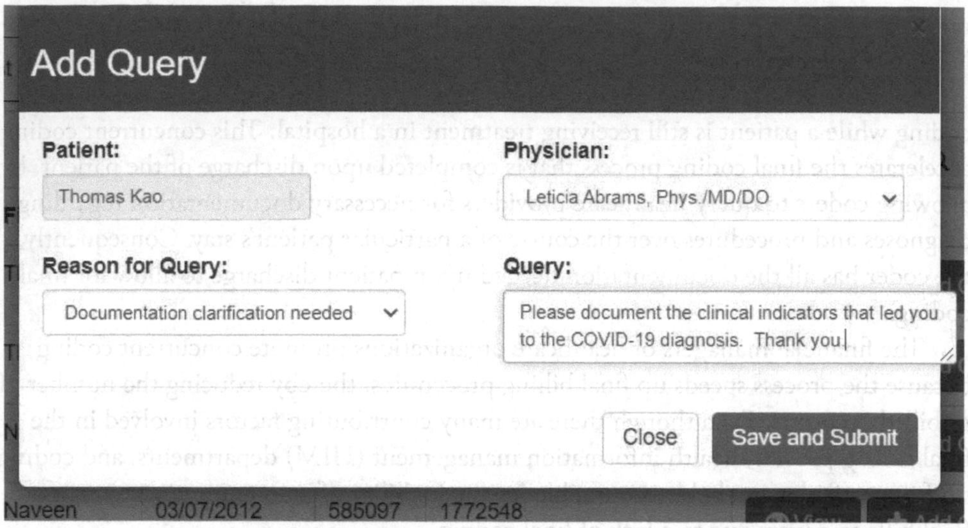

Add Query
Patient:
Thomas Kao
Physician:
Leticia Abrams, Phys./MD/DO
Reason for Query:
Documentation clarification needed
Query:
Please document the clinical indicators that led you to the COVID-19 diagnosis. Thank you
Close
Save and Submit
Naveen 03/07/2012 585097 1772548

> **EXPAND YOUR LEARNING**
>
> To learn more about present on admission (POA) indicators and reduced Medicare reimbursement for hospital-acquired conditions, review the following websites:
>
> https://EHR3.ParadigmEducation.com/MedicarePOA
>
> https://EHR3.ParadigmEducation.com/MedicareHAC

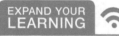

Computer-Assisted Coding Programs

Some EHR systems incorporate **computer-assisted coding (CAC)** programs that automatically assign diagnosis and procedure codes based on electronic documentation, which can increase the productivity of a coder by up to 20%. However, the use of a CAC program does not mean that the coding process is completely automated. When CAC programs are used, the coder assumes the role of a reviewer or an auditor. The coder must validate the codes, ensure that coding guidelines have been followed, and validate whether the coded diagnoses were **present on admission (POA)**, meaning that the patient had the diagnoses when they were admitted to the facility. All primary and secondary diagnoses require POA indicators to be reported on the Medicare claims of IPPS general acute care hospitals. POA indicator assignment is determined by the coder based on clinical documentation entered into the health record by the provider.

Coders must exercise care in assigning POA indicators. Medicare patients who experience diagnoses and conditions that are **hospital acquired**, meaning that they developed when the patient was an inpatient in the hospital, must not be reported as POA. The care and treatment of these hospital-acquired diagnoses and conditions (e.g., hospital-acquired pressure ulcer, urinary tract infection, or pneumonia) are typically not reimbursed by Medicare.

9.5 Internal and External Auditing for Coding Compliance

To verify that a healthcare facility is coding accurately and following guidelines, it is often audited, either externally or internally.

External Coding Audits

External companies and organizations routinely conduct audits to verify coding accuracy. These external companies and organizations include insurance companies, auditing companies hired by insurance companies, and Medicare and Medicaid auditors. The purpose of the audits is to ensure that coders followed coding guidelines and regulations in the assignment of diagnosis and procedure codes.

Insurance Audits

Insurance audits are conducted by insurance companies or auditing companies hired to review coding assignments on their behalf. These audits are routinely conducted for patient accounts that contain codes that are historically problematic for coders, resulting in a high error rate. Insurance company audits also focus on patient accounts or bills that exceed a specific threshold. For example, Cobalt Care might automatically conduct audits for any patient bill exceeding $100,000. Another insurance company may have a lower threshold of $80,000. Insurance companies also conduct more frequent coding audits of healthcare organizations that have historically had a higher coding error rate.

Recovery Audit Contractor Program

The goal of the Recovery Audit Contractor (RAC) program is to identify improper payments made for healthcare services provided to Medicare beneficiaries and to take actions to prevent these improper payments from occurring in the future. These improper payments include both overpayment and underpayment due to inaccurate coding. Any healthcare provider that bills Medicare Part A (inpatient services) or B (outpatient services) may be audited under the RAC program. These providers include hospitals, physician practices, nursing homes, home health agencies, durable medical equipment supplies, and any other provider or supplier that bills Medicare Part A or B charges. The Tax Relief and Health Care Act of 2006 required that a national RAC program be in place by January 1, 2010. The RAC program has resulted in the return of more than $10 billion to the Medicare program. For example, in 2019 alone, more than $89 million was returned to the Medicare fund.

Internal Coding Audits

The best way for a healthcare provider to avoid having to repay insurance companies or Medicare for inaccurate coding and billing is to reduce the risk of coding errors. How can a healthcare provider accomplish this?

- Conduct internal coding audits—Instead of waiting for external organizations to identify coding errors, providers should routinely conduct their own audits to identify coding problem areas. EHR reporting capabilities can greatly enhance the auditing process, because reports can be quickly generated to the level of specificity desired by the auditor.

- Intensive coder training—As problematic coding scenarios are identified with internal audits, providers should conduct coder training to reduce coding errors.

- Reaudit—Following coder training, the provider should reaudit the coding areas that were the subject of the coder training to ensure that coding accuracy has improved.

Tutorial 9.1

Coding a Patient's Record

Go to your online course to launch Tutorial 9.1. As an RHIT, practice coding a patient's record using the EHR Navigator.

CHECKPOINT 9.2

1. List three ways in which the EHR benefits the coding process.

   a. _____

   b. _____

   c. _____

2. True/False: A successful healthcare organization uses upcoding to ensure that the best DRG is selected for billing. Explain why you chose *true* or *false*.

   _____

   _____

   _____

Chapter Summary

Electronic health record (EHR) systems are revolutionizing the reimbursement, clinical coding, and billing processes. Some of the benefits of EHR implementation include easy access to clinical records by the coding and billing staff, more efficient methods of coding health records, a streamlined physician query process, improved documentation by providers, and improved fiscal management of healthcare organizations.

Nomenclature refers to a system of common clinical and medical terms, with codes to represent diseases, procedures, symptoms, and medications. SNOMED CT is a standardized vocabulary of clinical terminology used by healthcare providers for clinical documentation and reporting and is considered the most comprehensive healthcare terminology in the world. Another common nomenclature system is MEDCIN.

Classification systems are used for reimbursement, research, decision making, public health, quality improvement, resource utilization, and healthcare policy and payment. The types of classification systems used depend on the types of services one is coding. Common coding classification systems include International Classification of Diseases (ICD), Current Procedural Terminology (CPT®), Healthcare Common Procedure Coding System (HCPCS), *Diagnostic and Statistical Manual of Mental Disorders*, Fifth Edition (DSM-5), and Current Dental Terminology (CDT).

ICD-10 was implemented in the United States in October 2015. ICD-11 will likely be implemented in the United States around 2025.

CPT® is the classification system that describes medical, surgical, and diagnostic services and is used to report the procedures and services rendered to patients, including all surgical, radiologic, and anesthetic procedures, as well as other diagnostic screenings, such as laboratory and pathology studies. CPT® is published by the American Medical Association (AMA) and is updated annually in January.

HCPCS, the Healthcare Common Procedure Coding System, is divided into Levels I and II. Level I is composed of CPT® codes and is used to bill physician services and procedures. Level II is primarily used to bill for products, supplies, and services not included in the CPT® codes, such as ambulance services, durable medical equipment, prosthetics, orthotics, and supplies. HCPCS codes are published annually by the CMS.

CDT is the Current Dental Terminology nomenclature that is used to report all dental services. DSM-5 is published by the American Psychiatric Association and is used as a crosswalk to ICD-10 to bill for mental health services. Crosswalking is the act of translating a code in one code set to a code in another code set.

To assist with the coding process, a coder may use a clinical encoder software program and classify patients by their diagnosis-related group (DRG). IPPS is the Medicare inpatient prospective payment system that reimburses acute care hospitals for the treatment of Medicare patients. Concurrent coding is the task of coding while a patient is still receiving treatment in a hospital. Patient accounts not able to be final billed to the insurance company or responsible party because of a lack of final coding, insurance verification, or other data errors are considered discharged not final billed (DNFB).

As a coder navigates the EHR to accurately assign diagnosis and procedure codes, they must confirm they have enough information to accurately apply official coding guidelines. If not, they should initiate a physician query, a request to add documentation to the EHR and clarify a diagnosis or procedure. Coders must be vigilant and not engage in upcoding, the illegal practice of using higher paying but inaccurate DRGs for the purpose of increasing reimbursement. Unintentional upcoding is considered abuse, and intentional upcoding is considered fraud.

Computer-assisted coding (CAC) programs automatically assign diagnosis and procedure codes based on electronic documentation. In practice, coders verify the CAC code assignments to ensure accurate coding, including the correct assignment of present on admission (POA) codes, which indicate diagnoses that are present upon admission to the hospital as opposed to hospital-acquired conditions developed during a patient's stay.

Checks and balances are as important in an EHR environment as they are in a paper environment. Coders must follow official coding guidelines, and physicians and healthcare providers must thoroughly and accurately document procedures and diagnoses. External coding audits are conducted by insurance companies, auditing companies hired by insurance companies, and Recovery Audit Contractors (RAC) for Medicare to verify coding accuracy and compliance.

Review and Assessment

The following Review and Assessment activities are also available online in the Cirrus online course. Your instructor may ask you to complete these activities online. Cirrus also provides access to flash cards, a crossword puzzle, and practice quizzes to help strengthen your understanding of the chapter content.

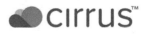

Acronyms/Initialisms

Study the following acronyms discussed in this chapter. Go to the online course for flash cards of the acronyms and other chapter key terms.

ADA: American Dental Association

AHA: American Hospital Association

AHIMA: American Health Information Management Association

AMA: American Medical Association

APA: American Psychiatric Association

CAC: computer-assisted coding

CDC: Centers for Disease Control and Prevention

CDT: Current Dental Terminology

CMS: Centers for Medicare & Medicaid Services

CPT®: Current Procedural Terminology

DNFB: discharged not final billed

DRG: diagnosis-related group

DSM-5: *Diagnostic and Statistical Manual of Mental Disorders*, Fifth Edition

HCPCS: Healthcare Common Procedure Coding System

HIM: health information management

ICD: International Classification of Diseases

IPPS: inpatient prospective payment system

POA: present on admission

RAC: Recovery Audit Contractor

SNOMED CT: Systematized Nomenclature of Medicine Clinical Terms

WHO: World Health Organization

Check Your Understanding

To check your understanding of this chapter's key concepts, answer the following questions.

1. The following are all examples of classification systems *except:*

    a. MEDCIN.

    b. International Classification of Diseases (ICD).

    c. Current Procedural Terminology (CPT®).

    d. *Diagnostic and Statistical Manual of Mental Disorders,* Fifth Edition (DSM-5).

2. Which of the following classification systems is used to code outpatient procedures and inpatient and outpatient provider services?

    a. Current Dental Terminology

    b. ICD-10-CM

    c. DSM-5

    d. CPT®

3. How does the implementation of an EHR system affect the process of coding health records?

    a. It allows for more efficient coding.

    b. It increases the accuracy of code assignments.

    c. It eliminates the physician query process.

    d. It allows for more efficient coding and increases the accuracy of code assignments.

4. When was ICD-10 implemented in the United States?

    a. October 1, 2012

    b. January 1, 2013

    c. January 1, 2014

    d. October 1, 2015

5. When is ICD-11 likely to be implemented in the United States?

    a. 2025

    b. 2020

    c. 2018

    d. Never

6. True/False: The term *nomenclature* refers to a standardized method of assigning codes to diagnoses and procedures.

7. True/False: Concurrent coding is an easy process to perform with paper records but is more difficult with an EHR system.

8. True/False: The RAC audits have *not* been successful in returning money to the Medicare fund.

9. True/False: Healthcare providers are best served by waiting for external auditors to show them where their coding problems exist.

10. True/False: The use of standardized classification systems has a direct impact on health care.

Go on the Record

To build on your understanding of the topics in this chapter, complete the following short-answer activities.

1. List and describe three purposes of diagnostic and procedural coding.

2. Discuss the differences between *nomenclature* and a *classification system*.

3. Define *clinical encoder* and discuss how this software program assists coding professionals.

4. List three ways in which the electronic health record (EHR) system improves work processes for a coder.

5. Define *physician query* and describe how the process is automated with the EHR system.

Navigate the Field

To gain practice in handling challenging situations in the workplace, consider the following real-world scenarios and identify how you would respond to each.

1. You are a coder for Northstar Medical Center. While coding diagnoses for a discharged patient's encounter, you notice that the attending physician has documented that the patient has type 1 diabetes mellitus, and a consulting

physician has documented that the patient has type 2 diabetes mellitus. How would you handle this discrepancy?

2. As the lead coder for a large physician practice, you notice that a couple of the coders are not following the official coding guidelines. What steps should you take to ensure accurate coding?

Think Critically

Continue to think critically about challenging concepts and complete the following activities.

1. As the supervisor of coding at a large teaching hospital, you are concerned about the new interns and residents who rotate through the hospital every year. You have noticed that their documentation is not complete enough for coders to accurately code. What should you do to rectify this situation that is ongoing as the new interns and residents rotate through the organization?

2. Conduct an internet search to identify two clinical encoders that can be interfaced with EHR systems. After examining the components of each system, write a proposal to the coding manager of Northstar Physicians that identifies the program you would select and discusses the reasoning behind your choice.

Make Your Case

Consider the scenario and then complete the following project.

As the coding manager for a hospital, you have been asked by the vice president of finance to prepare a short presentation for hospital administrators that addresses how the hospital's EHR system has benefited the coding process of the hospital.

Explore the Technology

EHRNAVIGAT✚R   *Complete the EHR Navigator practice assessments that align to each tutorial and the assessments that accompany Chapter 9 located in the online course.*

Chapter **10** Managing Insurance, Billing, and Reimbursement

Learning Objectives

10.1 Define *health insurance* and understand the concepts related to health coverage.

10.2 Discuss the evolution of health insurance.

10.3 Define individual and group insurance plans.

10.4 Differentiate between fee-for-service, managed care, and value-based insurance plans.

10.5 Define and discuss different types of government-sponsored health plans.

10.6 Discuss the importance and methods of verifying insurance.

10.7 Define *practice management* and explain how it relates to billing and electronic office billing systems.

10.8 Discuss how EHRs affect billing processes.

10.9 Demonstrate billing processes utilizing EHR software.

10.10 Demonstrate use of an electronic office billing system.

10.11 Demonstrate insurance claims processing.

10.12 Demonstrate use of practice management reports.

In 2016, there were 12,871,500,000 medical claims transactions annually, or about 39 transactions per year for every American. It is estimated that physicians in the United States leave approximately $125 billion on the table each year because of poor billing practices. The electronic health record (EHR) reduces the time and resources needed for manual charge entry, resulting in more accurate billing and reduction in lost charges. As with any business, to be successful, a healthcare organization must be financially stable. The financial stability of a healthcare organization results from the careful management of the health insurance, billing, and reimbursement process. In this chapter, we will explore the concepts of health insurance, billing, and reimbursement, and the role of the EHR in managing these transactions.

To understand health insurance, billing, and reimbursement, it is first important to understand **revenue cycle management**. The Healthcare Financial Management Association (HFMA) defines the revenue cycle as "all administrative and clinical functions that contribute to the capture, management, and collection of patient service revenue." The revenue cycle begins with the admission or registration of a patient and ends with collection and posting of payments. Figure 10.1 shows the revenue cycle management process. A healthcare organization that has a well-managed revenue cycle will experience a timelier, increased cash flow, which in turn translates into higher revenue.

Figure 10.1   Revenue Cycle Management

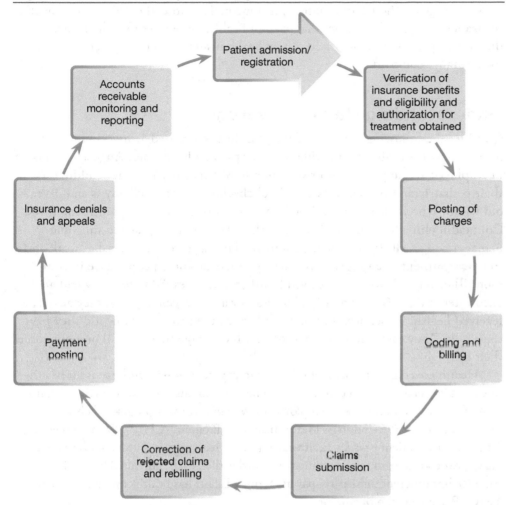

After patient admission or registration, the next step in revenue cycle management is to verify insurance benefits and eligibility. As you learned in Chapter 4, **admission/registration clerks** (also called *patient access specialists*) are generally responsible for entering insurance information into the EHR system at the time the patient is admitted to an inpatient hospital or scheduled for treatment at an outpatient facility or physician's office. Following insurance data entry, the admission/registration clerk or **insurance verifier** must confirm the patient's insurance coverage with the insurance company. The purpose of this insurance verification process is twofold: (1) to ensure that the patient has active coverage and (2) to determine important billing aspects of the insurance plan, such as the guarantor, guarantor information, covered dependents, copayments, deductibles, and any other limitations or payment rules. The verification process will be explored later in this chapter.

10.1 Health Insurance

You are likely familiar with the concept of insurance because you most likely have car insurance, homeowner's insurance, or life insurance. With any type of insurance, an individual makes a specified number of consistent payments called a **premium** to a company in exchange for payment if something occurs, such as a car accident, death, storm damage to a house, or healthcare treatment. Therefore, the definition of **health insurance** is a type of insurance that pays for healthcare services that are incurred by the insured person(s). In our discussion of health insurance, the third-party payer is the insurance company.

Understanding Health Coverage

Consider the following scenarios. Samuel Elliott is a retired army captain who recently saw his healthcare provider for unexplained headaches. Angela Singh is an unemployed single parent with two children. She recently took her children to their pediatrician for their back-to-school checkups. Hazel Bellamy is an 83-year-old widow who is also a retired librarian. Hazel just made an appointment at the Coumadin clinic for a blood check. Matthew Foltz is a 25-year-old full-time manager at a small, family-owned company. He was recently injured at work and sought treatment at an urgent care facility. What do these people have in common? They have all recently received healthcare services. Whether they had an encounter at a physician's office, a hospital, or an emergency room, they all received healthcare services and then a bill from the provider. How did they pay their bills? They each had some type of health coverage that paid all or a portion of their bills.

Health coverage is the legal entitlement to payment or reimbursement for healthcare costs, generally under a contract with a health insurance company, a group health plan offered in connection with employment, or a government program such as Medicare, Medicaid, or the Children's Health Insurance Program (CHIP). When someone other than the patient pays for healthcare services, that entity is referred to as a **third-party payer**. In the group of scenarios discussed earlier, each individual has health coverage but different third-party payers. Samuel Elliott has health coverage through TRICARE, a federal program for retired military. Angela Singh has Medicaid, a state-administered health insurance program for low-income families and children. Hazel Bellamy has Medicare, a federal health insurance program for people who are age 65 or older. And Matthew Foltz is insured by a traditional health insurance company, in which his mother is the subscriber through her employer. Each of these types of health coverage will be discussed further in this chapter.

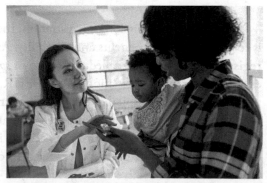

A checkup with a pediatrician can be covered by private insurance, Medicare, or the Children's Health Insurance Program (CHIP).

Evolution of Health Insurance

Over the course of the past century, there have been many significant advancements in the health insurance industry in the United States. The Affordable Care Act (ACA) has been the most recent, major legislative change in health insurance, but the discussion about a national health insurance system for Americans goes back much further.

Insurance Timeline

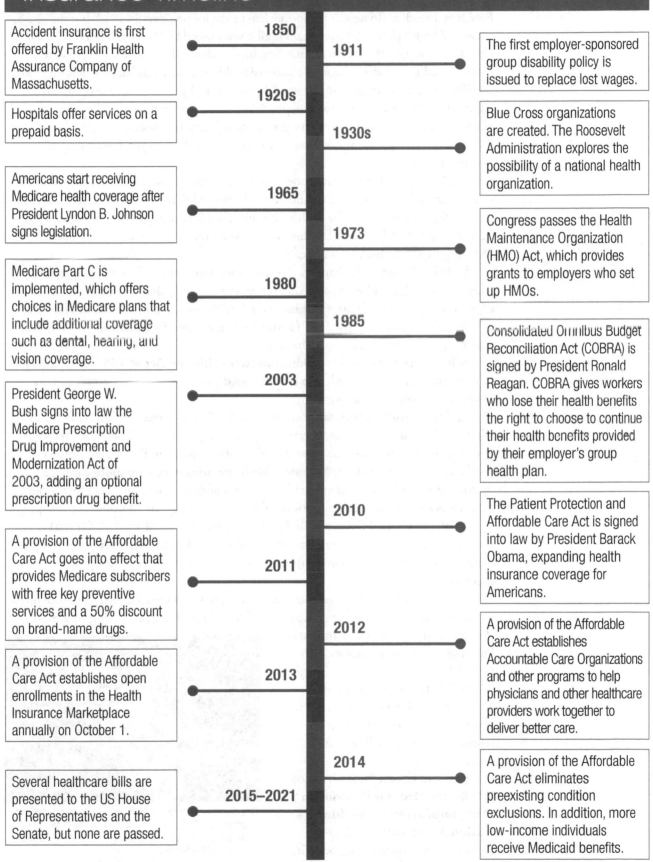

1850 — Accident insurance is first offered by Franklin Health Assurance Company of Massachusetts.

1911 — The first employer-sponsored group disability policy is issued to replace lost wages.

1920s — Hospitals offer services on a prepaid basis.

1930s — Blue Cross organizations are created. The Roosevelt Administration explores the possibility of a national health organization.

1965 — Americans start receiving Medicare health coverage after President Lyndon B. Johnson signs legislation.

1973 — Congress passes the Health Maintenance Organization (HMO) Act, which provides grants to employers who set up HMOs.

1980 — Medicare Part C is implemented, which offers choices in Medicare plans that include additional coverage such as dental, hearing, and vision coverage.

1985 — Consolidated Omnibus Budget Reconciliation Act (COBRA) is signed by President Ronald Reagan. COBRA gives workers who lose their health benefits the right to choose to continue their health benefits provided by their employer's group health plan.

2003 — President George W. Bush signs into law the Medicare Prescription Drug Improvement and Modernization Act of 2003, adding an optional prescription drug benefit.

2010 — The Patient Protection and Affordable Care Act is signed into law by President Barack Obama, expanding health insurance coverage for Americans.

2011 — A provision of the Affordable Care Act goes into effect that provides Medicare subscribers with free key preventive services and a 50% discount on brand-name drugs.

2012 — A provision of the Affordable Care Act establishes Accountable Care Organizations and other programs to help physicians and other healthcare providers work together to deliver better care.

2013 — A provision of the Affordable Care Act establishes open enrollments in the Health Insurance Marketplace annually on October 1.

2014 — A provision of the Affordable Care Act eliminates preexisting condition exclusions. In addition, more low-income individuals receive Medicaid benefits.

2015–2021 — Several healthcare bills are presented to the US House of Representatives and the Senate, but none are passed.

History of National Health Insurance and Medicare

A discussion regarding how to deal with health insurance for Americans was part of President Theodore Roosevelt's platform when he ran for president in 1912, but the idea for a national health plan didn't gain steam until it was pushed by President Harry S Truman. On November 19, 1945, seven months into his presidency, Truman sent a message to Congress, calling for the creation of a national health insurance fund open to all Americans.

The plan Truman envisioned would provide health coverage to individuals, paying for typical expenses such as physician visits, hospital visits, laboratory services, dental care, and nursing services. Although Truman fought to get a bill passed during his term, he was unsuccessful, and it was another 20 years before Medicare became a reality.

President John F. Kennedy made his own unsuccessful push for a national healthcare program for seniors after a national study showed that 56% of Americans over the age of 65 were not covered by health insurance, but it wasn't until 1965—after legislation was signed by President Lyndon B. Johnson—that eligible Americans started receiving Medicare health coverage.

In 1972, President Richard M. Nixon signed into law the first major change to Medicare. The legislation expanded coverage to include individuals under the age of 65 with long-term disabilities and individuals with end-stage renal disease (ESRD).

In 1973, Congress passed the **Health Maintenance Organization (HMO) Act**, which provided grants to employers who set up HMOs.

When Congress passed the **Omnibus Reconciliation Act of 1980**, it expanded home health services. The bill also brought **Medigap**—or Medicare supplemental insurance—under federal oversight.

In 1982, **hospice services** for the terminally ill were added to a growing list of Medicare benefits. That same year, other legislation gave those eligible for Medicare coverage more options on the private market when Medicare Part C, also known as *Medicare Advantage*, was implemented. Medicare Advantage gave more coverage options in the private insurance market and also added options such as prescription drug coverage for Medicare subscribers who wished to pay for additional coverage.

The Consolidated Omnibus Budget Reconciliation Act of 1985 (COBRA) is a health benefit act that Congress passed in 1986 requiring an employer to extend group health coverage to a terminated employee and their dependents at group rates for a specified period.

In 1996, Congress required most employer-sponsored group health insurance plans to accept transfers from other group plans without imposing a preexisting condition clause as a part of the Health Insurance Portability and Accountability Act (HIPAA).

In 2001, Congress expanded Medicare benefits to cover younger people with amyotrophic lateral sclerosis (ALS) upon diagnosis of the disease.

President George W. Bush signed into law the **Medicare Prescription Drug Improvement and Modernization Act of 2003**, adding an optional prescription drug benefit.

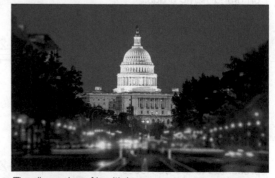

The discussion of health insurance has taken place in Washington, D.C., for decades, from the creation of Medicare to the Affordable Care Act (ACA) to possible changes in the future.

Until that time, about 25% of those receiving Medicare coverage did not have a prescription drug plan.

In 2019, the federal government covered 37% of Americans' healthcare costs. This is up from 26% in 2013. In 2019, private health insurance spending covered 31% of Americans' healthcare costs. National health spending is projected to grow at an average annual rate of 5.4% from 2019 to 2028 and to reach $6.2 trillion by 2028. Among major payers, Medicare is expected to experience the fastest spending growth (7.6% per year from 2019 to 2028), largely as a result of having the highest projected enrollment growth.

Today, Medicare continues to provide insurance coverage for qualified individuals over the age of 65 and those with certain predetermined conditions. By the end of 2020, 62.8 million Americans were covered by Medicare (up from just under 50 million in 2014), and 76.5 million Americans were covered by Medicaid (up from 67 million in 2014). It is clear from these statistics that the enrollment in government-funded healthcare programs continues to increase significantly.

Affordable Care Act

Federal legislation that has significantly affected the healthcare and insurance industries is the **Affordable Care Act (ACA)**. It was enacted in March 2010, with the goal of providing quality, affordable health care for all Americans. This comprehensive law was enacted in two parts: the **Patient Protection and Affordable Care Act** was signed into law on March 23, 2010, and was amended by the **Health Care and Education Reconciliation Act** on March 30, 2010. The name *Affordable Care Act* refers to the final, amended version of the law.

The ACA provides Americans with better health security by putting in place comprehensive health insurance reforms that:

- Expand coverage

- Hold insurance companies accountable

- Lower healthcare costs

- Guarantee more choice

- Enhance the quality of care for all Americans

To accomplish this, the ACA required immediate improvements in healthcare coverage for all Americans, preserved and expanded insurance coverage, and made insurance coverage available for all Americans. Provisions of the ACA continued to effect changes in health coverage from 2011 through 2014.

Insurance Terminology

Insurance can be a difficult topic to navigate. It is important to be familiar with the different terms used when discussing insurance to give you a better understanding of health insurance concepts.

A subscriber is the person whose insurance coverage is used for acute or outpatient care. This is the person who usually pays for the health insurance (insurance premiums) and/or whose employment makes them eligible for enrollment in a health insurance plan. Again, using our group of insured individuals, Samuel Elliott and Hazel Bellamy are the subscribers for their health insurance. Angela Singh is the subscriber for herself and her two children, and Matthew's mother is the subscriber for his health insurance coverage.

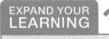

EXPAND YOUR LEARNING

Watch the video found at https://EHR3.ParadigmEducation.com/ACA-Video to experience an overview of the ACA.

EXPAND YOUR LEARNING

Have you ever thought about what goes into a medical bill? Many people find medical bills to be very complicated. The video "What Goes into a Medical Bill?" at https://EHR3.ParadigmEducation.com/MedicalBill-Video helps explain the components of a medical bill.

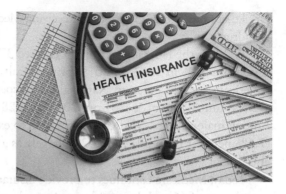

The insurance premium is the amount that the subscriber pays to the insurance company. The money is usually paid in regular installments, such as monthly, in exchange for insurance coverage.

Coinsurance is the insured person's share of the costs of a covered healthcare service, calculated as a percentage (for example, 20%) of the allowed amount for the service. The insured individual pays coinsurance plus any portion of the deductible they still owe. For example, if the plan's allowed amount for an office visit is $100 and the individual has met their deductible, the coinsurance payment of 20% would be $20. The plan pays the rest of the allowed amount.

A **copayment** is a fixed amount that an insured individual pays for a covered healthcare service, usually at the time the service is provided. For example, an individual may pay $15 for a visit to a physician. The amount can vary by the type of covered healthcare service, such as office visits, emergency room visits, or prescription medications.

The **out-of-pocket amount** includes expenses for medical care that are not reimbursed by the insurance company. Out-of-pocket costs include deductibles, coinsurance, and copayments for covered services plus all costs for services that are not covered.

The **allowed amount** is the maximum amount on which payment is based for covered healthcare services. The allowed amount is how much the insurance carrier has agreed to pay for the visit and is negotiated between the insurance carrier and the provider. This amount may also be referred to as *eligible expense*, *payment allowance*, or *negotiated rate*. If the healthcare provider charges more than the allowed amount, the insured individual may have to pay the difference.

The **benefit year** is the year of insurance benefits coverage under an individual health insurance plan. January 1 to December 31 is a typical benefit year, although many plans may have benefit years that do not align with the calendar year, such as April 1 to March 31.

A cap on the benefits the insurance company will pay in a year is called the **annual limit**. These caps are sometimes placed on particular services, such as prescriptions or hospitalizations. Annual limits may be placed on the dollar amount of covered services or on the number of visits that will be covered for a particular service. After an annual limit is reached, the insured individual must pay all associated healthcare costs for the rest of the year.

A cap on the total lifetime benefits an individual may receive from the insurance company is called a **lifetime limit**. An insurance company may impose a total lifetime dollar limit on benefits (such as a $1 million lifetime cap) or limits on specific benefits (such as a $200,000 lifetime cap on organ transplants or one gastric bypass per lifetime), or a combination of the two. After a lifetime limit is reached, the insurance plan may no longer pay for covered services. The ACA created policies that changed the ways some insurance companies handle lifetime limits.

The **guarantor** is the individual responsible for payment. An example might be a woman who obtains health insurance coverage through her employer for herself as well as her spouse and children. In such an example, the woman is the guarantor or subscriber, and the spouse and children are **covered dependents**.

A **deductible** is the amount an insured individual must pay out of pocket before the insurance will pay. This payment must be met before insurance coverage can be applied to healthcare services. For example, a family insurance plan may have a $25 copayment every time a parent takes their sick child to the pediatrician. That same family may have a deductible of $800 a year for healthcare services such as laboratory tests, x-rays, and hospitalizations before their insurance provider pays the remaining balance of any services rendered. Once the bill has been submitted to the insurance company, the deductible is calculated. The insurance company sends payment to the healthcare facility and a copy of the explanation of benefits (EOB) to the guarantor. The EOB describes the details of how the insurance company paid the healthcare bill. The healthcare facility subsequently bills the guarantor for the remaining balance of the bill that the insurance company did not pay.

Classifying Insurance Plans

Insurance plans are classified as either group health insurance plans or individual health insurance plans. An **individual health insurance plan** is an insurance plan that an individual purchases for themselves and/or their family. For example, John Smith's employer does not offer a group health insurance plan for its employees, so John purchases an individual health insurance plan to provide coverage for himself and his family. A **group health insurance plan** provides healthcare coverage to a specific group of people, typically based on an employer. For example, employees of ABC Chemical Manufacturing are the specific group of people that are eligible to sign up for the group health insurance plan offered by the company. Group health insurance plans typically cost less than individual plans as the employer pays a portion of the health insurance premium for their employees.

Traditionally, health insurance plans have been fee-for-service plans in which the healthcare provider is reimbursed for every test, procedure, and service they provide. The fee-for-service healthcare plans have proven to be too expensive for insurance companies as there is no incentive for the healthcare provider to manage the number and types of services performed, making it difficult for an insurance company to estimate or manage costs. Managed health insurance plans, or managed care plans, have replaced most fee-for-service plans in an effort to reduce costs by giving subscribers choices in their health care that impose certain rules or restrictions. Examples of managed care plan rules include limited choices in the selection of a healthcare provider, required referrals from a primary care physician to receive treatment from a specialist, prior authorization for surgical procedures or admission to a hospital, and so on. There are three basic types of managed care plans: health maintenance organizations (HMOs), preferred provider organizations (PPOs), and point of service (POS). Coverage is determined by in-network or out-of-network use.

Health Maintenance Organization

A **health maintenance organization (HMO)** is a type of health insurance plan that usually limits coverage to include care only from physicians who work for or contract with the HMO. It generally will not cover out-of-network care except in an emergency. An HMO may require individuals to live or work in its service area to be eligible for coverage.

As discussed in Chapter 7, a *care plan*, also known as a *treatment plan* or *plan of care*, is a patient's road map to better health, developed and executed by the entire clinical team in conjunction with the patient. A new approach to health care is called *integrated care*.

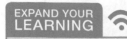

EXPAND YOUR LEARNING

Mental health is an important aspect of integrated care. Watch this video to learn how psychologists are playing a vital role in integrated care: https://EHR3 .ParadigmEducation .com/IntegratedCare.

Integrated care is the systematic coordination of health care. According to the World Health Organization, integrated care brings together inputs, delivery, management, and organization of services related to diagnosis, treatment, care, rehabilitation, and health promotion. In other words, the care plan focuses on the immediate needs of a patient within one setting, while integrated care involves the coordination of care across settings and beyond the scope of the initial visit or admission. HMOs often provide integrated care and focus on prevention and wellness.

Preferred Provider Organization

A **preferred provider organization (PPO)** is a type of health plan that contracts with medical providers, such as hospitals and physicians, to create a network of participating providers. Individuals pay less if they use providers that belong to the plan's network. They can use physicians, hospitals, and providers outside of the network for an additional cost.

Point of Service Plan

Point of service (POS) plans are considered to be a hybrid of HMOs and PPOs. The POS plans are considered to be the most flexible managed care insurance plans as they are less restrictive in the choice of providers and networks. For example, members do not have to choose an in-network physician, but they do need a referral from their primary care physician to go out of network. Another benefit of the POS plans is that the national network of providers is available to members when they are traveling. POS plans are more flexible than HMOs and typically cost less than PPOs, making POS plans a good choice for many individuals looking for lower-cost insurance without sacrificing choice.

Value-Based Plan

While most health insurance plans have transitioned from a fee-for-service basis to a managed care model, some insurance companies and other payers are now transitioning to value-based health insurance plans. With value-based plans, healthcare providers are still reimbursed for the services they provide, but they also receive incentive payments or reductions in payments based on patient outcomes. Value-based plans are structured so that the healthcare providers delivering the highest quality care will have the best patient outcomes and, therefore, receive the highest reimbursement. Medicare has several value-based programs in place such as the hospital readmission reduction program, the hospital acquired conditions program, the skilled nursing value-based program, and the home health value-based program. Medicare and other payers are expected to continue to develop more value-based programs in the future.

Consolidated Omnibus Budget Reconciliation Act

The **Consolidated Omnibus Budget Reconciliation Act (COBRA)** is a federal law that may allow individuals to temporarily keep health coverage after their employment ends, they lose coverage as a dependent of the covered employee, or another qualifying event occurs. If a person elects COBRA coverage, they pay 100% of the premiums, including the share the employer used to pay, plus a small administrative fee.

Insurance Classification of Healthcare Providers

Insurance coverage and costs are determined by the relationship of the insurance plan and the healthcare providers. In this regard, healthcare providers are separated into two categories: in-network and out-of-network.

In-Network

In-network includes providers or healthcare facilities that are part of a health plan's group of providers with which it has negotiated a discount. Insured individuals usually pay less when using an in-network provider, because those networks provide services at a lower cost to the insurance companies they have contracts with.

Out-of-Network

Out-of-network usually refers to physicians, hospitals, or other healthcare providers who are considered nonparticipants in an insurance plan (usually an HMO or a PPO). Depending on an individual's health insurance plan, expenses incurred from services provided by out-of-network health professionals may not be covered or may be only partially covered by an individual's insurance company.

Let's review some examples to make this concept clearer.

- ABC City Hospital is located in a large metropolitan area in which there are nine hospitals within a 20-square-mile area. Cobalt Care, a private payer, reduces costs of health care for the PPO plan it offers by contracting with only four of the nine hospitals in the area. ABC City Hospital is not one of the four hospitals that Cobalt Care has contracted with, so ABC City Hospital is considered out of network. A patient with the Cobalt Care PPO plan would most likely not want to receive healthcare services at ABC City Hospital, or the patient would likely be responsible for the entire hospital bill.

- Eloise Davis has healthcare insurance through an ApolloHealth HMO plan. Eloise should check the listing of physicians who have a contract with the ApolloHealth HMO plan before trying to schedule an office visit.

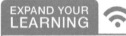

EXPAND YOUR LEARNING

Healthcare services and treatment in the United States can be quite expensive, as you may know from personal experience. Visit https://EHR3 .ParadigmEducation .com/FairHealth to identify the average costs of treatment.

CHECKPOINT 10.1

1. Name the type of health insurance plan that usually limits coverage to care from physicians who work for or contract with the insurance organization.

   _____

2. Name the type of health plan that contracts with medical providers, such as hospitals and physicians, to create a network of participating providers.

   _____

3. Name the federal law that may allow individuals to temporarily keep health coverage after employment ends.

   _____

Government-Sponsored Healthcare Programs

The US government sponsors five major healthcare programs: Medicare, Medicaid, TRICARE, CHAMPVA, and workers' compensation. There are specific eligibility requirements for each of these programs.

Medicare

Medicare is a federal health insurance program for people who are aged 65 or older and certain younger people with disabilities. It also covers people with end-stage renal disease (permanent kidney failure requiring dialysis or a transplant, sometimes called *ESRD*). Medicare has four parts: Part A, Part B, Part C, and Part D.

Part A Hospital Insurance Medicare **Part A** (hospital insurance) helps cover inpatient care in hospitals, including critical access hospitals and skilled nursing facilities (not custodial or long-term care). It also helps cover hospice care and some home health care. Most people don't pay a premium for Part A because they or their spouses have already paid for it through their payroll taxes while working. Beneficiaries must meet certain conditions to receive these benefits.

Part B Medical Insurance Medicare **Part B** (medical insurance) helps cover physicians' services and outpatient care. It also covers some other medical services that Part A doesn't cover, such as physical and occupational therapies and some home health care. Part B helps pay for covered services and supplies when they are medically necessary. Most people pay a monthly premium for Part B.

Medicare Part C Medicare **Part C** is also known as *Medicare Advantage Plans*, or *MA Plans*. These plans are offered through private companies approved by the Centers for Medicare & Medicaid Services (CMS). People who select a Medicare Advantage Plan will have Medicare Part A and Part B through their Advantage Plan and not CMS.

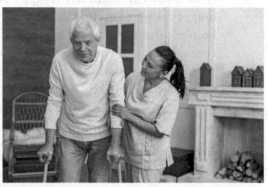

Medicare Part A helps cover inpatient care, skilled nursing facility care, and some home health care for people aged 65 or older.

Medicare Part D Medicare **Part D** is a program that helps pay for prescription drugs for Medicare beneficiaries who have a plan that includes Medicare prescription drug coverage. There are two ways to get Medicare prescription drug coverage: through a Medicare Prescription Drug Plan or a Medicare Advantage Plan that includes drug coverage. Both these plans are offered by insurance companies and other private companies approved by Medicare.

Medicaid

Medicaid is a state-administered health insurance program for low-income families and children, pregnant women, the elderly, people with disabilities, and in some states, other qualified adults. The federal government provides a portion of the funding for Medicaid and sets guidelines for the program. States also have choices in how they design their programs, so Medicaid benefits vary state by state and may have a different name in your state.

CHAMPVA and TRICARE

Due to the similarity between CHAMPVA (Civilian Health and Medical Program of the Department of Veterans Affairs) and the Department of Defense (DoD) TRICARE program (sometimes referred to by its old name, *CHAMPUS*), the two are often mistaken for each other. **CHAMPVA** is a comprehensive healthcare benefits program in which the Department of Veterans Affairs (VA) shares the cost of covered healthcare services and supplies with eligible beneficiaries. **TRICARE** is a DoD regionally managed healthcare program for active duty and retired members of the uniformed services, their families, and survivors.

Workers' Compensation

Workers' compensation is an insurance plan that employers are required to have to cover employees who get sick or injured on the job. Workers' compensation is managed by state governments, and rules and guidelines vary from state to state.

States will typically reimburse injured employees covered by workers' compensation with four types of payment, which include income replacement benefits, healthcare treatment, mileage reimbursement, and burial and death benefits.

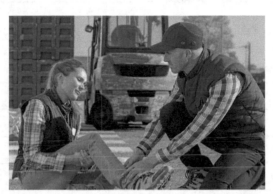

For those who are injured while on the job, workers' compensation can provide income replacement benefits.

Income Replacement

Benefits With income replacement benefits, states categorize the lost income of injured employees in one of four ways. These include **temporary total disability (TTD) benefits, temporary partial disability (TPD) benefits, permanent total disability (PTD) benefits**, and **permanent partial disability (PPD) benefits**. TTD benefits are paid when an employee has been injured at work and cannot perform their work duties. TPD benefits are paid when an employee works in a reduced capacity but cannot work to the same extent as they could before their injury or illness. PTD benefits are paid when the worker's injury permanently prevents the worker from returning to their former occupation. PPD benefits are paid when medical maximum improvement has been achieved and a worker may be able to work in some capacity, but the injury has caused damage for an indefinite period and they cannot return to their old occupation. As mentioned previously, benefits vary from state to state. For example, an injured worker in Ohio qualifying for TTD benefits would be paid for 12 weeks at 72% of the preinjury average weekly wage, and after the first 12 weeks, the worker would receive 66% of the weekly wage. If this injured worker qualified for the same workers' compensation benefits in California, the worker would receive approximately 66% of the preinjury average weekly wages for the entire covered period.

Healthcare Treatment
With the workers' compensation payment for **healthcare treatment**, the medical provider who treats the work-related injury or illness will be paid directly by the patient's employer's insurer.

Mileage Reimbursement
An employee injured at work who must travel to their medical appointments will receive **mileage reimbursement** from their employer for the mileage cost and for some of the wages they lose while in transit to and from and during their appointments.

Burial and Death   Dependents of an employee who dies from a work-related illness or injury are entitled to **burial and death benefits**. Death benefits are used to replace a portion of the employee's lost income due to the work-related illness or injury. A surviving spouse, minor children, and other dependents of the deceased employee may receive eligible death benefits. Death benefits are typically 75% of the employee's average weekly wages. Burial benefits may be paid to the person who paid for the deceased employee's burial expenses.

CHECKPOINT 10.2

1. Name the five major healthcare programs that are government sponsored.

   _____

   _____

   _____

   _____

2. Name the federal health insurance program for people who are aged 65 or older and for certain younger people with disabilities.

   _____

3. List the four types of payment covered by workers' compensation.

   _____

   _____

   _____

   _____

Verification of Insurance Coverage and Benefits

Major insurance plans have web pages for online eligibility requests (called *eligibility databases*) to determine coverage and benefits for their subscribers. In addition, providers may choose to partner with vendors that provide online responses to queries about all major insurance plans. Medicare and Medicaid also have online eligibility databases for providers to query their patients' eligibility, benefits, and in the case of Medicare, the number of coverage days in categories such as inpatient and skilled nursing facility. The Medicare eligibility database application is called the **HIPAA Eligibility Transaction System (HETS)**. The application provides access to Medicare beneficiary eligibility data in a real-time environment. Figure 10.2 is an example of a portion of a typical response from a search in the HETS. The actual response would continue for several additional pages.

Due to the difficulty of deciphering the HETS response, many providers choose to subscribe to a third-party vendor for Medicare inquiries. These vendors provide the data in a format that is easier to read.

See Table 10.1 for information on where to find coverage and benefits for veterans' and Medicaid subscribers.

In Chapter 4, you learned how to read an insurance card as presented by a patient and how to enter this information into the EHR. Figure 10.3 shows an example of a Medicare subscriber's insurance card.

EHR systems have a listing of the insurance plans that the provider accepts and from which they will receive reimbursement. Figure 10.4 illustrates the drop-down screen of accepted insurance providers in the EHR Navigator.

A provider of healthcare services must be eligible to receive reimbursement from an insurance payer, as not all healthcare providers are able to receive reimbursement from all insurance payers.

Figure 10.2 HETS Eligibility Response

```
□0000004511□
ISA*00* *00* *ZZ*CMS *ZZ*SUBMITTERID *150127*0758*^*00501*111111111*0*P*|~
GS*HB*CMS*SUBMITTERID*20150127*07580000*1*X*005010X279A1~
ST*271*0001*005010X279A1~
BHT*0022*11*TRANSA*20150127*07582355~
HL*1**20*1~
NM1*PR*2*CMS*****PI*CMS~
PER*IC**UR*http://www.cms.gov/HETSHelp/*UR*http://www.cms.gov/center/provider.asp~
HL*2*1*21*1~
NM1*1P*2*IRNAME*****XX*1234567893~
HL*3*2*22*0~
TRN*2*TRACKNUM*ABCDEFGHIJ~
NM1*IL*1*LNAME*FNAME*M***MI*123456789A~
N3*ADDRESSLINE1*ADDRESSLINE2~
N4*CITY*ST*ZIPCODE~
DMG*D8*19400401*F~
DTP*307*RD8*20150101-20150327~
EB*6**30~
DTP*307*RD8*20150101-20150108~
EB*I**41^54~
EB*1**88~
EB*1**30^10^42^45^48^49^69^76^83^A5^A7^AG^BT^BU^BV*MA~
DTP*291*D8*20050401~
EB*C**30*MA**26*1260~
```

Table 10.1 Coverage and Benefits

Benefits Program	Contact Information	Website
Veterans	US Department of Veterans Affairs (VA) 1-800-827-1000	www.va.gov
TRICARE	1-866-773-0404	www.tricare.osd.mil
Medicaid	Contact each state medical assistance (Medicaid) office.	www.medicaid.gov

Figure 10.3 Medicare Card

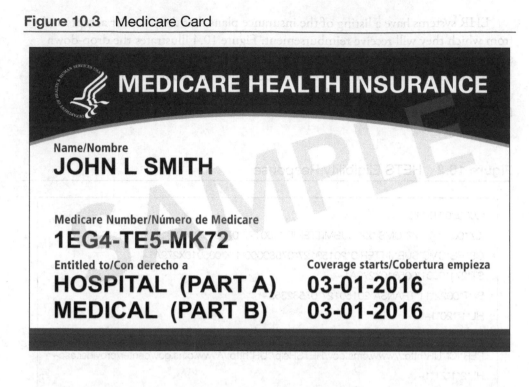

Figure 10.4 Insurance Companies in EHR Navigator

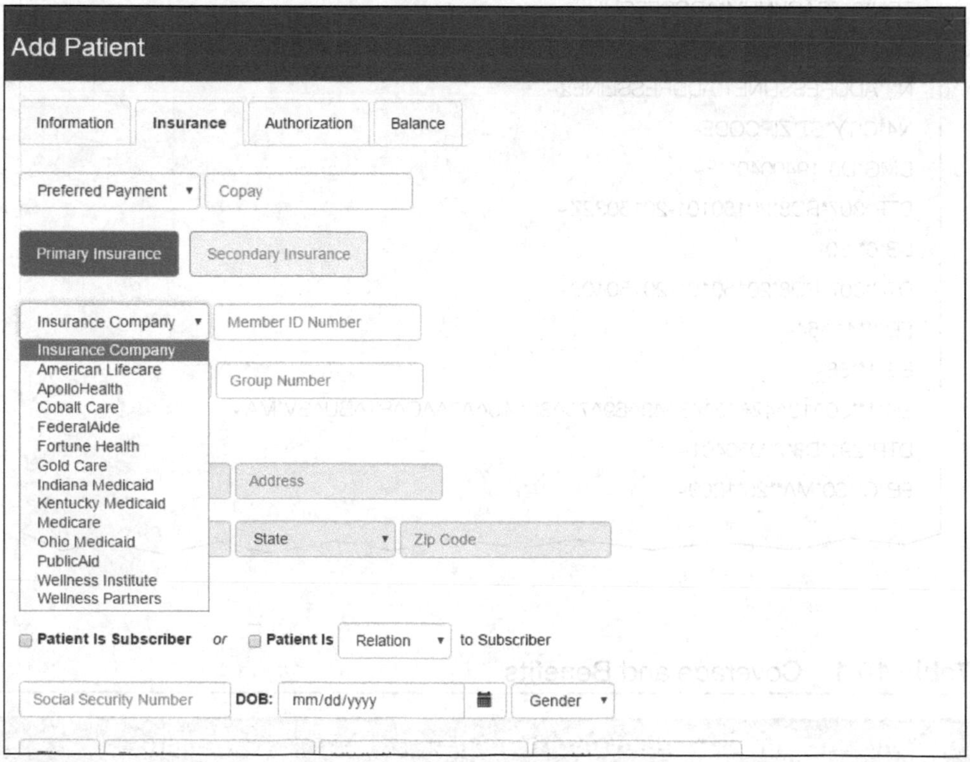

10.2 The Billing Process

Practice management is the day-to-day operations of a medical practice. An important function in a medical practice is the coding and billing for medical services rendered to patients.

The billing aspect of a medical practice is intricate and includes claims processing, claims management, revenue management, and reporting. Successful practice management in today's medical practice most often uses an electronic office billing system. Electronic office billing systems are used to process insurance claims. Billing staff members also need to follow up on the claims that have been billed and learn how to manage the revenue cycle. Electronic office billing systems include many practice management reports that are useful to the practice managers and owners, which will be discussed in this chapter in greater detail.

As you learned in Chapter 4, accurate data gathering must begin before or upon the delivery of healthcare services. This typically begins at the time the patient is scheduled for a visit or treatment. Patient data—including demographics, insurance, and payment information—must be updated to ensure accurate billing and reimbursement. The method of payment (such as self-payment or insurance) must be verified and entered into the EHR system.

Following the provision of healthcare treatment or services, a healthcare provider should receive payment for these services.

It is imperative that all staff of a healthcare provider, such as a physician's office or hospital, understand the importance of the coordination of timely and accurate patient data entry, billing, and reimbursement. Receipt of monies due for services rendered is required to keep a healthcare organization financially stable and viable.

Electronic Billing

An EHR system may have a billing software component built in, or the EHR system may interface with a separate billing software program. The EHR Navigator has billing software built directly into the EHR system, so there is no need for separate billing software to interface with the EHR system. Built-in billing software is the preferred method because potential communication problems between the EHR system and the billing software are eliminated.

The **electronic superbill** is an itemized form that allows charges to be captured from a patient visit. The provider selects the appropriate reason for the visit and treatment rendered. A superbill typically consists of provider information, patient demographic and insurance information, and details regarding the visit, such as the diagnosis and procedure codes.

The process of entering medical codes into the billing system is called **charge entry**. Staff members can enter charges they are responsible for or that the provider missed during the electronic superbill entry, via the *Add Charges* button.

Once charge entry is complete, electronic claims are produced for insurance reimbursement for patients who have insurance coverage, and bills are produced for patients who do not have insurance coverage.

It is important that a provider's billing staff understand basic insurance terms and how to effectively navigate an electronic billing system.

Figure 10.5 shows an example of a superbill, also known as an *encounter form*, that may be used in an orthopedic office. The master encounter form includes the set fee schedule for the physician's office. Prior to the EHR, a paper superbill was completed by the provider. Now, the superbill is an EHR function, and paper forms are only used when the EHR system is unavailable.

Figure 10.5 Encounter Form

Patient Identification			Insurance Identification		
Date:			COMPANY NAME:		
Name:			Insurance #:		
Student ID #:					
DOB:		Gender:	Provider name/NPI:		
Confidential visit today? ☐ Yes ☐ No		SHQ needed today? ☐ Yes ☐ No	Provider signature:		

OFFICE VISIT			ON-SITE LAB TESTS		
ESTAB	NEW		X	CPT	DESCRIPTION
99211		Minimal eval.			No labs given
99212	99201	Problem focused		80061	Lipid panel
99213	99202	Expanded problem focused		81000	Urinalysis – dip stick
99214	99203	Detailed		81001	Urinalysis, auto. – microscopy
	99204	Comprehensive, mod. complexity, 45 min.		81002	Urinalysis, non-auto. – no microscopy
99215	99205	Comprehensive, high complexity		81003	Urinalysis, auto – no microscopy
99354	99354	*Add-on code to 99215 or 99205* Prolonged service; with patient contact; beyond 30-74 min.		81015	Urine – microscopic only

EPSDT WELL CHILD EXAM / PREVENTIVE MEDICINE				81025	Urine pregnancy test-by visual color
ESTAB	NEW	Consider use of Modifier 25 (write in +25 after code)		82270	Guiac, occult blood
99391	99381	Infant		82465	Cholesterol, total
99392	99382	1-4 years		82947	Glucose; quantitative; blood
99393	99383	5-11 years		82948	Glucose fingerstick
99394	99384	12-17 years		82962	Glucose monitoring device
99395	99385	18+ years		84703	hCG preg. test (urine) – qualitative

NUTRITION				85013	Hematocrit
97802		Medical nutritional therapy, initial assessment and intervention, individual, each 15 min		85018	Hemoglobin
97803		Medical nutritional therapy, re-assessment and intervention, individual, each 15 min		86308	Mono-spot screen
				86677	H. pylori antibody

PSYCHIATRIC THERAPEUTIC PROCEDURES			87210	Wet mount (e.g., saline) for infectious agents
90832	Psychotherapy, 30 minutes with patient and/or family member		87430	Streptococcus, group A (culture nonbillable)
90833	Psychotherapy, 30 minutes with patient and/or family member when performed with an evaluation and management service - add-on code		87491	Urine CT/GC – amplified probe nonbillable
90834	Psychotherapy, 45 minutes with patient and/or family member		87880	Streptococcus, group A (rapid strep test)
90836	Psychotherapy, 45 minutes with patient and/or family member when performed with an evaluation and management service - add-on code		Q0091	PAP smear, obtaining/preparation **Man. care only**
90837	Psychotherapy, 60 minutes with patient and/or family member		Q0111	Web prep, obtaining/preparation
90838	Psychotherapy, 60 minutes with patient and/or family member when performed with an evaluation and management service - add-on code		92567	Tympanometry – impedance testing

MEDICATIONS, SUPPLIES, AND DURABLE MEDICAL EQUIPMENT					PROCEDURES	
					10060	I&D simple
J0170	Adrenaline, epinephrine up to 1 ml	J7603	Albuterol, unit dose form, 1 mg		10120	I&D of foreign body, subcutaneous (simple)
J0560	Penicillin G, up to 600,000 units	A4614	Peak flow meter, hand-held		11730	Nail avulsion
J0570	Penicillin G, up to 1,200,000 units	A4266	Diaphragm device		11740	Evacuation of subungual hematoma
J0580	Penicillin G, up to 2,400,000 units	A4261	Cervical cap for contraceptive use		11750	Excision of nail and nail maxtix, partial or complete, for permanent removal
J0696	Ceftriaxone 250 mg. IM per vial	A4267	Condom, male			
J1055	Depo Provera 150 mg. IM	A4268	Condom, female		12001	Suturing – specify body part:
J1056	Medroxyprogesterone	A4269	Spermicidal agent		12031	Layer closure of wounds of scalp, axillae, trunk, and/or extremities (excluding hands and feet) 2.5 cm
J2550	Promethazine HCl, injection up to 50 mg	J8499 U1	Plan B or similar emergency contraception			
J7300	Intrauterine copper contraceptive	J7307	Etenogestrel contraceptive implant system		16000	Initial tx – first-degree burn (local), doc. % coverage and depth
J7302	Levonorgesterel-releasing intrauterine (Mirena)	S4989	IUD other than above (Progestacert)			
J7303	Hormone-containing vaginal ring (Nuvaring	S4993	Contraceptive pills for birth control		17110	Wart removal
J7304	Hormone-containing patch (OrthoEvra)	Q0144	Azithromycin oral powder 1 gm **Man. care only**		26641	Closed tx of carpometacarpal (thumb) dislocation
J7602	Albuterol, concentrated form, 1 mg				28190	Removal of foreign body, foot, subcutaneous
					29130	Application of finger splint (static)

IMMUNIZATIONS					30300	Removal of foreign body, intranasal	
IMMUNIZATION ADMINISTRATION					36415	Venipuncture	
90471	One immunization **Managed care only**	90472	Each additional vaccine **Managed care only**		54050	Destruction of lesion(s), penis	
VACCINATIONS					56501	Destruction of lesion(s), vulva	
90633	Hep A	90702	DT		57170	Diaphragm fitting	
90645	HIB(HbOC) [HibTITER]	90707	Measles, Mumps, Rubella		58300	IUD insertion	
90646	HIB(PRP-D) [ProHIBIT]	90712	Poliovirus		58301	IUD removal	
90647	HIB(PRP-OMP) [PedvaxHIB]	90713	IPV (polio)		69200	Removal foreign body from external auditory canal	
90648	HIB(PRP-T) ActHIB or Omni HIB]	90715	Tdap		69210	Removal impacted cerumen (one or both ears)	
90649 **HB**	HPV females 9-10 and 19-26	90716	Varicella SQ		87220	KOH for skin/hair/nails	
90649	HPV females 11-18	90718	Tetanus and Diphtheria (Td)		94640	Nebulizer treatment	
90657	Influenza (split virus 6-35 mo.)	90732	Pneumococcal polyvalent, SQ or IM		94010	Spirometry	
90658	Influenza (split virus 3 yrs+)	907033	Meningococcal (polysaccharide, SQ)				
90669	Pneumococcal conjugate, IM <5 yrs	90734	Meningococcal conjugate vaccine, sero-groups A, C, Y, and W-135 (tetravalent)				
90700	DTaP						
90701	DT	90744	Hep B 3 dose IM			TELEHEALTH SERVICE	
90660	Influenza virus vaccine, live, for intranasal use	90748	Heb B/Hib Combination IM		Q3014	Telehealth originating site facility fee	

FOLLOW-UP	REFERRAL
Return to EMC (follow-up date):	To:
To provider:	

DIAGNOSIS (ICD-9)
Code # and name

Northstar Medical Center

CMS-1500 and UB-04 Forms

Traditionally, insurance companies were billed for services provided in a physician's office using a paper billing form called the *CMS-1500*. The **CMS-1500** is a universal claim form accepted by Medicare, Medicaid, and most insurance payers. Figure 10.6 shows an example of the CMS-1500 claim form.

Figure 10.6   CMS-1500 (02-12) Universal Billing Form for
                  Physician Services

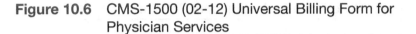

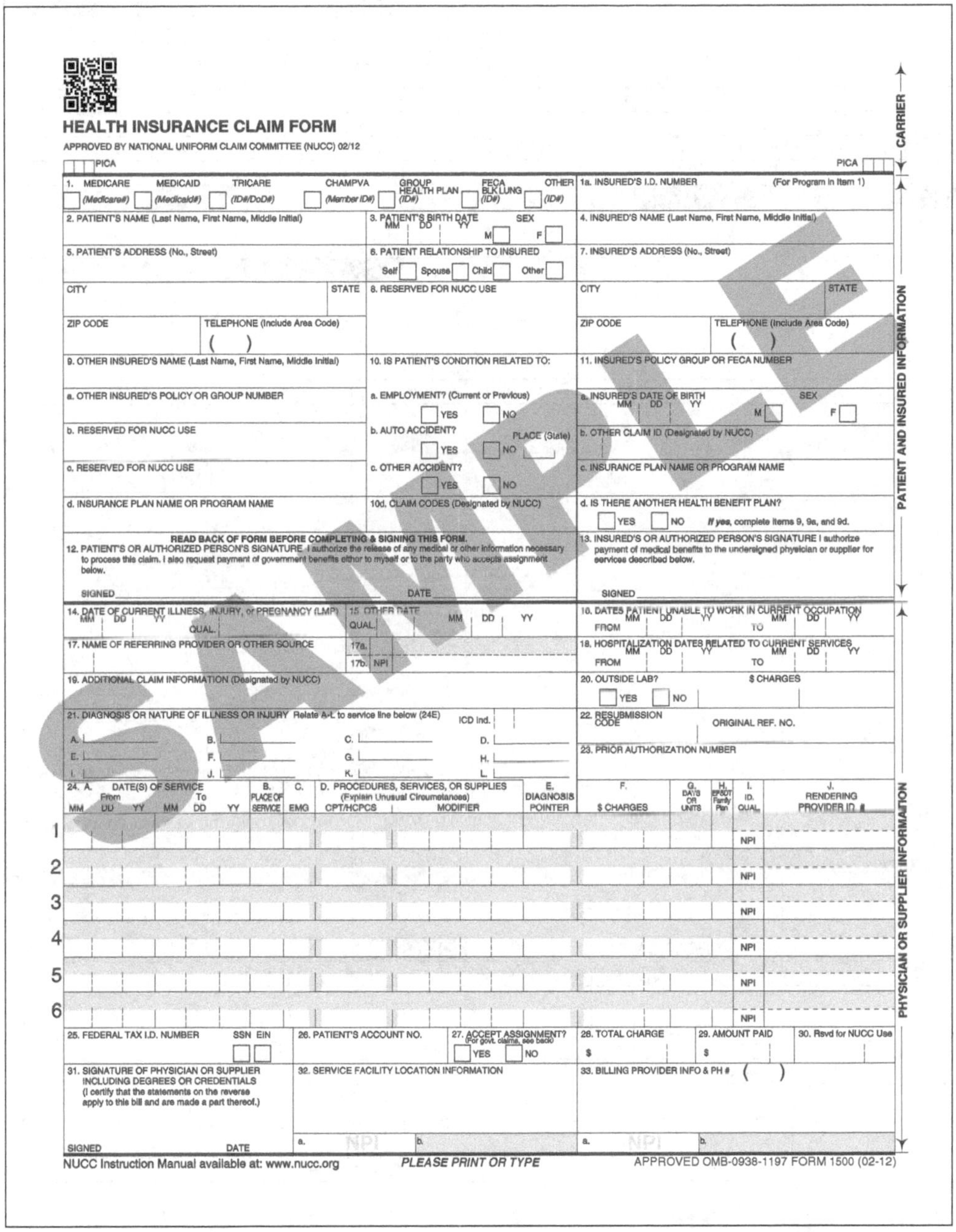

HIPAA regulations require that most claims now be processed electronically using the
HIPAA X12 837 Healthcare Claim, typically called the *837 Claim* or the *HIPAA Claim*.
The 837 Claim file is generated by the software and then transmitted to appropriate insurance payers. Depending on the volume of patients treated by the practice, claims may be filed weekly or even daily. Frequent claims processing should occur to keep cash flow steady.

In an inpatient facility, the UB-04 (also known as the *CMS-1450*) is the paper
form used to bill Medicare. It is also used for billing of institutional or hospital charges
to most Medicaid state agencies. The UB-04 contains pertinent information regarding
the patient's insurance coverage, medical provider, services provider, and diagnosis. It
also contains information that allows for the billing of outpatient services. Figure 10.7
illustrates a UB-04 form.

Figure 10.7 UB-04 (CMS-1450) Universal Billing Form for Institutional Providers

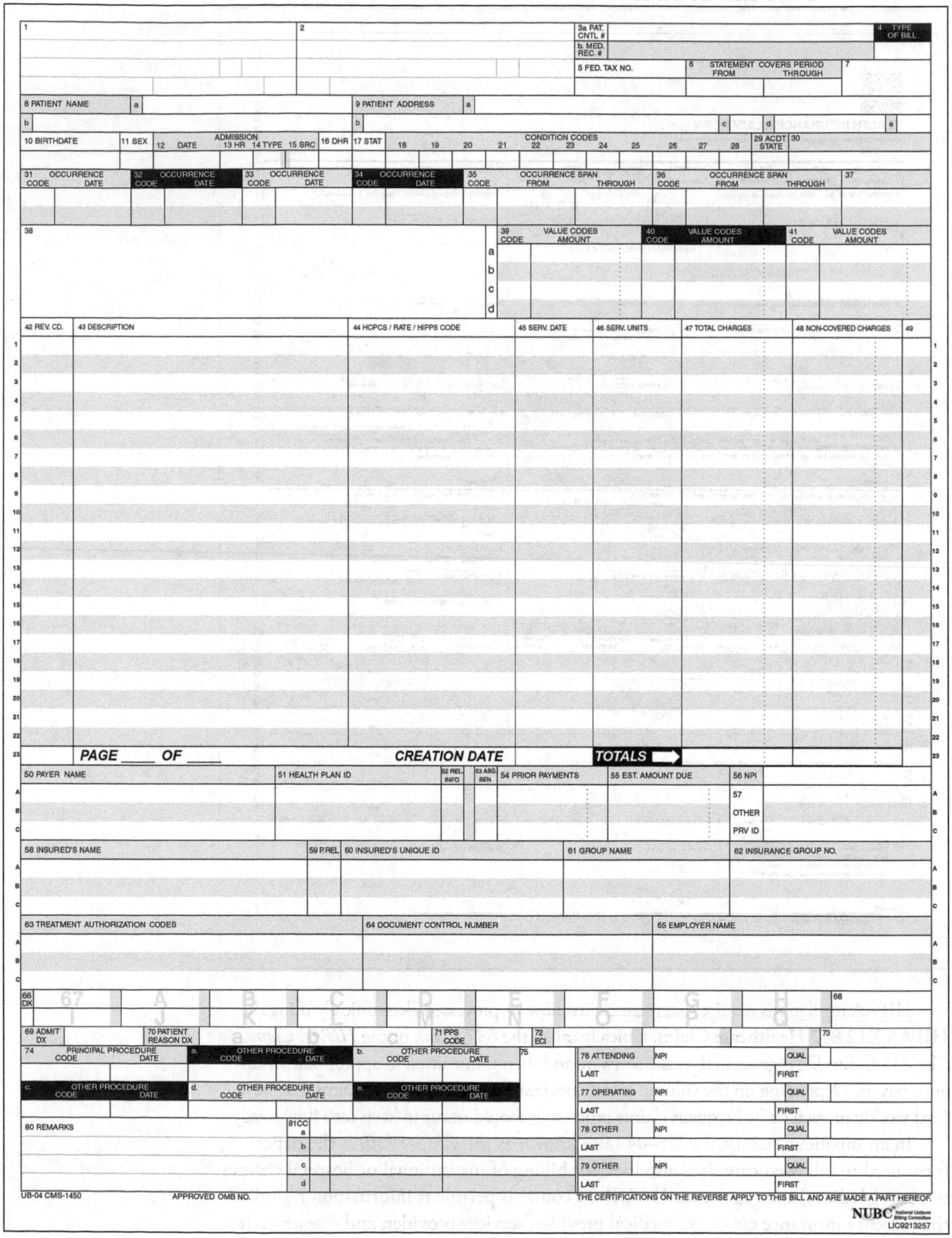
1
2
3a PAT. CNTL #
b. MED. REC. #
4 TYPE OF BILL
5 FED. TAX NO.
6 STATEMENT COVERS PERIOD FROM THROUGH
7
8 PATIENT NAME a
b
9 PATIENT ADDRESS a
b c d e
10 BIRTHDATE
11 SEX
ADMISSION 12 DATE 13 HR 14 TYPE 15 SRC
16 DHR
17 STAT
CONDITION CODES 18 19 20 21 22 23 24 25 26 27 28
29 ACDT STATE
30
31 OCCURRENCE CODE DATE
32 OCCURRENCE CODE DATE
33 OCCURRENCE CODE DATE
34 OCCURRENCE CODE DATE
35 CODE OCCURRENCE SPAN FROM THROUGH
36 CODE OCCURRENCE SPAN FROM THROUGH
37
38
39 CODE VALUE CODES AMOUNT
40 CODE VALUE CODES AMOUNT
41 CODE VALUE CODES AMOUNT
a b c d
42 REV. CD.
43 DESCRIPTION
44 HCPCS / RATE / HIPPS CODE
45 SERV. DATE
46 SERV. UNITS
47 TOTAL CHARGES
48 NON-COVERED CHARGES
49
1 2 3 4 5 6 7 8 9 10 11 12 13 14 15 16 17 18 19 20 21 22 23
PAGE ____ OF ____
CREATION DATE
TOTALS
50 PAYER NAME
51 HEALTH PLAN ID
52 REL. INFO
53 ASG. BEN.
54 PRIOR PAYMENTS
55 EST. AMOUNT DUE
56 NPI
57 OTHER PRV ID
A B C
58 INSURED'S NAME
59 P.REL
60 INSURED'S UNIQUE ID
61 GROUP NAME
62 INSURANCE GROUP NO.
A B C
63 TREATMENT AUTHORIZATION CODES
64 DOCUMENT CONTROL NUMBER
65 EMPLOYER NAME
A B C
66 DX
67 A B C D E F G H
I J K L M N O P Q
68
69 ADMIT DX
70 PATIENT REASON DX a b c
71 PPS CODE
72 ECI
73
74 PRINCIPAL PROCEDURE CODE DATE
a. OTHER PROCEDURE CODE DATE
b. OTHER PROCEDURE CODE DATE
75
76 ATTENDING NPI QUAL
LAST FIRST
c. OTHER PROCEDURE CODE DATE
d. OTHER PROCEDURE CODE DATE
e. OTHER PROCEDURE CODE DATE
77 OPERATING NPI QUAL
LAST FIRST
80 REMARKS
81CC a b c d
78 OTHER NPI QUAL
LAST FIRST
79 OTHER NPI QUAL
LAST FIRST
UB-04 CMS-1450
APPROVED OMB NO.
THE CERTIFICATIONS ON THE REVERSE APPLY TO THIS BILL AND ARE MADE A PART HEREOF.
NUBC National Uniform Billing Committee
LIC9213257

Tutorial 10.1   **EHR**NAVIGAT✛R

Populating a CMS-1500 Form

Go to your online course to launch Tutorial 10.1. Practice populating a CMS-1500 form.

Tutorial 10.2   **EHR**NAVIGAT✛R

Populating a UB-04 Form

Go to your online course to launch Tutorial 10.2. Practice populating a UB-04 form.

CHECKP✛INT 10.3

1. Define *practice management*.

   _____

2. Traditionally, insurance companies were billed for physician's services using *this* paper billing form.

   _____

3. Describe the 837 Claim file.

   _____

   _____

   _____

Benefits of Using an EHR for Billing Operations

Most EHR systems have a billing software component that may or may not be used by the healthcare organization. The decision to use the EHR's billing component depends on the sophistication of the organization's current billing software. Smaller healthcare organizations and physician practices are more likely to use the billing software component that comes with the EHR system that they implement. Hospitals and large physician practices are likely to already have a well-functioning billing system and may choose to interface it with the EHR system instead. An **interface** provides communication flow between two or more computer systems. If a healthcare organization chooses to interface the EHR system with the current billing or financial system, the patient record is easily accessible—which is an advantage to the billing staff. Regardless of which approach a healthcare organization chooses, an EHR system can have a positive influence on billing operations, including improved accuracy and efficiency of procedures.

Improved Accuracy

The implementation of an EHR system allows for better accuracy in healthcare claims. The software can check for billing errors as well as speed up the billing process. Faster billing typically improves cash flow for the healthcare facility. Using the EHR system for billing purposes may also eliminate having to chase down papers at the end of the business day. The system allows for daily charges to be reconciled and for staff to more easily determine what services and treatments were provided.

Improved Efficiency

In addition to improved accuracy, the use of an EHR system increases the efficiency of the billing process. No longer are patients and insurance companies provided with paper bills sent via the mail. EHR software

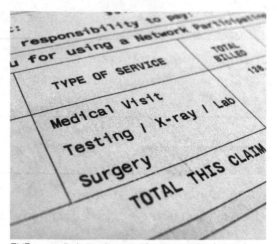

EHRs can eliminate the need for paper bills, improving efficiency of the billing process.

provides electronic billing and insurance forms, accesses the internet to securely send electronic bills or reminders to patients, submits claims to insurance companies and tracks their progress, checks for billing errors, provides data analysis tools related to medical office billing and finance, and more. All of these features allow for increased efficiency of the billing cycle, resulting in fewer rejected claims and a more robust monetary flow for the healthcare practice.

Superbills

As discussed earlier, a superbill (also known as an *encounter form*) is a staple of every physician office because it is a document that records the diagnosis and treatment for each patient at each visit. The content of superbills varies by healthcare organization and contains the common diagnoses and procedures charged by the healthcare organization. The superbill contains checkboxes next to the diagnoses, procedures, and associated International Statistical Classification of Diseases and Related Health Problems (ICD) and Current Procedural Terminology (CPT®) codes that are marked by the healthcare provider, such as the physician or nurse. Traditionally, a superbill has been a paper document that the patient carries from the check-in desk to the examination room and to areas of testing such as the laboratory and the radiology department. The electronic version of the superbill found in many EHR systems for use in the physician's office and outpatient setting looks very similar to the paper superbill that physicians and staff are used to. Figure 10.8 illustrates an electronic superbill. Figure 10.9 illustrates how charges are added to a superbill.

When used correctly, the superbill is a useful tool in coding compliance activities. (See Figure 10.10.) With the selection of the ICD and CPT® codes placed in the hands of the individual providing the healthcare service or treatment, coding should be accurate and consistent. When superbills are used, there must still be a review of the healthcare provider's documentation to ensure that the documentation supports the diagnoses and procedures selected on the superbill. A coder performs this review, and there must be frequent communication between the coder and the provider to ensure that the provider's superbill documentation and health record documentation are in sync.

Figure 10.8 Completed Electronic Superbill in the EHR Navigator

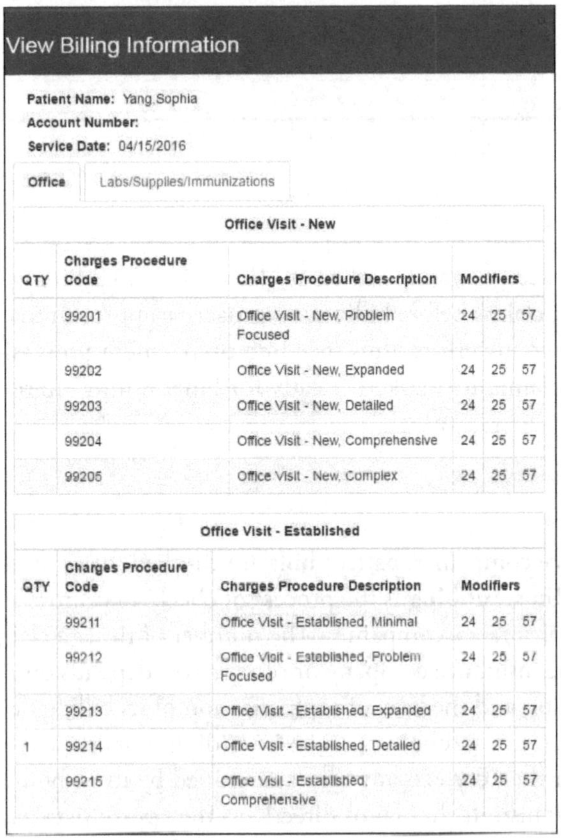

View Billing Information

Patient Name: Yang,Sophia
Account Number:
Service Date: 04/15/2016

Office | Labs/Supplies/Immunizations

Office Visit - New

QTY	Charges Procedure Code	Charges Procedure Description	Modifiers		
	99201	Office Visit - New, Problem Focused	24	25	57
	99202	Office Visit - New, Expanded	24	25	57
	99203	Office Visit - New, Detailed	24	25	57
	99204	Office Visit - New, Comprehensive	24	25	57
	99205	Office Visit - New, Complex	24	25	57

Office Visit - Established

QTY	Charges Procedure Code	Charges Procedure Description	Modifiers		
	99211	Office Visit - Established, Minimal	24	25	57
	99212	Office Visit - Established, Problem Focused	24	25	57
	99213	Office Visit - Established, Expanded	24	25	57
1	99214	Office Visit - Established, Detailed	24	25	57
	99215	Office Visit - Established, Comprehensive	24	25	57

Figure 10.9 Adding Charges to a Superbill in the EHR Navigator

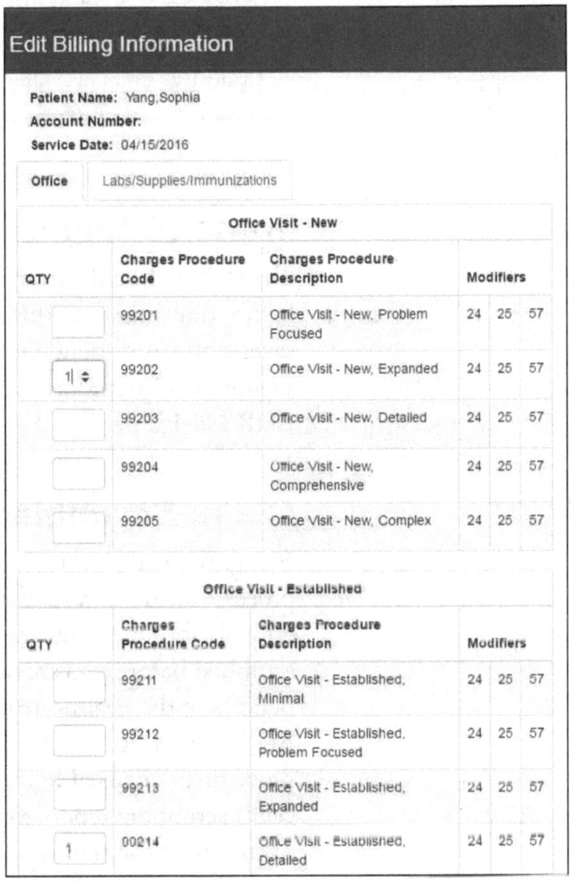

Edit Billing Information

Patient Name: Yang,Sophia
Account Number:
Service Date: 04/15/2016

Office | Labs/Supplies/Immunizations

Office Visit - New

QTY	Charges Procedure Code	Charges Procedure Description	Modifiers		
	99201	Office Visit - New, Problem Focused	24	25	57
1	99202	Office Visit - New, Expanded	24	25	57
	99203	Office Visit - New, Detailed	24	25	57
	99204	Office Visit - New, Comprehensive	24	25	57
	99205	Office Visit - New, Complex	24	25	57

Office Visit - Established

QTY	Charges Procedure Code	Charges Procedure Description	Modifiers		
	99211	Office Visit - Established, Minimal	24	25	57
	99212	Office Visit - Established, Problem Focused	24	25	57
	99213	Office Visit - Established, Expanded	24	25	57
1	99214	Office Visit - Established, Detailed	24	25	57

Figure 10.10 Electronic Superbill

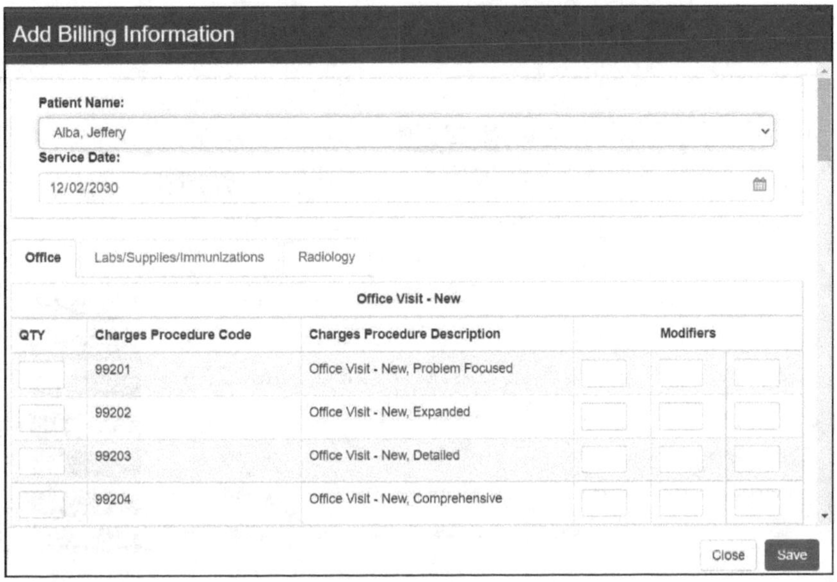

Add Billing Information

Patient Name:
Alba, Jeffery
Service Date:
12/02/2030

Office | Labs/Supplies/Immunizations | Radiology

Office Visit - New

QTY	Charges Procedure Code	Charges Procedure Description	Modifiers		
	99201	Office Visit - New, Problem Focused			
	99202	Office Visit - New, Expanded			
	99203	Office Visit - New, Detailed			
	99204	Office Visit - New, Comprehensive			

Close | Save

Tutorial 10.3

EHRNAVIGAT⊕R

Adding a Superbill

Go the online course to launch Tutorial 10.3. As a biller, practice adding a super-bill in the EHR Navigator.

Transmitting Claims

The claims should be reviewed for accuracy and marked as "Ready for Final Billing" before transmission. This review of claims before billing is a proactive approach that saves staff from spending time correcting errors, thus speeding up payment processing. Figure 10.11 demonstrates where claims are marked "Ready for Final Billing" in the EHR Navigator.

Claim Scrubbing

Before transmission to the insurance companies, patient bills are checked for errors via a process called *claim scrubbing*. **Claim scrubbing** is the process of checking claims for errors before transmitting them to insurance companies. The number of times a claim is scrubbed before transmission to the insurance company or other payer depends on the policies of the healthcare organization and the level of sophistication of its billing or EHR system. After performing the claim scrubbing process according to its policies and procedures, the healthcare provider then corrects any errors identified by its in-house claim scrubbing report and either transmits the claims directly to the appropriate payer or transmits the claims to a clearinghouse. A medical claims **clearinghouse** is a company that accepts electronic claims from healthcare providers, scrubs the claims, transmits the clean claims to the appropriate payer, and returns the claims that have errors to the healthcare provider. **Clean claims** are those without errors. Why don't

Figure 10.11   Ready for Final Billing in EHR Navigator

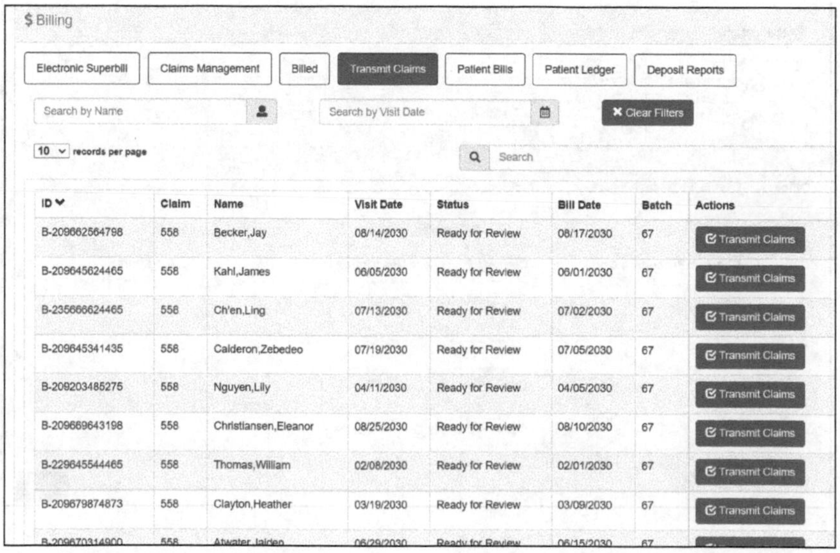

ID	Claim	Name	Visit Date	Status	Bill Date	Batch	Actions
B-209662564798	558	Becker,Jay	08/14/2030	Ready for Review	08/17/2030	67	Transmit Claims
B-209645624465	558	Kahl,James	06/05/2030	Ready for Review	06/01/2030	67	Transmit Claims
B-235666624465	558	Ch'en,Ling	07/13/2030	Ready for Review	07/02/2030	67	Transmit Claims
B-209645341435	558	Calderon,Zebedeo	07/19/2030	Ready for Review	07/05/2030	67	Transmit Claims
B-209203485275	558	Nguyen,Lily	04/11/2030	Ready for Review	04/05/2030	67	Transmit Claims
B-209669643198	558	Christiansen,Eleanor	08/25/2030	Ready for Review	08/10/2030	67	Transmit Claims
B-229645544465	558	Thomas,William	02/08/2030	Ready for Review	02/01/2030	67	Transmit Claims
B-209679874873	558	Clayton,Heather	03/19/2030	Ready for Review	03/09/2030	67	Transmit Claims
B-209670314900	558	Atwater,Jaiden	06/29/2030	Ready for Review	06/15/2030	67	

healthcare providers just scrub and transmit the claims themselves instead of having to pay a clearinghouse to do this for them? Most healthcare providers do not have claim scrubbing and transmission software sophisticated enough to perform the thousands of error checks, including billing rules, official coding guidelines, and specific insurance carrier rules required to ensure clean claims. In addition, with the hundreds of insurance companies and payers, all with their own billing and claims requirements, it is a monumental job to keep up with all the billing regulations and requirements. Smaller healthcare organizations, including most physician practices, do not have the resources, including software and staff to perform the same functions as a clearinghouse; therefore, the clearinghouses play a significant role in facilitating fast, accurate billing and reimbursement.

The healthcare providers that perform claim scrubbing in house utilize their EHR and billing systems to perform a set of edits on the claims that are ready to be final billed. In the EHR Navigator, you can run reports that show which claims contain errors and then correct those errors for final billing.

Tutorial 10.4   EHRNAVIGAT⊕R

Running a Claim Scrubbing Report and Editing the Claims

Go to the online course to launch Tutorial 10.4. As a biller, practice running a claim scrubbing report. Then identify the errors on the report and correct them in the EHR Navigator.

Final Billing

Following transmission of the clean claim, also known as the *final bill*, to the payer, the EHR system automatically updates to reflect the name of the payer, date, and amount billed. The billing supervisor of the physician practice receives a report automatically delivered to an email address that lists the accounts that were final billed.

When the review of claims is complete and the claims have been marked for final billing, the claims are electronically transmitted to payers or the clearinghouse, and patient bills are printed and mailed or emailed. Since the bills have already been reviewed and marked for final billing, they are in a holding file awaiting the electronic transfer. To accomplish this, the medical biller needs to select the *Transmit Claims* button in the EHR Navigator. The claims that are transferred electronically are sent to either the appropriate insurance payer or the clearinghouse. Amounts that are the patient's responsibility are either printed for postal mailing or generated and sent via email, depending on the patient's preference. In the EHR Navigator, this is accomplished by selecting the *Patient Bills* button.

Payments and Adjustments

Once a claim has been final billed, payers will review the claims and process payments to providers for treatment rendered. Upon receipt of payments, providers update patient accounts with payment information. Figure 10.12 reflects an insurance payment.

Figure 10.12 Payment Dialog Box

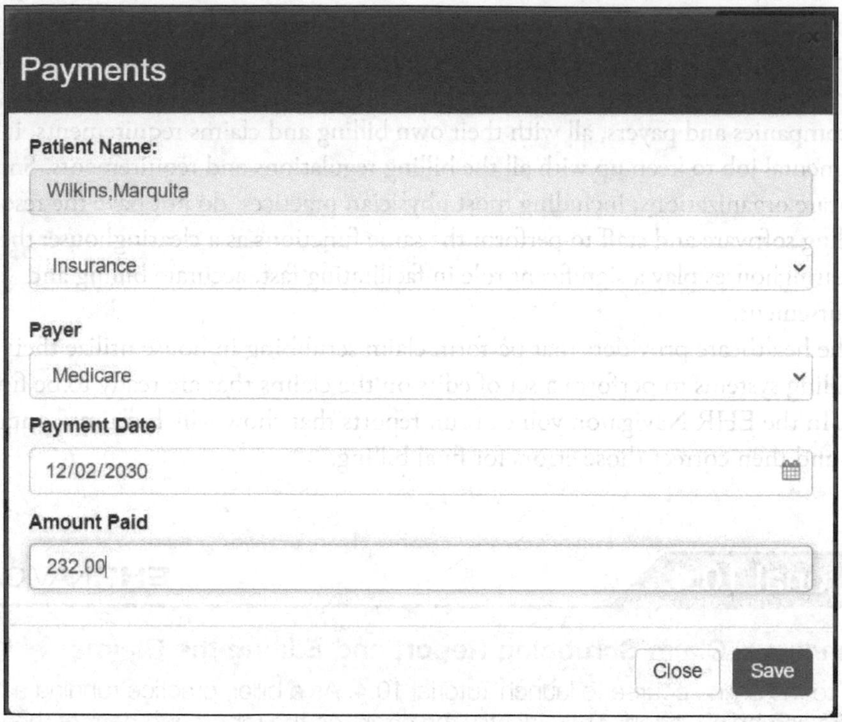

Payments

Patient Name:

Wilkins,Marquita

Insurance

Payer

Medicare

Payment Date

12/02/2030

Amount Paid

232.00

Close   Save

In addition to posting payments to patients' accounts, providers will post adjustments as well, for many reasons, including bad debt write-off, charged in error, credit, credit adjustment, discount, insurance adjustment, insurance overpayment, Medicare write-off, patient write-off, and professional courtesy. Figure 10.13 reflects an insurance adjustment.

Figure 10.13 Insurance Adjustment

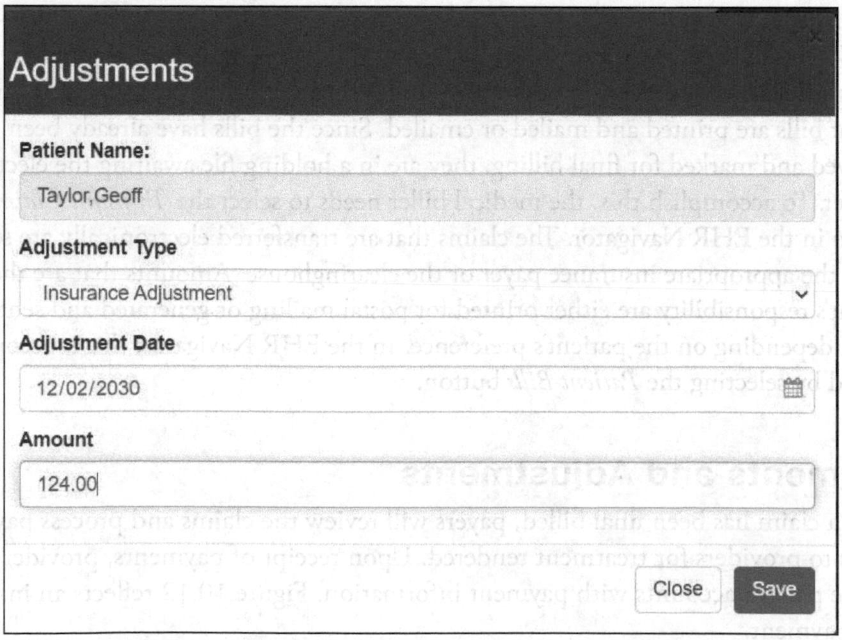

Adjustments

Patient Name:

Taylor,Geoff

Adjustment Type

Insurance Adjustment

Adjustment Date

12/02/2030

Amount

124.00

Close   Save

10.3 Reimbursement Methodology

Reimbursement is the act of compensating a person for services rendered. In the healthcare industry, medical providers treat patients before receiving payment. Fees may not be collected before the patient receives treatment because the necessary treatment is not yet known. There are many different reimbursement methods within health care. The following section reviews the most common methods.

Fee-for-Service Reimbursement

Fee-for-service is a reimbursement method that requests payment for each service or procedure. Each service or procedure has a set fee or charge. Providers are reimbursed only the allowed amount as listed on the third-party payer fee schedule.

Fee Schedules

A **fee schedule** is a price list of services and procedures. Each payer has its own customized fee schedule. However, many healthcare providers base their fees on the **CMS Medicare Physician Fee Schedule (MPFS)**. Medicare uses the **resource-based relative value scale (RBRVS)** to create the MPFS. The RBRVS sets fees for CPT® and HCPCS codes. To calculate the value of a service or procedure, the RBRVS uses three factors:

1. **Relative value units (RVUs)** calculated for three components:

   - Work RVUs—the amount of work needed to render the treatment

   - Practice expense RVUs—the expense to the practice to facilitate the treatment

   - Malpractice RVUs—the risk of malpractice associated with the treatment

2. **Geographic practice cost indices (GPCI)** are adjustments applied to the RVUs to account for variations in the costs of practicing medicine in specific geographic regions.

3. **Conversion factor (CF)** is a fiscal year monetary amount that is adjusted annually and is derived from a formula set by the US Congress to convert the GPCI into a dollar amount that reflects several elements:

   - The category of services (medical, surgical, or nonsurgical)

   - The percentage of changes to the Medicare Economic Index

   - Physician expenditures

   - Access to health care

   - Quality of health care

Examples of the calculations are provided in Tables 10.2 and 10.3.

Table 10.2   Example of a National (Standard) RVU Calculation

CPT®/HCPCS Code	RVU Component			Total RVUs
	Work	**Practice Expense**	**Malpractice**	
49540	$10.74	$6.18	$2.51	$19.43

Table 10.3 Calculation of RVUs for Los Angeles, California, and Red Banks, Mississippi, Using GPCI

City	CPT®/HCPCS Code	RVU Component GPCI Value			Total RVUs
		Work	Practice Expense	Malpractice	
Los Angeles, CA	49540	$11.24	$7.17	$2.28	$20.69
Red Banks, MS	49540	$10.74	$5.34	$1.53	$17.61

The national RVU calculation provides the base value for CPT® and HCPCS codes. Table 10.1 shows the use of the RVU formula for code 49540, *Repair lumbar hernia*. The three RVU components—work, practice expense, and malpractice—are given set values. The values are added to determine the national (standard) RVUs for the procedure: $10.74 + $6.18 + $2.51 = $19.43.

However, a procedure performed in a major metropolitan area such as Los Angeles, California, will have higher work, practice expenses, and malpractice costs than the same procedure in a smaller city, such as Red Banks, Mississippi. The RVU calculation is geographically adjusted by the GPCI (informally referred to as the *gypsy*). Table 10.2 compares the RVUs for the two cities for code 49540, calculated as:

> Los Angeles = $11.24 + $7.17 + $2.28 = $20.69
> Red Banks = $10.74 + $5.34 + $1.53 = $17.61

To convert the GPCI into a dollar amount, the total RVU value is multiplied by a monetary CF. CFs differ based on the category of services (medical, surgical, or nonsurgical).

Using a CF of 35.7547 and the values in Table 10.2, the fees for code 49540 in Los Angeles and Red Banks are calculated by multiplying their respective GPCI-adjusted, total RVUs by the CF:

> Los Angeles = $20.69 × 35.7547 = $739.76
> Red Banks = $17.61 × 35.7547 = $629.64

Rounding the results to the nearest penny shows that the procedure has a Medicare monetary value of $739.76 in Los Angeles and $629.64 in Red Banks.

The MPFS lists RVUs on the CMS website. The MPFS is updated on April 15 of each year. The formulas used to establish RVUs and GPCIs are published in the *Federal Register*, the US government's daily publication of final and administrative regulations for federal agencies. Coders reference the *Federal Register* to stay current on changes that affect healthcare regulations and Medicare.

Health insurance companies base their fees on the MPFS. Physician's offices may also use the MPFS to establish a fixed fee schedule for the office, which lists all services and procedures offered at that practice. However, the fees set by the practice do not determine reimbursement amounts from third-party payers. Hospitals compile all procedures, services, supplies, and drugs that are billed to insurance payers into a computer database called a **hospital chargemaster**. Most hospital chargemasters include several thousand line items that are reviewed and updated annually by a medical coder who has the title of chargemaster. Physician's offices incorporate their most common procedure and diagnosis codes into the superbill.

Posting payments, insurance appeals, and collections is the last step in the billing or revenue cycle. At this point in the revenue cycle, the focus is on making sure the healthcare organization receives the correct amount of reimbursement for the treatment and services rendered. When insurance companies do not pay correctly, healthcare organizations go through an appeals process to request additional payment from the insurance companies. When individuals owe the healthcare organization monies and do not pay in a timely manner, the healthcare organizations initiate a formal collections process.

Consider This

Let's look at CPT® code 20610, *Arthrocentesis, aspiration and/or injection, major joint or bursa (e.g., shoulder, hip, knee, subacromial bursa); without ultrasound guidance.* Code 20610 may be reported for the removal of fluid from a major joint or bursa. It may also be reported for the injection of drugs into a major joint or bursa. Physician's offices typically accept patients with Medicare, Medicaid, and commercial insurance. The physician, who is contracted with the payers, has access to the fee schedules for each payer. The following is a list of the payers' fees for code 20610 as well as the office fee:

Payers' Fee Schedule for Code 20610:

Medicare	$61.14
Medicaid	$58.12
Commercial payer	$78.28

Physician's Office Fee Schedule:

Code 20610 $85.00

The fee schedule shows that each payer has a different allowable fee for code 20610. The commercial payer fee represents a single amount despite the range of fees set by the many different commercial payers that all have their own fee schedules. Rather than looking up the exact fee for each payer, billing is expedited if the physician's office has one set fee for code 20610, typically set a few dollars above the highest listed fee on the commercial payers' fee schedules. If the fee is set lower than what is listed on the fee schedule, and the reimbursement is approved, the payer will pay only the amount requested. In our example, the physician's office sets a fee of $85.00 for code 20610.

10.4 Practice Management Reports

Frequent and routine monitoring of billing and collections reports is necessary to ensure that the practice is receiving the correct monies owed. One such report is the **billing/payment status report**. This report lists the status of every patient account, allowing the billing staff to identify claims that need to be billed or rebilled and insurance payers that need to be contacted regarding lack of payment. Figure 10.14 illustrates the billing/payment status report in the EHR Navigator. Payments from payers may come in the form of electronic funds transfer or a check. The billing supervisor receives a **remittance advice (RA)** report that lists the patient's information and amount paid by Medicare or another payer to the physician practice.

Figure 10.14   Billing/Payment Status Report

Billing/Payment Status Report:

Patient Account Number	Patient Name							
Date	Procedure	Amount	Policy 1	Policy 2	Policy 3	Guarantor	Adjustments	Balance
1772559	Wang, Tabitha							
	1. Fortune Health							
	2.							
	3.							
10/12/2030	99212	45.00	-25.00*	0.00*	0.00*	Not Billed	-10.00	10.00
8/27/2030	99213	60.00	12/6/2009	0.00*	0.00*	Billed	0.00	60.00
							SubTotal:	70.00
							Unapplied Payments and Adjustments:	0.00
							Case Balance:	70.00
1772568	Ortiz, Marco							
	1. Gold Care							
	2.							
	3.							
6/25/2030	99213	60.00	Billed	Not Billed	0.00*	Billed	0.00	60.00
							SubTotal:	60.00
							Unapplied Payments and Adjustments:	60.00
							Case Balance:	0.00
							Patient Reference Balance:	60.00
								60.00
							Report Balance:	**$130.00**

Tutorial 10.5

EHRNAVIGAT⊕R

Posting a Payment from a Remittance Advice

Go to the online course to launch Tutorial 10.5. As a billing supervisor, practice posting a payment from a remittance advice using the EHR Navigator.

Production Reports

The EHR system is able to generate valuable financial and statistical **production reports** to assist the practice manager with budgeting and revenue management. These reports assist the practice manager in daily, weekly, monthly, and yearly financial reconciliations of billed charges, receipts, and adjustments. Reports should be generated and reviewed routinely by the practice manager for opportunities to improve the management of practice revenues and expenses, as well as billing, accounts receivable, and collections processes. Let's take a look at some of these reports.

Production by Provider Report

The **production by provider report** shows how many patients are treated within a specified period by each provider in a practice, along with the revenue generated. These are important statistics to track over time and may be used for a variety of reasons, including the following:

- Calculating provider salaries if based on the number of patients treated
- Calculating the number of appointment slots needed for each provider
- Scheduling staff
- Ordering supplies

Figure 10.15 is a sample production by provider report, illustrating the incoming revenue for each provider. This report reflects both month-to-date and year-to-date totals. In the first column, you see the ID number of the provider; the second column is the

Figure 10.15 Production by Provider Report

Production by Provider:
Date: 11/01/2030 - 11/30/2030

Doctor ID	Doctor ⌄	Month To Date			Year to Date		
		Charges	Payments	Adjustments	Charges	Payments	Adjustments
1	Corners, Bonnie	$150	$15	$0	$150	$15	$0
2	Merck, Colotta	$42	$10	$0	$42	$10	$0
10	Connor, Marcia	$175	$100	$0	$175	$100	$0
15	Roman, Silvia	$42	$20	$0	$1746	$595	$0
16	Dapkins, Thomas	$150	$20	$0	$1672	$320	$0
17	Hill, Geoff	$42	$50	$0	$1142	$340	$0
22	Petterson, Opal	$42	$50	$0	$409	$240	$0
24	Goldman, Ryan	$150	$50	$0	$300	$65	$0
27	Goodson, Michelle	$375	$15	$0	$525	$25	$0
28	Montague, Roberta	$150	$50	$0	$150	$50	$0
29	Kyee, Nicolas	$42	$30	$0	$1938	$897	$47
30	Feltner, Alana	$150	$0	$0	$2362	$795	$0
31	Turrell, Avis	$150	$50	$0	$1454	$505	$0
32	Gertz, Lester	$150	$0	$0	$2716	$510	$0
33	Vandenbosch, Ricardo	$80	$10	$0	$80	$10	$0
34	Holzer, Gregory	$150	$50	$0	$2971	$770	$0
35	Dowling, Linda	$150	$70	$0	$4552	$1135	$25

name of the provider; then there are three columns for month-to-date totals and three columns for year-to-date totals. The first of these three columns in each section reflects the amount of charges generated. The second column reflects the amount paid. The third column reflects adjustments that were made to the patient's account. There are many reasons for adjustments, such as refunds or overpayments, differences between the amount billed and the allowed amount per the insurance contract, and nonpayment by a patient.

Calculating Provider Salaries If a provider's salary at Northstar Physicians is based partially or totally on how much revenue is produced by the provider, you would use the Payments column to calculate the provider's salary since that is the actual revenue that was received. In the previous example, if we look at the year-to-date totals, Dr. Lester Gertz would earn the highest salary. Dr. Alana Feltner would earn the lowest salary, since she generated the least amount of revenue for the practice.

Calculating Appointment Slots and Scheduling Staff Using this same report, an office manager is able to see at a glance which providers need the most appointment slots available for scheduling and the most scheduled medical assistants and staff available to assist them.

Ordering Supplies Because the use of supplies would also be expected to fluctuate with the amount of patient activity, an office manager is able to use this report to gauge supply use and ordering.

Production by Procedure Report

The **production by procedure report** reflects the number of procedures performed during a specific period along with the associated revenue. Figure 10.16 is an example of one page of a production by procedure report. This report lists the CPT® code that was billed along with the description of the CPT® code, the associated charge for the procedure, the number of procedures performed during the period specified, the total amount billed, the expected payment amount to be received, the actual payment

Figure 10.16 Production by Procedure Report

	Production by Procedure Report-Summary: Report includes Data From: 11/01/2030 Through: 11/30/2030							
CPT Procedure Code ✔	Procedure Description	Charge	Number of Procedures Performed	Total Billed Amount	Expected Payment Amount	Actual Payment Amount	Actual Adjustment
80048	Metabolic panel, basic	$80	20	$1600	$848	$752	$22
81000	UA	$90	17	$1530	$895	$635	$0
85025	CBC, w auto differential	$42	33	$1386	$-11	$1397	$12
87088	Urine culture	$380	15	$5700	$4985	$715	$0
99201	Office Visit - New, Problem Focused	$150	10	$1500	$995	$505	$0
99204	Office Visit - New, Comprehensive	$375	11	$4125	$3745	$380	$0
99212	Office Visit - Established, Problem Focused	$150	74	$11100	$8190	$2910	$75
99213	Office Visit - Established, Expanded	$175	13	$2275	$1715	$560	$0
Totals:			193	$21864	$21362	$7854	$109

amount that was received, and the actual adjustment in the patients' accounts that needed to be made. Another useful data sort would be by *actual payment amount*. A **data sort** is arranging data in a particular sequence, from high to low or low to high.

Figure 10.17 illustrates the production by procedure report sorted in ascending numerical order by CPT® code. However, another useful data sort of this report would be by number of procedures performed, in descending order, so the practice manager would be able to report the most common procedures performed by the practice. In this report, you can see the most common procedure performed/billed by the practice is 99212, *Office Visit—Established Patient 10 minutes*.

Figure 10.18 is an example of the production of procedure report sorted by actual payment amount. This report shows that the most revenue for the month of June was generated by CPT® procedure code 99213, *Office Visit—Established Patient 15 minutes*.

Figure 10.17 Production by Procedure Report Sorted by Procedure

	Production by Procedure Report-Summary: Report includes Data From: 06/01/2030 Through: 06/30/2030							
CPT Procedure Code	Procedure Description ✔	Charge	Number of Procedures Performed	Total Billed Amount	Expected Payment Amount	Actual Payment Amount	Actual Adjustment
88141	Cervical Pap Smear	$31.36	49	$1,537.62	$922.57	$872.40	$665.22
99212	Office Visit-Established Patient 10 minutes	$110.00	309	$33,990.00	$20,394.00	$19,420.00	$14,570.00
99213	Office Visit-Established Patient 15 minutes	$160.00	283	$45,280.00	$27,168.00	$25,723.00	$19,557.00
99214	Office Visit-Established Patient 25 minutes	$260.00	55	$14,300.00	$8,580.00	$8,450.00	$5,850.00
99215	Office Visit-Established Patient 40 minutes	$305.00	108	$32,940.00	$19,764.00	$19,140.00	$13,800.00
99211	Office Visit-Established Patient 5 minutes	$54.00	200	$10,800.00	$6,480.00	$6,320.00	$4,480.00
99201	Office Visit-New Patient 10 minutes	$92.00	0	$0.00	$0.00	$0.00	$0.00
99202	Office Visit-New Patient 20 minutes	$180.00	46	$8,280.00	$4,968.00	$5,110.00	$3,170.00
99203	Office Visit-New Patient 30 minutes	$250.00	38	$9,500.00	$5,700.00	$5,610.00	$3,890.00
99204	Office Visit-New Patient 45 minutes	$355.00	18	$6,390.00	$3,834.00	$3,800.00	$2,590.00
99205	Office Visit-New Patient 60 minutes	$441.00	12	$5,292.00	$3,175.20	$3,250.00	$2,042.00
87070	Throat Culture	$173.00	58	$10,034.00	$6,020.40	$5,110.00	$4,924.00

Figure 10.18   Production by Procedure Report Sorted by Actual Amount

CPT Procedure Code	Procedure Description	Charge	Number of Procedures Performed	Total Billed Amount	Expected Payment Amount	Actual Payment Amount ✔	Actual Adjustment
				Production by Procedure Report-Summary: Report Includes Data From: 06/01/2030 Through: 06/30/2030			
99201	Office Visit-New Patient 10 minutes	$92.00	0	$0.00	$0.00	$0.00	$0.00
99215	Office Visit-Established Patient 40 minutes	$305.00	108	$32,940.00	$19,764.00	$19,140.00	$13,800.00
99212	Office Visit-Established Patient 10 minutes	$110.00	309	$33,990.00	$20,394.00	$19,420.00	$14,570.00
99213	Office Visit-Established Patient 15 minutes	$160.00	283	$45,280.00	$27,168.00	$25,723.00	$19,557.00
99205	Office Visit-New Patient 60 minutes	$441.00	12	$5,292.00	$3,175.20	$3,250.00	$2,042.00
99204	Office Visit-New Patient 45 minutes	$355.00	18	$6,390.00	$3,834.00	$3,800.00	$2,590.00
99202	Office Visit-New Patient 20 minutes	$180.00	46	$8,280.00	$4,968.00	$5,110.00	$3,170.00
87070	Throat Culture	$173.00	58	$10,034.00	$6,020.40	$5,110.00	$4,924.00
99203	Office Visit-New Patient 30 minutes	$250.00	38	$9,500.00	$5,700.00	$5,610.00	$3,890.00
99211	Office Visit-Established Patient 5 minutes	$54.00	200	$10,800.00	$6,480.00	$6,320.00	$4,480.00
99214	Office Visit-Established Patient 25 minutes	$260.00	55	$14,300.00	$8,580.00	$8,450.00	$5,850.00
88141	Cervical Pap Smear	$31.38	49	$1,537.62	$922.57	$872.40	$665.22

Production by Insurance Report   Another useful production report is a **production by insurance report**. This report reflects the amount of revenue generated by each insurance carrier. As you can see by the sample report found in Figure 10.19, Kentucky Medicaid has generated the most charges for Northstar Physicians year to date. While the amount of charges can indicate the insurer that generates the most revenue, charges alone cannot be used interchangeably with term revenue. Each insurer may include payment specifics of discounts, or payment and charge caps that will impact the amount of charges that translate to revenue.

Figure 10.19   Production by Insurance Report

Company ID ✔	Company	Month To Date			Year to Date		
		Charges	Payments	Adjustments	Charges	Payments	Adjustments
1	American Lifecare	$NaN	$360	$12	$1404	$NaN	$12
2	Cobalt Care	$3090	$1125	$25	$4250	$1310	$25
3	PublicAid	$579	$370	$0	$979	$400	$0
4	ApolloHealth	$1496	$305	$0	$1871	$375	$0
5	FederalAide	$545	$250	$0	$795	$250	$0
6	Medicare	$1352	$640	$0	$2032	$680	$0
7	Wellness Partners	$NaN	$360	$0	$1928	$480	$0
8	Fortune Health	$1769	$555	$0	$2539	$620	$0
9	Gold Care	$1372	$325	$0	$1727	$355	$0
10		$470	$275	$25	$920	$300	$25
11	Ohio Medicaid	$501	$195	$0	$876	$225	$0
12	Indiana Medicaid	$2153	$780	$0	$3053	$900	$0
13	Kentucky Medicaid	$4173	$870	$47	$4643	$1072	$47
14	Wellness Institute	$2056	$385	$0	$2511	$455	$0
Totals:		$NaN	$6795	$109	$29528	$NaN	$109

Production by Insurance:
Date: 11/01/2030 - 11/30/2030

Running Production Reports

Go to the online course to launch Tutorial 10.6. Practice running various production reports in the EHR Navigator.

CHECKP✛INT 10.4

1. Why is a billing/status report generated?

_____

_____

2. Name and describe a report that may assist the practice in revenue cycle management.

_____

_____

3. Describe why a production by provider report is used.

_____

_____

_____

Day Sheets

Besides production reports, which may be generated for different periods and focus, there are several other reports that are useful in practice management. One such report is a day sheet. A **day sheet** is a report of practice activity for a 24-hour period that is used to reconcile patient accounts on a daily basis to ensure that no fraud, abuse, or theft is occurring. To accomplish this daily reconciliation or balancing, the most common type of day sheet used is the **patient day sheet** (Figure 10.20). The format of a patient day sheet may vary but usually contains the patient's name and account number, a description of the activity (such as charge, payment, or adjustment), the provider, the transaction code (such as the CPT® code for a charge, type of payment, or reason for adjustment), the amount, and end-of-report totals. Figure 10.20 illustrates the way different criteria can be selected to show various day sheets in the EHR Navigator.

Two other day sheet reports that may prove useful with a practice's daily activity reconciliation are the payment day sheet and the procedure day sheet. The **payment day sheet** is similar to the patient day sheet, except that it lists only the payments made during the 24-hour period. Likewise, the **procedure day sheet** is similar to the patient day sheet but lists only the procedures charged during the 24-hour period.

Running Day Sheets

Go to the online course and launch Tutorial 10.7. Practice running various day sheets in the EHR Navigator.

Figure 10.20 Patient Day Sheet Report

Patient Day Sheet -- Report Date: 12/02/2030

Patient Account Number ⌄	Name	Activity	Transaction Date	Diagnosis	TX Code	Amount
1772573	Jennifer Bari	Adjustment	12/02/2030	N39	99214	-31
1772544	Tyler Mulligan	Adjustment	12/02/2030	R21	99213	-26
1772500	Vance Donaldson	Adjustment	12/02/2030	I10	99213	-16
1772503	Lily Nguyen	Adjustment	12/02/2030	B35 .1.99213		-45
1772563	Henry Tran	Adjustment	12/02/2030	J01	99212	-15
1772513	Todd Jackson	Adjustment	12/02/2030	J44.9	99214	-5
1772573	Jennifer Bari	Adjustment	12/02/2030	R32	90714	-8
1772569	Kenji Wantabe	Adjustment	12/02/2030	E10.9	99213	-22
1772541	Stephanie Miller	Adjustment	12/02/2030	Q05.8	97010	-18
1772519	Simona Brushfield	Adjustment	12/02/2030	Z23	99213	-25
1772540	Bette Goldman	Adjustment	12/02/2030	I10	90782	-20
1772532	Sophia Yang	Charge	12/02/2030	Z00.00	97010	-25
1772551	Rhonda Taylor	Charge	12/02/2030	E66.9	99214	-15
1772531	Mason Fernandez	Charge	12/02/2030	A53.9	97010	-20
1772561	Benjamin Fowler	Charge	12/02/2030	I70.501	90781	-20
1772506	Miguel Esparza	Charge	12/02/2030	A54.21	90714	-30
1772543	Franklin Romero	Charge	12/02/2030	K57.32	90714	-15
1772568	Marco Ortiz	Charge	12/02/2030	K57.32	99213	-26
1772519	Simona Brushfield	Charge	12/02/2030	I10	90782	-25

Deposit Reports

Two types of deposit reports may be generated daily, weekly, monthly, and yearly for the deposits made from insurance payers and from patient payments. The reports reflect the totals for payments made in cash, checks, credit cards, and electronic direct deposit. The **deposit report** may be filtered by several categories as noted below. A filter limits the records that are included in the report. For example, if the deposit report is filtered by the *Payer Type of Patient*, then only the payments made by patients would be included in the report, whereas payments from insurance companies would not be included.

Filters on this report include the following:

- *Payment Date: From* and *To*
- *Payer Type: Insurance* or *Patient*
- *Payer: All Insurance Payers or Patients* or *Specific Insurance Payer or Patient*
- *Provider:* A specific provider or all providers

A typical deposit report is illustrated in Figure 10.21.

Patient Ledger

The **patient ledger** is a report that reflects the patient's financial status in summary and/or in detail. Charges, ledger notes, billings, payments, and adjustments are all shown in both the summarized and detailed status. The status of each charge is listed, as well as insurance payments that have been made and the amount for which the patient or guarantor is responsible. Figure 10.22 shows a patient ledger.

Patient Aging Report

A **patient aging report** is an accounts receivable report that shows how long patients have owed money to the practice. A provider's staff may use this report to follow up with patients regarding payment of past-due balances. This report is separated by the length of time outstanding, such as 15 days, 21 days, 30 days, 45 days, 60 days, over 90 days, or over 120 days. A typical patient aging report is shown in Figure 10.23.

Figure 10.21　Deposit Report

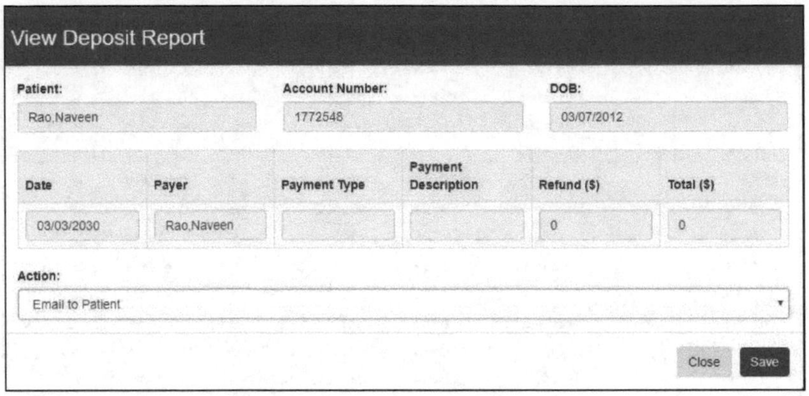

Figure 10.22　Patient Ledger

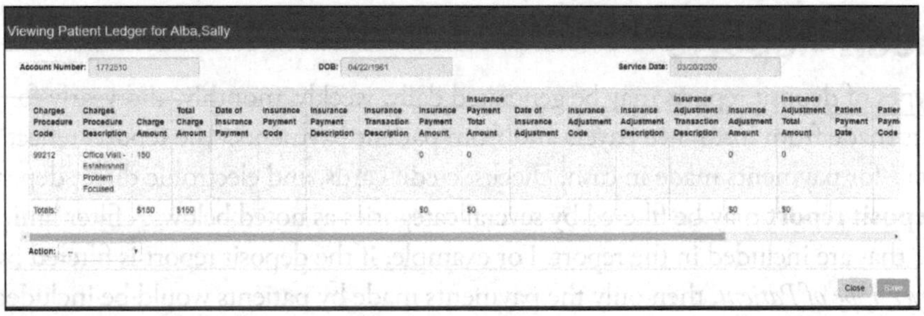

Figure 10.23　Patient Aging Report

Medical Record # ˅	Patient Account #	Last Name	First Name	Current 0-30 days	31-60 days	61-90 days	91-120 days	121+ days	Total Balance Due
585108	1772559	Wang	Tabitha	$0.00	$15.00	$0.00	$0.00	$0.00	$15.00
585109	1772560	Chan	Brian	$0.00	$0.00	$20.00	$0.00	$0.00	$20.00
585110	1772561	Fowler	Benjamin	$0.00	$0.00	$0.00	$0.00	$0.00	$0.00
585111	1772562	Santos	Sebastian	$0.00	$55.00	$0.00	$0.00	$0.00	$55.00
585112	1772563	Tran	Henry	$0.00	$0.00	$0.00	$80.00	$0.00	$80.00
585113	1772564	Blackwater	Jake	$0.00	$0.00	$66.00	$0.00	$0.00	$66.00
585114	1772565	Yang	Mia	$0.00	$0.00	$0.00	$0.00	$55.00	$55.00
585115	1772566	Tambe	Sandeep	$0.00	$10.00	$0.00	$0.00	$0.00	$10.00
585116	1772567	Singh	Manhesh	$25.00	$0.00	$30.00	$0.00	$0.00	$55.00
585117	1772568	Ortiz	Marco	$0.00	$120.00	$0.00	$25.00	$0.00	$145.00
585118	1772569	Watanabe	Kenji	$0.00	$0.00	$0.00	$0.00	$0.00	$0.00
585119	1772570	Saito	Minako	$0.00	$0.00	$48.00	$50.00	$0.00	$98.00
585121	1772571	Walker	Marjorie	$10.00	$0.00	$0.00	$0.00	$0.00	$10.00
585121	1772572	Oberg	Ingrid	$0.00	$0.00	$40.00	$0.00	$0.00	$40.00
585122	1772573	Bari	Jennifer	$0.00	$0.00	$0.00	$240.00	$0.00	$240.00
585123	1772574	Smith	Emmanuel	$0.00	$30.00	$0.00	$0.00	$0.00	$30.00
585124	1772575	Castanza	Joyce	$25.00	$0.00	$0.00	$0.00	$0.00	$25.00
585125	1772576	Smith	Nathaniel	$0.00	$75.00	$0.00	$0.00	$0.00	$75.00
585126	1772577	Smith	Emmanuel	$0.00	$15.00	$0.00	$0.00	$0.00	$15.00
Totals				$60.00	$320.00	$204.00	$395.00	$55.00	$1,034.00

Chapter Summary

Healthcare service providers must have accurate insurance information to be able to accurately bill for their services. Health insurance is a type of insurance that pays for healthcare services that are incurred by the insured person(s). The discussion of national health insurance has been going on for many decades and includes the creation of Medicare and the Affordable Care Act (ACA). There are many third-party payers with which medical billers will work. These include government-sponsored plans (such as Medicare, Medicaid, CHAMPVA, TRICARE, and workers' compensation), private payers, and self-funded health plans. Patient insurance eligibility and coverage is verified to ensure accurate insurance information for billing. There are many detailed steps the billing staff must perform in the practice to ensure accurate and timely payment for healthcare treatment and services. Most healthcare providers are required to electronically transmit claims to insurance payers. The practice billing system that is part of the EHR or that interfaces with the practice's EHR assists in billing and claims processing as well as revenue cycle management. The electronic superbill is used by providers to document the treatment and procedures that are to be billed. Standard practice management reports must be generated and monitored routinely.

Review and Assessment

The following Review and Assessment activities are also available online in the Cirrus online course. Your instructor may ask you to complete these activities online. Cirrus also provides access to flash cards, a crossword puzzle, and practice quizzes to help strengthen your understanding of the chapter content.

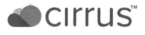

Acronyms/Initialisms

Study the following acronyms discussed in this chapter. Go to the online course for flash cards of the acronyms and other chapter key terms.

ACA: Affordable Care Act

ALS: amyotrophic lateral sclerosis

CF: conversion factor

CHAMPVA: Civilian Health and Medical Program of the Department of Veterans Affairs

CHIP: Children's Health Insurance Program

COBRA: Consolidated Omnibus Budget Reconciliation Act

DoD: Department of Defense

EOB: explanation of benefits

ESRD: end-stage renal disease

GPCI: geographic practice cost indices

HETS: HIPAA Eligibility Transaction System

HFMA: Healthcare Financial Management Association

HIPAA: Health Insurance Portability and Accountability Act

HMO: Health Maintenance Organization (Act)

MA: Medicare Advantage

MPFS: Medicare Physician Fee Schedule

POS: point of service

PPD: permanent partial disability

PPO: preferred provider organization

PTD: permanent total disability

RA: remittance advice

RBRVS: resource-based relative value scale

RVU: relative value unit

TPD: temporary partial disability

TTD: temporary total disability

VA: Veterans Affairs

Check Your Understanding

To check your understanding of this chapter's key concepts, answer the following questions.

1. The following are all considered government-sponsored healthcare programs *except*

   a. TRICARE.

   b. Medicare.

   c. UnitedHealth.

   d. CHAMPVA.

2. Medicare Part A helps cover all of the following *except*

   a. inpatient care in hospitals.

   b. physician's office visits.

   c. critical access hospital care.

   d. skilled nursing facility care.

3. Which of the following is *not* a goal of the Affordable Care Act?

   a. expand coverage

   b. limit choice

   c. lower healthcare costs

   d. enhance quality of care

4. In 2013, the federal government accounted for paying which percentage of the healthcare costs of Americans?

   a. 26%

   b. 40%

   c. 50%

   d. 20%

5. Which of the following describes TRICARE?

   a. a healthcare program for active-duty and retired uniformed services members and their families

   b. an insurance plan that employers are required to have to cover employees who get sick or injured on the job

c.   a state-administered health insurance program for low-income families and children

d.   a program that helps pay for prescription drugs for people with Medicare

6.   True/False: The definition of *health coverage* is "a type of insurance that pays for healthcare services that are incurred by the person(s) that are insured."

7.   True/False: A managed care plan is a type of insurance offered by a carrier who has negotiated and contracted with healthcare providers to provide healthcare services for their subscribers.

8.   True/False: Medicare Part A helps cover physicians' services and outpatient care.

9.   True/False: An HMO is a type of health insurance plan that usually limits coverage to care from physicians who work for or contract with the HMO.

10.   True/False: COBRA is a federal law that may allow individuals to temporarily keep health coverage after their employment ends.

11.   True/False: The electronic superbill is how charges are captured for a patient visit.

12.   True/False: Insurance claims should be filed monthly.

13.   True/False: Office managers may choose to bill insurance companies either via paper or electronically.

14.   True/False: The *Add Charges* screen does *not* provide an opportunity to enter charges that were missed.

15.   True/False: A patient aging report is a listing of all patients' ages and dates of birth.

16.   True/False: There are two types of deposit reports: insurance payers and patient payments.

17.   Three production reports that are useful in managing a practice include production by

a.   patient, procedure, and provider.

b.   provider, procedure, and insurance.

c.   guarantor, insurance, and Medicare.

d.   patient aging, insurance, and provider.

18.   Which of the following reports is used to reconcile a practice's daily activity?

a.   patient ledger

b.   insurance manual

c.   patient day sheet

d.   patient aging report

19. All of the following data elements are found on the patient ledger *except*

    a. a diagnosis code.

    b. a date of service.

    c. a procedure code.

    d. patient marital status.

20. It is necessary to reconcile accounts on a daily basis for all of the following reasons *except*

    a. fraud.

    b. abuse.

    c. theft.

    d. privacy.

Go on the Record

To build on your understanding of the topics in this chapter, complete the following short-answer activities.

1. Explain the difference between in-network and out-of-network providers.

2. List the five comprehensive health insurance reforms of the ACA.

3. Discuss the difference between coinsurance and copayment.

4. Give an example of a government-sponsored health program and a private payer.

5. What are the major differences between Medicare and Medicaid?

6. Explain how charges are captured for a patient visit.

7. Before the transmission of claims, what procedure should be completed?

8. Discuss two reasons why production reports are used.

9. Explain the difference between a patient day sheet and a payment day sheet.

10. Describe the patient aging reports.

Navigate the Field

To gain practice in handling challenging situations in the workplace, consider the following real-world scenarios and identify how you would respond to each.

1. You are the medical biller for a large physician practice and experience frequent difficulties deciphering eligibility responses from Medicare's HETS. What might you suggest to the supervisor of your billing department that would help you and the other billing staff obtain Medicare insurance verifications that are easier to read?

2. You are the office manager of a physician practice, and you would like your staff to become more familiar with Medicare. Search the Medicare Learning Network and identify a training program that you would like your staff to review.

Here is the website for your reference: https://EHR3.ParadigmEducation.com/MLNch9Activity.

3. You are the office manager for a large physician practice, and for the past week, the daily deposits have not matched the day sheets. Why should you be concerned?

4. You are a medical assistant in a small rural physician practice, and you have noticed that the physician you work with has, in your opinion, been marking the electronic superbill incorrectly. For example, the physician has been spending 10 minutes with the patient yet marks 99205 new PT Level 5. How would you address this with the physician?

Think Critically

Continue to think critically about challenging concepts and complete the following activities.

1. Apply the knowledge that you have gained about healthcare insurance, and research current articles about the future of health insurance in the United States. Summarize your findings in a two-page paper.

2. Compare and contrast the workers' compensation coverage and benefits in your home state with two other states of your choice. The following website will likely assist with your review: https://EHR3.ParadigmEducation.com/WorkersComp.

3. You are a medical assistant working for a physician practice that currently outsources its medical billing. Because of the high cost of outsourcing, the physicians have decided to bring the medical billing process in house. Since you are interested in the position, you have been asked to write the job description. Based on the knowledge acquired in this chapter, write a detailed job description for a medical biller.

4. Go to the Medicare Learning Network (MLN) Suite of Products and Resources for Billers at https://EHR3.ParadigmEducation.com/MLNBillers and explore the Medicare Learning Network. Identify three resources that you would find useful if you were a medical biller. Prepare a one-page summary of your findings.

Make Your Case

Consider the scenario and then complete the following project.

1. As the office manager, you have been asked to prepare a presentation for your office on HIPAA regulations as related to electronic billing.

2. Describe the main components of the Affordable Care Act. You may find the following website helpful in your research: https://EHR3.ParadigmEducation.com/ACAComponents.

Explore the Technology

Complete the EHR Navigator practice assessments that align to each tutorial and the assessments that accompany Chapter 10 located in the online course.

EHRNAVIGAT🜨R

Chapter 11 Data Management

Field Notes

" With the shift to value-based reimbursement, there are several quality measures our providers are expected to meet. Our EHR automatically captures which patients fall into which measure and indicates whether the measure has been satisfied. This allows us to ensure that as many patients are meeting the measures as possible. Not only does this have a positive financial impact on our organization, but it also allows our providers to quickly identify and reach out to some of their more at-risk patients. "

– Ryan Jeska, Senior EHR Clinical Analyst

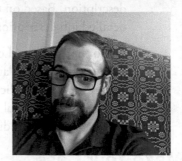

Learning Objectives

11.1 Identify data elements in the electronic health record.

11.2 Identify primary and secondary data sources.

11.3 Discuss the concepts and standards of data integrity.

11.4 Define and identify data dictionary elements.

11.5 Define and explain the term *data mapping*.

11.6 Explain how data collection and tools are used in maintaining health data.

11.7 Identify data sets, databases, and indices used in health care.

11.8 Define and explain the term *data warehouse*.

11.9 Explain data governance.

11.10 Identify the eight principles of data quality management.

11.11 Examine the role that data plays in decision making.

11.12 Discuss big data in health care.

11.13 Define and differentiate *informatics* and *health informatics*.

Data is invaluable in every industry, because data turns into information, and information is priceless if managed and analyzed appropriately. The healthcare industry is experiencing an enormous accumulation of data and information captured by the electronic health record (EHR). Whether you are a medical assistant entering a patient's vital signs, a physician entering assessments and diagnoses, a nurse scanning medication barcodes and documenting the results of medication administration, a lab technician entering information about a blood draw, or a coder entering diagnosis and procedure codes, you are helping to build a repository of a patient's health information within the EHR.

The data and information from the EHR play a critical role in health care because they can be analyzed to create personalized care and improve the quality and delivery of health care. Furthermore, data and information are used by healthcare organizations, state and federal agencies, public health organizations, and research organizations to make decisions regarding expansions in service, public policy, and medical protocols—and more importantly, influencing the quality of the care and the services provided.

Recall that in Chapter 2, you learned that data plays a vital role in the health record. This chapter will provide a more in-depth examination of data, its importance in the EHR, its role in healthcare organizations, the roles of healthcare providers in the creation of data, and how this data is used.

11.1 Data Elements

Data is defined as descriptive or numeric attributes of one or more variables. Often the term *data* is referred to as a *data element* in the EHR. A data element can be one single detail. In the EHR, examples of data elements include date of birth, race, ethnicity, gender, and laboratory test results. In Chapter 2, you learned that data is collected and analyzed to become information. To expand on this idea, data elements are combined into meaningful information about a specific group of patients. Data is stored in the EHR, personal health record, databases, and registries, which will be explored later in this chapter.

11.2 Internal and External Data

There are two types of data used in health care to improve the quality of care as well as to facilitate decision making. They are internal data and external data. **Internal data** is data that is accessed from within the healthcare organization. An example of internal data may be patient financial information. **External data** is data that comes from outside the organization. Sources of external data include Centers for Medicare & Medicaid Services (CMS) and Hospital Compare.

Hospital Compare is part of the CMS's Hospital Quality Initiative. The goal of Hospital Compare is to provide data to examine how well a hospital delivers quality care and how healthcare organizations can improve. An example of data from Hospital Compare is the readmission rate after a hip or knee replacement by state. The data may be used to compare two health-care organizations.

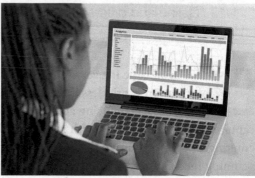
Internal data is accessed within the healthcare organization.

Data Sources

There are two kinds of data sources: primary and secondary. These sources are important to recognize when using and reporting data. Primary data is the original collection or original data found in the health record. Secondary data sources are data that is collected by someone else or data that already exists. It is important to use a combination of the two data sources, primary and secondary, to help researchers predict outcomes based on available data.

Primary Data

Primary data sources are data and information from the patient's EHR. For example, data entered into the EHR in the course of treating the patient would be considered a primary source of data. Types of primary data sources found in the EHR include administrative data, clinical notes, diagnosis and procedure codes, and laboratory procedures. Primary data may be used to document a patient visit and to bill insurance.

Secondary Data

Secondary data sources are indexes and registries. The data is extracted from the patient's health record and reported to external organizations such as cancer registries to capture the number of patients treated for cancer or vital statistics to capture the number of births. Secondary data can be used for research, marketing, and public health monitoring, such as the number of cases of COVID-19 or influenza.

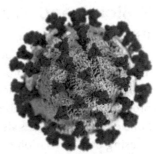

Secondary data can help monitor public health issues, such as the spread of the COVID-19 virus.

CHECKPOINT 11.1

1. Name four data elements.

   a. _____

   b. _____

   c. _____

   d. _____

2. What is the difference between primary and secondary data sources?

   _____

   _____

   _____

   _____

11.3 Data Integrity

Data integrity refers to the accuracy, completeness, and reliability of data. The EHR includes data from multiples sources, including primary and secondary sources. When data is generated by multiple sources, it increases the likelihood that errors will be present in the EHR. Data integrity can be compromised when the content of the data element is entered incorrectly or when the EHR system protections do not work properly. For example, a nurse does not enter a patient's medication allergy correctly in the EHR, which results in an alert that does not work correctly or is ignored. The result of incorrect data is that the patient may be harmed. To prevent incorrect data, policies and procedures for data standards should be implemented.

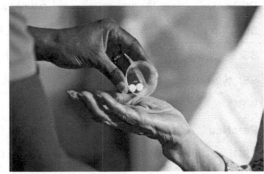

If data is entered into the EHR incorrectly, medication errors can occur.

Standards

Data standards are agreed-upon definitions and formats of data. Interoperability is a key component to data standards. Chapter 1 explains interoperability in relation to the EHR. Chapter 1 also addresses common data standards such as Health Level 7 International (HL7). Data standards are important for bringing data into a common format to allow for sharing, which aids in patient care. Data standards help create the exchange, transfer, and transmission of data between systems.

EXPAND YOUR LEARNING

Events both big and small can trigger trends that will impact health care in the future. Read this article from AHIMA about the impact of the coronavirus pandemic on health information management:

https://EHR3
.ParadigmEducation
.com/HealthDataTrends.

Policies and Procedures

Policies are principles or guidelines that are agreed upon by the organization. **Procedures** are methods used to put policies into action within the healthcare organization. Together, policies and procedures provide an explanation to employees of the healthcare organization about how to handle data operations. Policies and procedures provide a framework to identify the data standards for a healthcare organization. Policies and procedures also detail the use of data, such as the policies and procedures of using data in relation to privacy and confidentiality.

Data Dictionary

A **data dictionary** is a document that describes the content, format, and structure of data elements within a database. A data dictionary is important to data standards because it provides a way to prevent inconsistencies, define elements and their meanings, provide consistency, and enforce data standards. Common data elements that may be found in a data dictionary include the data field name, definition, data type, format, data field size, and data values. See Table 11.1 for an example of a data dictionary entries for each variable, its value, and its description. In an EHR, the data that is entered needs to be consistent among users. The *Variable Name* is the label for the variable. The *Value* identifies the type of data that is entered, and the *Description* explains the data that is entered by the user.

Table 11.1 Example of a Data Dictionary Table

Table List of Candidate Values		
Variable Name	**Value**	**Description**
SurgID	varchar	surgery identifier
SurgTime	date	date of surgery
PtID	varchar	patient identifier
SurgType	varchar	{CABG, HERNIA, HIP, KNEE}
SSI	integer	{0 for absent, 1 for present}
SSI_type	varchar	{superficial, deep, organ}
WBC	number	highest wbc postop day 3-30
PercNeu	number	highest % neutrophils post op day 3-30
ESR	number	highest ESR postop day 3-30
CRP	number	highest CRP (in mg/dL) postop day 3-30
Fever	number	highest temp (in Fahrenheit) postop day 3-30
Cx_Sent	integer	whether a culture was sent postop day 3-30
Cx_Pos	integer	whether postop cx was positive
Path_Org	varchar	S. aureus, P. aeruginosa, enterobacteriaceae, etc.
Cx_Site_Match	integer	for example, culture site hip for hip operation
Re_Admit	integer	readmission on postop day ____; null if no readmission

Data Mapping

Data mapping is a special type of data dictionary. Data mapping is a method that is used to connect data from one system to data of another system. Data is analyzed in the original or source system to match data in the other or target system. Mapping the data is key to accurate data connection. Data mapping can be matched through the data dictionary or data sets. There can be challenges with data mapping when the source and target data do not match. An example of when this issue may arise is when the source system uses SNOMED CT terms but the target system requires ICD-10 codes.

Data Collection

As discussed in Chapter 7, data collection is important to capture and maintain the accuracy and completeness of data. Data collection consists of both manual and automated data collection. The collected information can then be shared to provide quality care to the patient. Manual data collection is data collected by a staff member or entered by the patient. Manual data collection can take place through a paper or digital form completed by an employee or the patient. Automated data collection uses technology to scan paper content, such as paper health records and images, and then translate or convert that to electronic data and files in the EHR.

CHECKPOINT 11.2

1. Explain why policies and procedures are important to data standards.

2. Why is a data dictionary important to data standards?

3. Explain *data mapping*.

11.4 Data Sets

A **data set** is a structured collection of related data elements. These data elements have standard definitions to provide consistent information for all users. Data sets used in health care are frequently created to relate to a specific area of health care, such as inpatient care, outpatient care, long-term care, and home health care. Healthcare data sets are also frequently used for clinical areas, such as cardiology, gastroenterology, and pediatrics. Several data sets that are commonly used in health care are defined next.

Uniform Hospital Discharge Data Set

Initially discussed in Chapter 4, the Uniform Hospital Discharge Data Set (UHDDS) began with 14 data elements and applied only to acute care hospitals. Since then, 6 additional data elements have been added for a total of 20 data elements. These data elements are required by the US Department of Health and Human Services (HHS) to be extracted and reported for Medicare and Medicaid inpatients only. Querying is the common process used to identify and match information in the patient's record to required data elements. However, most hospitals extract the UHDDS for all inpatients, as this information is vital for organizational planning. Use of the UHDDS made the implementation of the prospective payment system possible for acute care hospitals.

In 2006, long-term care hospitals (LTCHs) or long-term acute care hospitals (LTACs) were required to use the UHDDS to facilitate implementation of the LTCH prospective payment system. The UHDDS has been revised over the years to accommodate changes in data required by users and agencies.

Uniform Ambulatory Care Data Set

As presented in Chapter 4, the US National Committee on Vital and Health Statistics recommended a data set for ambulatory care records. These 16 data elements represented the uniform minimum basic data set for ambulatory records. This basic data set for ambulatory records was revised and titled the Uniform Ambulatory Care Data Set (UACDS). Like the UHDDS, the UACDS contains data elements that identify the patient, provider, place, and reason for the encounter as well as the services provided and patient disposition.

Minimum Data Set

The Minimum Data Set (MDS) is a core set of screening, clinical, and functional status elements required to be completed for all residents of nursing homes certified by Medicare or Medicaid. some of these core data elements from the MDS are listed below. The MDS is part of the Resident Assessment Instrument (RAI). The primary purpose of the RAI tool is to identify resident care problems that are addressed in an individualized care plan; however, use of the RAI has expanded. Data collected from MDS assessments is used for the Skilled Nursing Facility Prospective Payment System (SNF PPS) Medicare reimbursement system and many state Medicaid reimbursement systems. Data is also used for monitoring the quality of care provided to nursing home residents. A sampling of the Minimum Data Set Version 3.0 Resident Assessment and Care Screening is illustrated in Figure 11.1.

Minimum Data Set Core Elements:

- Facility provider numbers
- Type of provider
- Type of assessment
- Unit certification or licensure designation
- Preadmission screening and resident review
- Identification information

- Hearing, speech, and vision
- Cognitive patterns
- Mood
- Behavior
- Preferences for customary routine and activities
- Functional status
- Functional abilities and goals

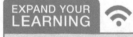

EXPAND YOUR LEARNING

Visit this Medicare site showing data that allows consumers to compare nursing homes:

https://EHR3
.ParadigmEducation
.com/NursingHome.

- Bladder and bowel
- Active diagnoses
- Health conditions
- Swallowing/nutritional status
- Oral/dental
- Skin conditions
- Medications
- Special treatments, procedures, and programs
- Restraints
- Participation in assessment and goal setting
- Care area assessment summary
- Correction request
- Assessment administration

Figure 11.1 Minimum Data Set Version 3.0 Resident Assessment and Care Screening

Resident ______________ Identifier ______________ Date ______________

MINIMUM DATA SET (MDS) - Version 3.0
RESIDENT ASSESSMENT AND CARE SCREENING
Nursing Home Comprehensive (NC) Item Set

Section A	**Identification Information**
A0050. Type of Record	
Enter Code ☐	1. **Add new record** → Continue to A0100, Facility Provider Numbers 2. **Modify existing record** → Continue to A0100, Facility Provider Numbers 3. **Inactivate existing record** → Skip to X0150, Type of Provider
A0100. Facility Provider Numbers	
	A. National Provider Identifier (NPI): ☐☐☐☐☐☐☐☐☐☐ **B. CMS Certification Number (CCN):** ☐☐☐☐☐☐☐☐☐☐☐☐ **C. State Provider Number:** ☐☐☐☐☐☐☐☐☐☐☐☐☐☐☐
A0200. Type of Provider	
Enter Code ☐	**Type of provider** 1. **Nursing home (SNF/NF)** 2. **Swing Bed**
A0310. Type of Assessment	
Enter Code ☐☐	**A. Federal OBRA Reason for Assessment** 01. **Admission** assessment (required by day 14) 02. **Quarterly** review assessment 03. **Annual** assessment 04. **Significant change in status** assessment 05. **Significant correction** to **prior comprehensive** assessment 06. **Significant correction** to **prior quarterly** assessment 99. **None of the above**
Enter Code ☐☐	**B. PPS Assessment** **PPS Scheduled Assessments for a Medicare Part A Stay** 01. **5-day** scheduled assessment 02. **14-day** scheduled assessment 03. **30-day** scheduled assessment 04. **60-day** scheduled assessment 05. **90-day** scheduled assessment **PPS Unscheduled Assessments for a Medicare Part A Stay** 07. **Unscheduled assessment used for PPS** (OMRA, significant or clinical change, or significant correction assessment) **Not PPS Assessment** 99. **None of the above**
Enter Code ☐	**C. PPS Other Medicare Required Assessment - OMRA** 0. **No** 1. **Start of therapy** assessment 2. **End of therapy** assessment 3. **Both Start and End of therapy** assessment 4. **Change of therapy** assessment
Enter Code ☐	**D. Is this a Swing Bed clinical change assessment?** Complete only if A0200 = 2 0. **No** 1. **Yes**
Enter Code ☐	**E. Is this assessment the first assessment** (OBRA, Scheduled PPS, or Discharge) **since the most recent admission/entry or reentry?** 0. **No** 1. **Yes**

MDS 3.0 Nursing Home Comprehensive (NC) Corrected Version 1.14.0 DRAFT   Page 1 of 45

Outcomes and Assessment Information Set and OASIS-D

The **Outcome and Assessment Information Set (OASIS)** is a group of data elements that represent core items of a comprehensive assessment for an adult home care patient. OASIS is the basis for measuring patient outcomes to analyze and improve the quality of care for home care patients. Just like the previous data sets discussed in this section, OASIS is also a requirement of the Medicare and Medicaid certified home health agencies (HHAs). The use of OASIS data began in 1999, and since October 2000, OASIS has been used to reimburse HHAs for the care rendered to Medicare beneficiaries and participating states for Medicaid clients.

OASIS was updated in January 2019 and is now titled OASIS-D. The reason for the update is to meet requirements of the Improving Medicare Post-Acute Care Transformation (IMPACT) Act. OASIS-D increases standardization for pressure ulcer measure to replace the current standardized measure.

OASIS data regarding the assessment of the condition of the patient as well as treatment and services rendered are collected at the following time points:

- Start of care
- Resumption of care following inpatient facility stay
- Recertification within the last 5 days of each 60-day recertification period
- Other follow-up during the home health episode of care
- Transfer to an inpatient facility
- Discharge from home care
- Death at home

In 2017, CMS, with the goal of reducing the data collection burden for OASIS, identified OASIS items to eliminate from the data set. Data items were eliminated if they were not

- used to calculate a measure finalized for the Home Health Quality Reporting Program (HH QRP),
- used in the Home Health PPS,
- used in the survey process for Medicare certification,
- used to calculate a measure in the Home Health Value-Based Purchasing (HH VBP) demonstration,
- used as a critical risk adjustment factor, or
- incorporated into OASIS to fulfill a data category as part of the Conditions of Participation.

A few examples of the data elements that were eliminated include the following:

- Vision
- Ability to hear
- Understanding of verbal content
- Pressure ulcer assessment
- Formal pain assessment

The release OASIS-E was scheduled for May 2020, but due to the coronavirus pandemic, CMS delayed the release of the updated data set.

Data Elements for Emergency Department Systems

In 1997, the National Center for Injury Prevention and Control developed **Data Elements for Emergency Department Systems (DEEDS)**, which are uniform specifications for data entered into emergency department (ED) patient records. There are 156 data elements in this data set, and the number of data elements used to complete a patient's record will vary according to the complexity of the patient's problem and the extent of care rendered during the ED visit. DEEDS focuses on the detailed clinical condition of the patient along with a very thorough reporting of the treatments rendered, including all medications, which significantly increases the number of data elements as compared to the UHDDS and UACDS.

Essential Medical Data Set

The Essential Medical Data Set (EMDS) complements DEEDS, because it provides the data elements for the history of the emergency room patient, whereas DEEDS provides the data elements for the specific ED encounter by the patient.

11.5 Databases

A **database** is a collection of data that is organized in rows, columns, and tables. The data is indexed. **Indexes** in a database are used to find data without searching every row. The data is combined to form information that can be analyzed, managed, and updated. The EHR system is a database that collects the healthcare organization and patient data. Healthcare organizations use data from databases to improve delivery and quality of care. Many types of databases are used by healthcare organizations. A few of the most frequently used databases are HealthData.gov, the Healthcare Cost and Utilization Project, Medicare Provider Analysis and Review, and National Practitioner Data Bank.

HealthData.gov

HealthData.gov (shown in Figure 11.2) provides access to health data with the hope of improving healthcare quality. Healthcare data is collected from various sources, such as CMS, the Centers for Disease Control and Prevention (CDC), the US Food and Drug Administration (FDA), and the National Institutes of Health (NIH). The database is used by innovators who are developing new applications and services that can improve the quality and delivery of health care. The goal of HealthData.gov is to permit private sector innovators to access data collected by HHS.

The Healthcare Cost and Utilization Project

The **Healthcare Cost and Utilization Project (HCUP)** is a collection of databases that is sponsored by the Agency for Healthcare Research and Quality (AHRQ). The collection of databases contains data from state organizations, hospitals, private data organizations, and the federal government to create a national resource of encounter-level healthcare data. The database contains all payer encounter-level information dating back to 1988. HCUP contains a variety of databases, including the National Inpatient Sample (NIS), the Kids' Inpatient Database (KID), the Nationwide Emergency Department Sample (NEDS), the Nationwide Readmissions Database (NRD), the State Inpatient Databases (SID), the

Figure 11.2   HealthData.gov Site

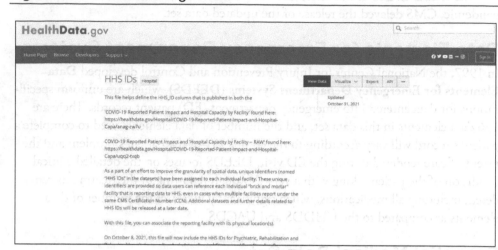

State Ambulatory Surgery and Services Databases (SASD), and the State Emergency Department Databases (SEDD). HCUP data is primarily used by researchers and policymakers; however, this data is publicly available. The collection of data is an information resource of patient-level healthcare data that is used to identify, track, and analyze trends in healthcare use, including access, quality, and outcomes.

Medicare Provider Analysis and Review

Medicare Provider Analysis and Review, known as MEDPAR, is a database that contains inpatient hospital and skilled nursing facility records for all Medicare beneficiaries. MEDPAR contains procedures, diagnoses, and diagnosis-related groups (DRGs); length of stay; beneficiary and Medicare payment amounts; and summarized revenue center charge amounts. The data is organized by state and then by DRG. The data fields include total charges, covered charges, Medicare reimbursement, total days, number of discharges, and average total days. This data set contains data on older patients, since they are most likely Medicare patients.

National Practitioner Data Bank

The **National Practitioner Data Bank (NPDB)** is a database that contains information on medical malpractice payments and actions against healthcare practitioners, providers, and suppliers. The database was established in 1986 by the US Congress to deter practitioner fraud and abuse and promote healthcare quality. A user of this database must be authorized to access the data. The data provides information on healthcare providers, including malpractice awards, loss of license, and exclusion from participation in Medicare or Medicaid. A healthcare organization accesses the NPDB prior to authorizing a healthcare provider to deliver care to patients. Other users of this database include professional societies and state and federal licensing and certification agencies. Healthcare providers may use this database to view their own information.

Data Warehouse

A **data warehouse** is a database that accesses data from multiple databases that are integrated to be used for analytic purposes. The data warehouse is viewed as the trusted source that brings together all the data from the EHR and other data generators and

EXPAND YOUR LEARNING

When analyzing data, it is important to examine how data is collected from hospitals, payers, primary care providers, specialists, pharmacies, public health organizations, and patients. Read the article "The Importance of Data Collection in Healthcare" to better understand the purpose of health data collection and how it is used for making decisions.
https://EHR3
.ParadigmEducation
.com/DataCollection

gathers them within the organization. The data from the warehouse can provide information on a single patient or a related group of patients. The goal of analyzing data from a data warehouse is to help healthcare practitioners and organizations provide better care.

Data Indices

The International Classification of Diseases (ICD) classification system was discussed in Chapter 9. Recall that ICD is an index that is used to classify and code all diagnoses, symptoms, and procedures in combination with a patient's inpatient or hospital care.

Current Procedural Terminology (CPT®) classification system was discussed in Chapter 9. Remember that CPT® is an index of medical, surgical, and diagnostic procedure codes used by healthcare providers in the delivery of outpatient care.

11.6 Data Registries

An EHR is used to collect various clinical and demographic data about each patient for every healthcare encounter. A data registry is more specific, as it is used to collect data about certain diseases or conditions. In the future, once interoperability between systems is in place, an EHR may populate the registry. Currently, technology is being developed to integrate registries into the EHR. Meanwhile, registries provide valuable information regarding the health status of patients.

The National Vital Statistics System is an example of data sharing in public health by collecting data from the National Center for Health Statistics (NCHS) and vital registration systems. State laws require birth certificates to be submitted for all births. Federal law requires the national collection and publication of births. A birth registry contains information about the newborn, mother and father, and health information. The registry contains information on live births, infant deaths, and fetal deaths.

Cancer Registries

A **cancer registry** is a collection of data focusing on cancer and tumor diseases. The data is collected by cancer registrars who gather and report information such as patient history, diagnosis, treatment, and status. The registry contains this information for every patient who has been diagnosed with cancer by a healthcare provider in the United States. Healthcare organizations are required to report new cancer cases to their state cancer registries. The data may be submitted electronically or by paper. The registry helps report cancer incidences as well as evaluate the patient's experience and the quality of treatment.

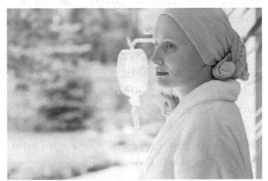

All patients with cancer in the United States are added to a cancer registry.

Clinical Trials

ClinicalTrials.gov is a registry that provides access to information on publicly and privately funded clinical studies. Clinical trials evaluate new laboratory findings that may advance diagnosis, treatment, or prevention in humans. A clinical trial is a study that uses human volunteers. These studies assign interventions based on a plan and then evaluate the health effect and outcome. The registry is maintained by the National Library of Medicine at the NIH. Clinical trials can be based on new treatments, different drugs, or changes in diet.

Trauma Registries

A **trauma registry** includes the collection, storage, and reporting of patient trauma data. Trauma data that is collected for the registry is based on serious bodily injury. An example of trauma that may be reported would be a person who is seriously injured in a car accident and whether the patient was wearing a seat belt. The registry collects data about an injured patient who meets specific criteria. The data consists of demographic, injury, and trauma outcome data. The registry helps analyze injuries, establish prevention programs, evaluate major trauma outcomes, and support research and education.

Immunization Registries

An **immunization registry** includes patient data on various immunizations. Healthcare clinics can report confidential vaccination data about their patients to public health agencies. Immunization registries are important tools to help remind patients when vaccines are past due and to consolidate immunization records for patients who may have multiple healthcare providers. This is accomplished with the help of the Immunization Information System (IIS), a database that consolidates all immunization doses administered by participating providers. Inclusion in the IIS database is voluntary, and participants are informed about the IIS, what information is provided, and how it will be used. The IIS combines information from different sources into a single record so that immunization records can be shared with schools and day cares for example. This helps to track when immunizations are due and when children get only the vaccinations they need.

11.7 Information Governance

One of the major challenges in the management of healthcare information is creating an effective framework for the access and use of healthcare data. This framework is known as **information governance** and includes the policies, procedures, and processes for data and information creation, storage, access, use, analysis, archival, and deletion.

Information governance is a relatively new concept in health care. It took the implementation of EHR systems for many healthcare executives to recognize the vast amount of data and information available to their organizations and the need for governance of this data and information. Healthcare executives typically turn to their information technology (IT) departments and/or health information management (HIM) departments for assistance with information governance.

An effective information governance system should include the following components:

- Data governance committee

- Strategic plans for using and expanding data

- Management of data quality

- Appropriate access to data

- Resources for users to correctly interpret the data

Data Governance Committee

One of the first steps in establishing a data governance program is to create a data governance committee made up of a broad representation of the organization's stake-holders. A broad representation promotes the establishment of processes, policies, and procedures that apply to the organization, avoiding those that are narrow in scope. For example, if only IT and HIM staff serve on the data governance committee, many clinical needs could be ignored, whereas including representatives from clinical departments enhances the committee's membership.

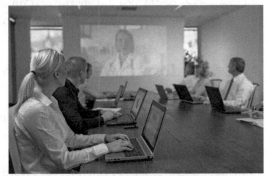

All departments in a healthcare facility should be represented on a data governance committee.

Strategic Plans for Using and Expanding Data

The data governance program should be a fluid program that is constantly growing and changing to meet the needs of the organization. The healthcare organization often uses a strategic plan to drive the data governance program. A **strategic plan** is an organization's process of defining its direction by including goals or objectives and a sequence of steps to achieve each goal and objective. Establishment of strategic plans, both short term and long term, helps keep the data governance program on track and relevant to the needs of the organization.

Management of Data Quality

In the discussion of the importance of data quality earlier in this chapter, you learned how important it is to an organization to have accurate data. A successful data governance program should have specific auditing programs in place to ensure data accuracy. A key data auditing program that will be discussed in Chapter 13 is a clinical documentation improvement (CDI) program. In addition to the auditing and correcting of clinical data, data quality auditing should also be conducted for financial and demographic data.

Appropriate Access to Data

As we have discussed in previous chapters, there is a need for data security as well as a process of minimum use in which each user of the organization's data has access to only the minimum amount of data necessary for completion of their job role. Considering the heightened focus on the security of health data in the daily news, there is a tendency to keep a tight control on all data. However, a well-functioning data governance program should encourage the use of data while keeping security protocols in mind. To facilitate appropriate access to data, an organization should consider merging committees dealing with IT privacy, security, and data governance.

Resources for Users to Correctly Interpret Data

Data users must have the necessary resources to correctly interpret data. Otherwise, poor decisions could result. For example, the concept of the data dictionary, which was discussed earlier in this chapter, is a perfect example of a necessary resource. Consider this example. The CEO of a hospital asks the director of radiology to provide the actual cost of a chest x-ray performed at the hospital over the past year. The director of radiology queries or performs a search of the database using specific criteria to request the number of chest x-rays performed on the admissions for the past year. By requesting data based on admissions, the director of radiology is missing the number of chest x-rays performed during the year on outpatients. The presence of a data dictionary would assist the director in accurately extracting the data needed to fulfill the request.

AHIMA Information Governance Principles for Healthcare

According to the American Health Information Management Association (AHIMA), the foundation of data and information governance is accomplished with the implementation of eight key principles. These eight key principles form the AHIMA Information Governance Principles for Healthcare (IGPHC) and are described here.

1. "Accountability: Designation or identification of a senior member of leadership responsible for the development and oversight of the IG Program.

2. Transparency: Documentation of processes and activities related to IG are visible and readily available for review by stakeholders.

3. Integrity: Systems evidence trustworthiness in the authentication, timeliness, accuracy, and completion of information.

4. Protection: Program protects private and confidential information from loss, breach, and corruption.

5. Compliance: Program ensures compliance with local, state, and federal regulations, accrediting agencies' standards and healthcare organizations' policies and procedures and ethical practices.

6. Availability: Structure and accessibility of data allows for timely and efficient retrieval by authorized personnel.

7. Retention: Lifespan of information is defined and regulated by a schedule in compliance with legal requirements and ethical considerations.

8. Disposition: Process ensures the legal and ethical disposition of information including, but not limited to, record destruction and transfer."

Source: Davoudi, Sion; Dooling, Julie A.; Glondys, Barbara; Jones, Theresa D.; Kadlec, Lesley; Overgaard, Shauna M.; Ruben, Kerry; Wendicke, Annemarie. "Data Quality Management Model (2015 Update)" Journal of AHIMA 86, no. 10 (October 2015): expanded web version.

CHECKPOINT 11.3

1. Explain the difference between a data set, database, registry, and index.

_____

_____

_____

2. List the eight principles of the AHIMA Information Governance Principles for Healthcare.

_____

_____

_____

11.8 Data and Decisions

There has been a great deal of information presented in this chapter about the importance of data in health care. Healthcare data is important for making decisions about patient care. Healthcare data provides information about patients, which can in turn identify treatments to improve and create patient-centered quality care. Analyzing a patient's data may also help to identify warning signs of serious illness to provide treatment at an early stage, which can also be less expensive. Other ways data influences decisions include helping to predict epidemics, cure diseases, and avoid preventable deaths.

Big Data

The term *big data* is often discussed in health care today. **Big data** refers to large data sets that are analyzed to reveal trends and patterns. Healthcare decisions are being made based on data. Big data is being used to learn as much as possible about the patient to pick up on warning signs as early as possible. This approach can lead to earlier treatment and decreased costs. A few of the ways in which big data is transforming health care include:

- Big data creates value for patients by making information personal and accurate.

- Big data improves quality of life to help treat and manage patients' current conditions.

- Big data reduces medical errors with evidence-based and personalized care.

- Big data provides cost effectiveness to healthcare facilities by helping to eliminate fraud and abuse.

- Big data improves innovation by analyzing data from past trials and current health trends.

Consider This

Healthcare organizations are large and complex. The healthcare industry has been slow to adopt the use of data to improve the quality and delivery of health care. The question is, how can healthcare organizations use data to improve the quality and delivery of health care?

Medication errors have been a big problem in the delivery of health care. Because humans can make errors, patients may end up with incorrect medications, which could lead to adverse effects. Using data can help reduce errors by analyzing the patient's health record and medication list. Analyzing the data could help flag any medications that appear to be out of place. Another way healthcare organizations could use data to improve delivery of care is by identifying high-risk patients. Currently, many patients still repeatedly use the ED. Using the ED for care increases the cost of health care and often does not lead to better outcomes. One way data could be used to improve outcomes for patients is by predicting high-risk patients, reducing ED visits, and offering patient-centric care.

(Continues)

Analyzing healthcare data could be used to reduce wait times. A clinic could track the wait time and overall visit time of patients. Analysts can look at procedures and healthcare providers to analyze efficiencies and identify holdups. The data from the EHR can alert staff if a patient has been waiting too long. Data can be used to identify and prevent security breaches. Data can also be used to analyze websites, tracking pages and application interfaces to catch attacks and analyze uncharacteristic access patterns as well as complete security forensics. Finally, data from wearable technology, if shared with healthcare providers, can improve patient engagement and outcomes. The data can be analyzed to help patients remain independent and reduce office visits. The EHR has become easier for healthcare professionals to access and use to analyze data. There is still room for improvement with analyzing the available data. What other ways do you think healthcare organizations can use data to improve the quality and delivery of health care?

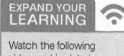

EXPAND YOUR LEARNING

Watch the following video on big data in health care:

https://EHR3 .Paradigm Education .com/BigData.

11.9 Informatics

Informatics is a growing and evolving multidisciplinary field that focuses on technology and information. **Informatics** is defined as the science of processing data for storage and retrieval. There are many subspecialties of informatics, including health care, pharmacy, public health, nursing, and biomedical research. The goal of informatics is to examine the data to serve as information to increase knowledge between individuals and groups.

Healthcare Informatics

Healthcare informatics is the study of managing health information. Healthcare informatics includes health systems such as the EHR, data standards such as HL7, terminologies including SNOMED CT, and health data collected through personal digital devices. Healthcare informatics is used to evaluate the patient's data to improve the quality and delivery of health care. You can now pursue a career specialization in health informatics as a health informatics specialist. A person working in this career specialty utilizes technology to analyze clinical and administrative data and works closely with providers to improve the quality and delivery of healthcare.

Chapter Summary

Data is invaluable in the healthcare industry. As healthcare providers enter patient data into the EHR, they are participating in the accumulation of vast amounts of data and information about patients, their health statuses, and treatments rendered.

Data is defined as descriptive or numeric attributes of one or more variables, and the term *data* is frequently referred to as a *data element* in the EHR. The two types of data that are used in health care to improve quality and care and to facilitate decision making are known as *internal* and *external data*. There are two kinds of data sources, primary and secondary. The accuracy, completeness, and reliability of this data in the EHR, also known as *data integrity*, is vital for organizations to achieve their goals of providing high-quality care and making good decisions for their patients. It is important for healthcare organizations to establish policies and procedures for their employees to follow regarding data usage and operations. A data dictionary is one such policy, as the data dictionary describes the contents, format, and structure of elements within a database. A data set is a structured collection of related data elements that have standard definitions. Healthcare data sets include UHDDS, UACDC, MDS, OASIS, DEEDS, and EMDS. Healthcare databases, a collection of data that is organized in rows, columns, and tables, include HealthData.gov, the Healthcare Cost and Utilization Project (HCUP), Medicare Provider Analysis and Review (MEDPAR), and National Practitioner Data Bank (NPDB). Data registries are databases focused on a collection of information about a specific condition or disease. Examples include cancer registries, birth registries, and trauma registries. A data warehouse is a database that accesses data from multiple databases to be used for analytic purposes. The goal of analyzing the data is to help healthcare providers and organizations provide better care.

One of the major challenges in the management of healthcare information is information governance, which is an effective framework for the access and use of healthcare data. An effective information governance system should include a data governance committee, strategic plans for using and expanding data, management of data quality, appropriate access to data, and resources for users to correctly interpret the data.

The term *big data* is often used in health care today, and it refers to the large data sets that are used to reveal trends and patterns, such as predicting epidemics, curing diseases, and avoiding preventable deaths.

Informatics is the science of processing data for storage and retrieval and is a growing and evolving multidisciplinary field that focuses on technology and information.

Review and Assessment

The following Review and Assessment activities are also available online in the Cirrus online course. Your instructor may ask you to complete these activities online. Cirrus also provides access to flash cards, a crossword puzzle, and practice quizzes to help strengthen your understanding of the chapter content.

Acronyms/Initialisms

Study the following acronyms discussed in this chapter. Go to the online course for flash cards of the acronyms and other chapter key terms.

AHRQ: Agency for Healthcare Research and Quality

CDC: Centers for Disease Control and Prevention

CDI: clinical documentation improvement

CMS: Centers for Medicare & Medicaid Services

DEEDS: Data Elements for Emergency Department Systems

EMDS: Essential Medical Data Set

FDA: US Food and Drug Administration

HCUP: Healthcare Cost and Utilization Project

HH QRP: Home Health Quality Reporting Program

HH VBP: Home Health Value-Based Purchasing

IGPHC: Information Governance Principles for Healthcare (AHIMA)

IMPACT: Improving Medicare Post-Acute Care Transformation (Act)

KID: Kids' Inpatient Database

LTAC: long-term acute care hospital

LTCH: long-term care hospital

MDS: Minimum Data Set

MEDPAR: Medicare Provider Analysis and Review

NCHS: National Center for Health Statistics

NEDS: Nationwide Emergency Department Sample

NIH: National Institutes of Health

NIS: National Inpatient Sample

NPDB: National Practitioner Data Bank

NRD: Nationwide Readmissions Database

OASIS: Outcomes and Assessment Information Set

PPS: Prospective Payment System

RAI: Resident Assessment Instrument

SEDD: State Emergency Department Databases

SASD: State Ambulatory Surgery and Services Databases

UACDS: Uniform Ambulatory Care Data Set

UHDDS: Uniform Hospital Discharge Data Set

Check Your Understanding

To check your understanding of this chapter's key concepts, answer the following questions.

1. Which of the following is an example of data integrity being compromised?

    a. A medication allergy was entered incorrectly in a patient's EHR.

    b. A medical coder selected the wrong principal diagnosis for billing.

    c. A health information management department staff member released a patient's record with a patient authorization.

    d. A physician entered an order for a lab test.

2. The MDS is a core set of screening, clinical, and functional status elements that is required to be completed for which of the following?

    a. All residents of nursing homes certified by Medicare and Medicaid

    b. All home health patients using Medicare or Medicaid as their payment source

    c. All Medicare and Medicaid patients, both inpatient and outpatient

    d. All inpatients and outpatients covered by Medicare or Medicaid

3. All of the statements about the Outcome and Assessment Information Set (OASIS) are true *except*

    a. OASIS is a requirement of Medicare and Medicaid.

    b. OASIS is a group of data elements that represent core items of a comprehensive assessment.

    c. OASIS is used to reimburse home health agencies.

    d. OASIS was updated in January 2019 to support measurement domains mandated by IMPACT.

4. The Healthcare Cost and Utilization Project is a collection of databases that is sponsored by the

    a. AHRQ.

    b. SID.

    c. HIMSS.

    d. CMS.

5. MEDPAR contains all the following data *except*

    a. diagnoses.

    b. procedures.

    c. social history.

    d. revenue center charge amounts.

6. NPDB is a database that contains information on which of the following?

    a. Medicare beneficiaries

    b. patients' vital statistics such as births and deaths

    c. cancer and tumor diseases

    d. medical malpractice payments against healthcare providers

7. A database that accesses data from multiple databases that are integrated to be used for analytic purposes is the definition of

    a. a data warehouse.

    b. external data sources.

    c. information governance.

    d. the Healthcare Cost and Utilization Project.

8. An organization's process of defining its direction by including goals or objectives and a sequence of steps to achieve each goal and objective is known as

    a. management of data quality.

    b. a data governance committee.

    c. a strategic plan.

    d. big data.

9. An effective information governance system should include all *except*

    a. appropriate access to data.

    b. management of data quality.

    c. data governance committee.

    d. data warehousing.

10. Documentation of processes and activities related to information governance need to be visible and readily available for review by stakeholders. This is one

of the eight key principles of the AHIMA Information Governance Principles for Healthcare and is called

   a. protection.

   b. transparency.

   c. availability.

   d. retention.

Go on the Record

To build on your understanding of the topics in this chapter, complete the following short-answer activities.

1. Explain the difference between the two types of primary and secondary data. Include examples of each data type.

2. Explain why standards, policies, and procedures are important elements of data integrity.

3. Describe three different data sets.

4. List and describe three registries.

5. Explain the components that should be included in an information governance system.

Navigate the Field

To gain practice in handling challenging situations in the workplace, consider the following real-world scenarios and identify how you would respond to each.

1. You are the chair of the Information Governance Committee at Northstar Medical Center. You have been asked to educate physicians on the importance of health information governance. Prepare an outline that lists the components of health information governance you will include in your training to the physicians.

2. You are the IT administrator. You have been instructed to create a data dictionary for Wellness Hospital. Create a table that identifies the field name, data type, and description for the following fields: patient first name, patient last name, date of birth, patient ID, diagnosis, admission date, discharge date, encounter type, procedure ID, clinical date, procedure code, antibiotic name, antibiotic dose, antibiotic frequency, vital sign temperature, lab ID, lab test name, and lab test result.

Think Critically

Continue to think critically about challenging concepts and complete the following activities.

1. You are a data analyst with Northstar Medical Center. You have been asked to review the National 2017 Emergency Department statistics to make some comparisons. Go to https://EHR3.ParadigmEducation.com/HCUPNET. Under *HCUP Products*, select *HCUPnet*. Then select *Get Quick Statistics Tables*. Select *Emergency Department*. Select *National*. Select *2018* for the year.

Select *No* for the question regarding data on specific diagnosis or condition. Then select *Create Analysis*. Select Accept. How are the statistics broken down? What type of statistics are included in the table? Is the information helpful? Submit the tables and explanation in a Word document.

2. Investigate an entry-level career focusing on healthcare data.

    a. Select an entry-level position that you might be interested in pursuing.

    b. Describe the position along with promotional and transitional career.

    c. Describe how data plays an important role in this career.

Make Your Case

Consider the scenario and then complete the following project.

You are presenting to Northstar Medical Center about a clinical trial you helped create. Create a presentation of your clinical trial. Go to https://EHR3.ParadigmEducation.com/ClinicalTrials. Select a condition/disease of your choice. Select *United States* for the country. Click *Search All Studies*. Review the possible clinical trials. Select a clinical trial that has a status of recruiting. Prepare a presentation that includes the following elements: title of clinical trial, purpose, study type, study design, summary of clinical trial, primary and secondary outcome measures, estimated enrollment, anticipated study start and completion date, eligibility, criteria, and location. Include any other information that is important to share about the clinical trial.

Explore the Technology

To expand your mastery of EHRs, explore the technology by completing the following online activities.

1. Perform an internet search and identify and explain three different ways data is collected with the EHR.

2. Locate the top 10 cancers in 2018 by going to https://EHR3.ParadigmEducation.com/USCS. Click *United States Cancer Statistics*. Click *Data Visualizations Tool*. Submit the graphs to your instructor by ethnicity. Is there anything that surprises you? Are there any interesting trends? Then search again to determine the states with the highest occurrences of cancer. Why do you think certain states have a high occurrence of cancer? Are there any trends you can identify from the data?

3. Conduct an internet search to identify how data collected through personal digital devices is improving health outcomes.

4. Research how health informatics is being used to improve the quality and delivery of health care.

Chapter **12** Data Analytics

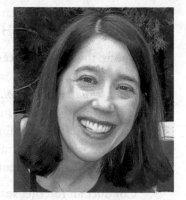

12.1 Define *data analytics*.

12.2 Explain the importance of data analytics in health care.

12.3 Identify the users of healthcare data analytics.

12.4 Define and discuss the types of data analytics used in health care.

12.5 Define *data mining*, *artificial intelligence (AI)*, and the *Internet of Things (IoT)*.

12.6 Discuss the importance of the management of information plan.

12.7 Discuss the steps of a data use strategy.

12.8 Describe the role of the EHR in data analytics.

12.9 Describe and discuss the many uses of data analytics.

12.10 Discuss how the EHR and data analytics contribute to healthcare reporting.

As you learned in Chapter 11, data is invaluable to the healthcare industry because data turns into information and information is priceless when managed and analyzed appropriately. The healthcare industry has experienced an explosion of data due to the implementation of EHR systems, so much so that organizing healthcare data into usable information has been a major challenge for the healthcare industry. In this chapter, we will discuss the uses of data analytics in healthcare, beginning with a definition.

12.1 Data Analytics

Data analytics is defined as the practice of exploring and manipulating data for the purposes of identifying new information that can be used to improve the operations of an organization. In health care, data analytics is used to improve the delivery of patient care, improve patient outcomes, identify populations and health conditions that are underserved, identify opportunities to reduce healthcare costs, and attempt to predict future healthcare needs and trends.

Healthcare providers, patients, payers, and other stakeholders are all invested in the goal of providing high-quality healthcare at the lowest cost. Data analytics is a tool for these interested parties to identify opportunities to better achieve this goal. In the past, most healthcare services were paid on a fee-for-service basis. As healthcare services were provided, they were paid for with little to no indication of what the cost might be for a specific patient with a particular disease or condition treated in a particular provider setting. As payment for healthcare services moves from this fee-for-service model to prospective systems and value-based care, there are more cost control measures in place, including reimbursement limits on the cost of care. Data analytics plays an important role in estimating and predicting the healthcare needs of the population as well as the estimated costs to providers and third-party payers. Using data analytics to budget and allocate money and services is key to the financial stability of all parties.

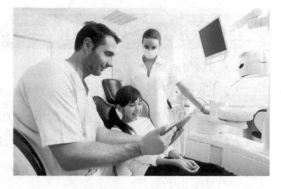

While financial stability is of utmost importance, one of the most exciting applications of data analytics is in the improvement of patient care. EHR systems allow providers to quickly and easily compile vast amounts of patient data to identify patterns and trends in the successful and unsuccessful provision of healthcare. With that information, clinicians can develop and refine clinical protocols to improve the quality of care. For example, by tracking the medication regimens and health outcomes of patients with a specific disease, providers can identify the most effective medications for that disease or condition.

Internal and External Users

Due to the complexity of the healthcare system, the number and types of users of healthcare data analytics is significant. There are both internal and external users. Internal users include employees working to ensure that the healthcare organization is providing the best care in the most cost-effective manner. This includes clinicians, financial managers, medical staff, risk managers, quality improvement staff, administrators, and the board of trustees. External users include government agencies that require reporting from healthcare organizations, accrediting bodies, public health agencies, and interested contracted companies.

Depending on the user and the purpose of the data use, access may be restricted to aggregate data. Aggregate data provides opportunities for data analysis without compromising patient confidentiality with the ability to identify patients. For example, internal users such as administrators and the board of trustees of the healthcare organization do not need to know the identity of individual patients when reviewing financial data by clinical departments, whereas internal users working on identifying opportunities to improve the quality of healthcare would need specific patient data to accomplish their goals. External users typically do not have access to individual patient data and receive information in aggregate. There are exceptions, however, when individual patient data is needed by external users. For example, when a state health department is investigating a patient complaint, they would obviously need access to specific patient information to determine whether the complaint is valid.

12.2 Types of Healthcare Data Analytics

There are several types of data analytics that are used to address the needs of the users of healthcare data. These include descriptive analytics, predictive analytics, and prescriptive analytics.

Descriptive Analytics

Descriptive analytics refers to using historical data to identify patterns and study trends in historical events. In health care, users performing descriptive analysis on a set of data look for patterns that could lead to opportunities for improvement in the quality, delivery, and cost of care. Consider an identified pattern of stable patients remaining in the ICU for long lengths of stay. A review of the patient data might demonstrate an opportunity to safely transfer patients from the ICU to a lower level of care. Descriptive analytics could serve as the basis for conversations among the medical staff and discharge planners and potentially result in better patient care outcomes as well as considerable cost savings.

Predictive Analytics

When the power of artificial intelligence is combined with historical data, users are able to conduct what is called *predictive analytics*. **Predictive analytics** in health care is the use of historical patient data with the application of statistical algorithms to identify expected future outcomes and trends in health care. Some examples of predictive analytics in health care include predicting the types of patients who are likely to be readmitted frequently to an inpatient hospital, predicting which patients are at high risk for self-harm, and identifying newborns who are most at risk to develop early-onset neonatal sepsis.

Consider This

Charlie is in the ICU on mechanical ventilation at Northstar Medical Center due to respiratory failure from a stroke he suffered two weeks ago. The physicians are speaking with the family about transferring Charlie to a long-term acute care hospital that has reported excellent patient outcomes for weaning patients off ventilators and providing rehabilitation services to help patients regain their independence. While Charlie's family is concerned about his impending discharge from the ICU for fear that his condition might deteriorate, they are comforted to learn that Northstar Medical Center uses predictive analytics that can estimate the probability of a patient's risk of death or readmission within 48 hours if they are discharged from the ICU.

Prescriptive Analytics

Prescriptive analytics also works with future predictions like predictive analytics. Prescriptive analytics also uses AI but takes predictive analytics a step further by identifying the best options for achieving future outcomes. **Prescriptive analytics** presents "what if" options to give decision-makers the opportunity to select the best option for the desired outcome. For example, prescriptive analytics can present suggested treatment plans for patients with end-stage renal disease to prevent or limit repeated admissions to the hospital. The suggested treatment plans are produced from an analysis of thousands of end-stage renal disease patient records. Healthcare providers may choose to select one of the suggested treatment plans for their patient.

As we continue our discussion of data analytics in health care, it is important to understand several key terms, including *data mining*, *artificial intelligence*, and the *Internet of Things*.

Data Mining

Data mining is the process of searching for and examining data to organize it into useful patterns and trends. The structured data in an EHR system can be mined quickly and easily because the fixed nature of structured data makes it possible to search, query, and quantify. Data mining of unstructured data is a more challenging process that researchers and developers are working to simplify. A wealth of information is buried in the narrative provider notes of an EHR, waiting to be manipulated and studied.

Artificial Intelligence

According to the Healthcare Information and Management Systems Society (HIMSS), **artificial intelligence (AI)** is defined as computer systems able to perform tasks that usually require human intelligence. AI is used by healthcare organizations to mine the patient data maintained in EHR systems. AI is also used to interpret and classify the clinical documentation found in EHR systems, including unstructured documentation such as provider progress notes and other free text documentation found in history and physical exams, consultation reports, discharge summaries, and so on.

Internet of Things

The **Internet of Things (IoT)** is new terminology used to describe networks of devices that can connect to share data. An IoT in health care is a network of patient data devices that are able to connect and share data. Some examples of IoT devices include sleep monitors, smart contact lenses, smart necklaces that identify whether medications have been taken as prescribed, vital signs monitors, glucose monitors, and sleep and safety monitors for infants. These devices have the capability of transmitting data to patients' healthcare providers who track and prevent acute and chronic diseases. For example, sleep monitors may register that a patient has sleep apnea. Sleep apnea is a disorder in which breathing starts and stops while sleeping. Depending on the severity, sleep apnea can make some chronic diseases worse, such as high blood pressure. Sleep apnea can even result in death due to cardiac arrest, so identifying this condition early with an IoT device could save lives. Additional IoT devices and uses are described in Chapter 14.

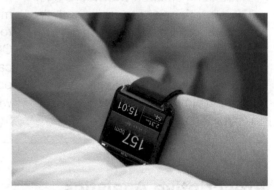

Smartwatches can be used to monitor heart rate, blood pressure, temperature, respiration, and other health indicators.

12.3 Management of Information Plan

With the amount of data being generated by EHR systems and all the technological systems used by a healthcare organization, an intentional and strategic plan to manage the organization's data and data needs must be developed and managed by an interdisciplinary group of the organization's stakeholders and data users. This **management of information plan** must encompass all technological systems used by the organization; all the data generated, used, and stored; and all the processes used to contribute to the flow of information. The plan should take into account all patient data as well as financial data, human resources data, and supply inventories. In addition to the internal flow of information, the flow of information to and from external organizations is another important consideration for information management planning. The management of information plan also considers the data and information required to support the contracts and relationships with outside providers and affiliates, contracted services, and payers. A tool that healthcare organizations might use to develop their management of information plan is a data use strategy.

Data Use Strategy

Although the value of information is well understood, unlocking that value is often a challenge due to the high volume of data and the challenges associated with collecting, organizing, and analyzing it. Developing a data use strategy can help businesses overcome these challenges and access the value of their data while efficiently using their resources.

A good data use strategy consists of eight steps, described in Figure 12.1.

Figure 12.1   Eight Steps to Develop a Data Use Strategy

1. Establish a Management of Information Team (MIT)—The establishment of an MIT is imperative for the successful management of an organization's data needs and uses. This team should be interdisciplinary with key stakeholders of the organization who are interested in working with data to achieve the goals of the organization.

2. Identify the data needs of the organization—The MIT should work with data users in the organization to identify the data needed. The MIT might begin this process with a survey and follow up with interviews and meetings to clarify the data needs.

3. Identify the data already being collected—Of the data needed by data users of the organization, what data are already being collected?

4. Identify gaps in data collection—Once the MIT has identified the data needs of the organization and the data that are already being collected, the gaps in data collection can be identified.

5. Identify strategies to gather data—Once the gaps in data collection have been identified, a strategy to gather the data can be developed.

6. Identify data storage needs—Data storage is one of the most important aspects of a data use strategy to ensure that data are safe, secure, and available when needed.

7. Develop a Management of Information Plan—A Management of Information Plan is developed by the MIT and is updated on an annual basis and more often as needed.

8. Implement the Management of Information Plan—The Management of Information Plan must be implemented in a strategic and organized fashion to ensure success.

CHECKPOINT 12.1

1. Computer systems able to perform tasks that usually require human intelligence is the definition of what?

2. List two examples of the IoT.

12.4 Role of the EHR in Data Analytics

The use of data analytics in health care is not a new concept. Clinicians, researchers, students, auditors, surveyors, and other interested parties have historically abstracted data from paper medical records to accomplish their work. EHR systems have taken healthcare data analytics to a new level because they make data more accessible, timely, and accurate.

Accessibility of Data

Consider how data was abstracted before the use of EHRs. In acute care hospitals, the health information management department (formerly the medical record department) staff were responsible for abstracting a minimum set of data from each patient's medical record. This minimum data set was prescribed and required to be abstracted from all hospital inpatient medical records as part of the accreditation standards of The Joint Commission, an organization that surveys and accredits hospitals and other types of healthcare facilities. The minimum data set included basic demographic patient information along with the patient's medical record number; diagnosis and procedure codes; names of the admitting, attending, and consulting physicians; length of stay; and discharge status. A minimum amount of clinical data was part of this data set and included such things as height, weight, and medications.

Before computers were widely used in health care, the data was documented on paper, scanned, and mailed to the Commission on Professional and Hospital Activities (CPHA), a data processing company for compilation. The data was compiled at the CPHA and basic reports were printed and mailed to the submitting hospital. These reports were basic indexes organized by physician, diagnosis, and operative procedure. The reports were primarily used to identify the patients of a particular population. For example, if a physician wanted to conduct a study of patients who had suffered a transient ischemic attack (TIA), a medical record department staff member would use the diagnostic index to identify the patients with the TIA diagnosis code and pull the individual paper medical records from the file shelves for the physician to review. Keep in mind that even after all the work of the initial abstracting and report generation, the physician conducting the study was basically starting their data analysis from scratch.

EHR systems have made data accessible in real time and available with just a few keystrokes, which is a monumental advance in healthcare data analytics. Consider the amount of time saved from manually reviewing and organizing data. Consider too the expediency with which data can now be accessed and used to make changes in healthcare treatment and services that could save patient lives.

Timely Data

As we have discussed throughout this text, one of the most significant advantages of using an EHR is the real-time updates to patient data stored in the EHR system. Individual data can be accessed as soon as it is entered in the EHR, and reports with data from an entire clinic can be generated in a more timely fashion from the EHR.

Volume of Data

As expected, with the implementation of EHR systems, the volume of patient data stored by healthcare organizations has grown exponentially. At the current rate of growth, big data for US health care will soon reach the zettabyte (10^{21} gigabytes) scale and, not long after, the yottabyte (10^{24} gigabytes). With an effective and well-maintained management of information plan, a large volume of data is an asset to an organization. However, if an organization does not have a good management of information plan in place, a large volume of data could be detrimental to an organization if bad decisions occur based on mismanagement of the data.

Accuracy of Data

EHR patient data are more accurate due to edits and parameters placed on data entry. Data must be entered according to the EHR system requirements. In addition, there are no transcription errors that are known to occur in the abstracting process from paper to computer records.

12.5 Uses of Data Analytics

Earlier in this chapter, we discussed the users of healthcare data. Now we will discuss some specific ways healthcare data are used.

Patient Care

Data analytics is used at the point of care to provide the best healthcare treatment as technology is leveraged to provide clinicians with the best information for:

- Diagnosis

- Optimal treatments

- Medication risks, benefits, indications, and contraindications

- Diagnostic test results reporting

The EHR system tools that support diagnosis, treatment selection, and medication selection have been explored in previous chapters. One of the EHR system point-of-care tools that support diagnostic test results reporting is clinical results reporting.

Clinical Results Reporting

Clinical results reporting, also known as **clinical outputs**, refers to an accumulation of relevant data points from a patient's EHR or many patients' EHRs organized for comparison and study. For example, a physician might run a cumulative report of the laboratory results of a patient to easily determine whether trends in laboratory values need to be addressed. The transcribed reports of an H&P as well as consultations and radiology reports are additional examples of clinical outputs. All clinicians involved in the patient's care can then use this data.

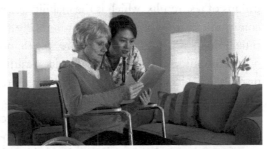

Clinical results reporting through the EHR allows for accurate and timely communication between healthcare providers and patients.

Clinical results reporting is an EHR system function that allows healthcare providers to view laboratory and diagnostic test results immediately, provided there is an interface between the clinical results system and the EHR. This feature satisfies one of the National Patient Safety Goals (NPSGs) of The Joint Commission. Hospitals accredited by The Joint Commission are required to comply with the NPSGs, which were established to help hospitals address specific areas of concern with regard to patient safety. The first set of NPSGs became effective on January 1, 2003, and the goals are updated annually by The Joint Commission based on the recommendations of the Patient Safety Advisory Group, a panel of widely recognized patient safety experts that includes nurses, physicians, pharmacists, risk managers, clinical

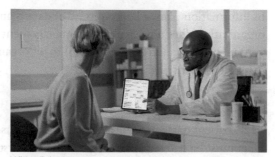

With clinical results reporting, clinicians are able to view and discuss lab results with patients immediately upon completion.

engineers, and other professionals with hands-on experience in addressing patient safety issues. Reporting the critical results of tests and diagnostic procedures in a timely manner has been included in the NPSGs since 2005 and is likely to remain on the list of NPSGs for many years.

According to surveyors from The Joint Commission, "There is an increased awareness that poor communication is at the heart of medical errors and lawsuits, which is why The Joint Commission is emphasizing the role of communication in critical value reporting." This goal is meant to ensure that laboratories report important clinical results to healthcare personnel in a timely manner, thereby allowing them to expediently treat patients. Hospitals must have policies and procedures in place that specify the time frame during which healthcare providers must be advised of test results that are considered critical. Each healthcare organization is responsible for specifying the values and circumstances that define a critical test result. These specifications should be clearly defined in facility policy and medical staff bylaws. For example, the hematocrit laboratory value might be considered critical if it were less than 18% or greater than 55% for an adult. A chest x-ray with a suspicious shadow may also be considered critical.

Automated Clinical Results Reporting   The clinical results reporting feature of EHR systems addresses a long-standing problem associated with phone and fax communications of test results, which is the inability for healthcare providers to receive these communications when they are not in their offices (such as weekends, holidays, and nighttime hours). When EHR systems are able to interface with laboratory computers and other computers that output test results, healthcare providers can use personal computers or mobile devices to access these test results and order medications, treatments, and further tests to address the reported results. This is an example of the **automatic method** of results entry and how it decreases the time from when a test is conducted to when the results are reported to the provider and when the provider can take action. The automated transfer of the results also reduces the likelihood of an error introduced during transcription. In addition, many EHR systems are able to generate email or text alerts to notify providers of critical test results or other important information.

Manual Method of Clinical Results Reporting   In an environment that does not have an EHR system interfaced with laboratory computers, the laboratory sends a printed report via fax to the prescriber's office, and then a staff member scans the report into the EHR. This is an example of the **manual method** of results entry. However, the preferred method for retrieving laboratory and test reports would be via automatic transmission or an interface between the laboratory systems and the EHR.

Eventually, most laboratory and other diagnostic company computers will be interfaced with all EHR systems, but this process will take time to accomplish. In the meantime, telecommunications continue to be the best way to obtain test results for facilities whose laboratory computers cannot interface or transfer clinical results. Until total interface and interoperability is achieved, scanning results is a manageable process and the best option available for some EHR users.

Tutorial 12.1   **EHR**NAVIGAT⊕R

Running a Diagnostic Test Report

Go to your online course to launch Tutorial 12.1. As an office manager, practice running and printing a diagnostic test report using the EHR Navigator.

Tutorial 12.2   **EHR**NAVIGAT⊕R

Viewing Clinical Results

Go to your online course to launch Tutorial 12.2. As a medical assistant, practice viewing a patient's lab results using the EHR Navigator.

Tutorial 12.3   **EHR**NAVIGAT⊕R

Signing a Scanned Diagnostic Report

Go to your online course to launch Tutorial 12.3. As a physician, practice signing a scanned diagnostic report using the EHR Navigator.

Quality Improvement

Arguably, the most important use of data analytics is in the improvement of the quality of healthcare. This involves improving patient outcomes and the patient experience as well as keeping patients safe. There are many stakeholders interested in improving healthcare quality, including patients, healthcare providers, payers, government agencies, public health agencies, and the public at large. The US Department of Health and Human Resources, Office of Disease Prevention and Health Promotion has healthcare quality initiatives focused on increasing patient safety through national action plans. Examples of these initiatives include pathways to safer opioid use, teaming up against healthcare-associated infections, and preventing adverse drug events.

Healthcare providers engage in quality improvement activities as a routine part of daily work. Good healthcare organizations are committed to providing the best care possible to their patients and use data analytics to target potential opportunities for improvement, such as reducing infections, increasing discharges to home, and improving patient call-light response times. In addition to internal quality improvement activities, many quality improvement activities of providers are prescribed by government programs and accrediting bodies. Let's take a look at some of these requirements.

The Joint Commission

Acute care hospitals are accredited by The Joint Commission. Failure to keep The Joint Commission accreditation status in good standing could result in a hospital's loss of

EXPAND YOUR LEARNING

Learn more about the health care quality initiatives of the Office of Disease Prevention and Health Promotion at https://EHR3 .ParadigmEducation .com/HealthcareQuality.

their Medicare provider number, meaning that the hospital would no longer be able to treat Medicare patients. This would be a significant loss of revenue for the hospital. The Joint Commission puts a great deal of focus on high-quality care and requires hospitals to report data regularly to prove adherence with The Joint Commission patient safety goals that are updated annually. Refer to Figure 12.2 for the 2020 NPSGs.

The Joint Commission also accredits other types of healthcare providers, including physician's offices, nursing homes, office-based surgery centers, behavioral health treatment facilities, home care providers, and assisted living facilities. All of these providers are required to participate in quality improvement activities to meet accreditation standards.

CMS Quality Reporting Requirements

As the largest payer of healthcare services in the United States, the Centers for Medicare & Medicaid Services (CMS) continuously seeks ways to improve the quality of healthcare. CMS manages quality programs that address many different areas of health care, including acute care hospitals, nursing homes, ambulatory surgery centers, home health agencies, long-term care hospitals, inpatient rehab hospitals, psychiatric hospitals, and outpatient facilities. CMS initiated many of these programs in response to legislation requiring quality improvement and monitoring. For example, the Hospital Readmissions Reduction Program (HRRP) is a quality initiative that tries to reduce readmissions to acute care hospitals for patients with conditions that typically result in readmissions. The six conditions that CMS monitors for readmissions include:

- Acute myocardial infarction

- Chronic obstructive pulmonary disease (COPD)

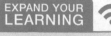

EXPAND YOUR LEARNING

The Joint Commission publishes the accreditation status and adherence with patient safety goals on a Quality Check website for the public to learn more about the healthcare providers in their area. Search for a hospital near you at https://EHR3 .ParadigmEducation .com/QualityCheck.

Figure 12.2 The Joint Commission 2020 National Patient Safety Goals

Hospitals depend on EHR patient data and data analytics to assist with The Joint Commission's reporting on the NPSGs.

2020 Safety Goals	Organizations Should	Implemented
Improve the accuracy of patient identification.	Use of Two Patient Identifiers	⊘
Improve the effectiveness of communication among caregivers.	Timely Reporting of Critical Tests and Critical Results	⊘
Improve the safety of using medications.	Labeling Medications	⊘
	Reducing Harm from Anticoagulation Therapy	⊘
	Reconciling Medication Information	⊘
Reduce the harm associated with clinical alarm systems.	Use Alarms Safely on Medical Equipment	⊘
Reduce the risk of health care-associated infections.	Meeting Hand Hygiene Guidelines	⊘
The organization identifies safety risks inherent in its patient population.	Identifying Individuals at Risk for Suicide	⊘
Universal Protocol	Conducting a Pre-Procedure Verification Process	⊘
	Marking the Procedure Site	⊘
	Performing a Time-Out	⊘

- Coronary artery bypass graft surgery

- Elective primary total hip arthroplasty and/or total knee arthroplasty

- Heart failure (HF)

- Pneumonia

Hospitals are required to report readmissions for these condition to CMS. See Figure 12.3 for an example of a report generated from the EHR Navigator that provides the readmissions for heart failure data needed to report to CMS.

Tutorial 12.4   **EHR**NAVIGAT⊕R

Running a Postoperative Readmission Report

Go to your online course to launch Tutorial 12.4. As an admission clerk, practice running and printing a postoperative readmission report using the EHR Navigator.

Hospital Readmissions of Postoperative Patients

In addition to the required CMS reporting of readmissions, hospitals monitor readmissions within 48 hours of all postoperative patients to identify potential quality concerns. Figure 12.4 is an example of such a report.

In addition to required reporting, CMS encourages healthcare providers to participate in many quality improvement initiatives and has a website dedicated to sharing quality information. Healthcare organizations and stakeholders are encouraged to sign up for regular updates from this CMS site.

Figure 12.3 Hospital Readmissions Report

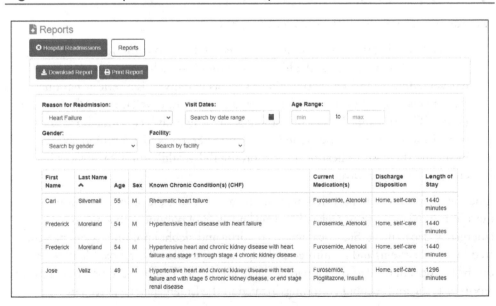

First Name	Last Name ∧	Age	Sex	Known Chronic Condition(s) (CHF)	Current Medication(s)	Discharge Disposition	Length of Stay
Carl	Silvernail	55	M	Rheumatic heart failure	Furosemide, Atenolol	Home, self-care	1440 minutes
Frederick	Moreland	54	M	Hypertensive heart disease with heart failure	Furosemide, Atenolol	Home, self-care	1440 minutes
Frederick	Moreland	54	M	Hypertensive heart and chronic kidney disease with heart failure and stage 1 through stage 4 chronic kidney disease	Furosemide, Atenolol	Home, self-care	1440 minutes
Jose	Veliz	49	M	Hypertensive heart and chronic kidney disease with heart failure and with stage 5 chronic kidney disease, or end stage renal disease	Furosemide, Pioglitazone, Insulin	Home, self-care	1296 minutes

Figure 12.4 Readmissions of Postoperative Patients

Northstar Medical Center
Readmissions of Post-Operative Patients
12/02/2030

Procedure	# Adm	# Readm	% Readm ∨
Amputation of lower extremity	693	187	27%
Debridement of wound, burn or infection	1155	211	19%
Coronary Artery Bypass Graft (CABG)	4515	722	16%
Colorectal Resection	525	74	14%
Percutaneous Coronary Angioplasty (PTCA)	1911	248	13%
Excision, lysis peritoneal adhesions	399	48	12%
Heart valve procedures	1617	194	12%
Incision and Excision of the Central Nervous System	378	42	11%
Skin graft	567	62	11%
Treatment, fracture or dislocation of lower extremity	1239	124	10%
Partial excision, bone	798	80	10%
Spinal fusion	231	208	9%
Laminectomy, excision intervertebral disc	1113	89	8%
Hip Replacement, total and partial	1953	137	7%
Oophorectomy, unilateral or bilateral	1365	109	6%

Tutorial 12.5   **EHR**NAVIGAT⊕R

Generating a Hospital Readmissions Report
Go to your online course to launch Tutorial 12.5. As a data analyst, practice running a report of the hospital readmissions related to heart failure.

Drug and Alcohol Poisonings

According to the National Institute on Drug Abuse,

> In 2019, nearly 50,000 people in the United States died from opioid-involved overdoses. The misuse of and addiction to opioids—including prescription pain relievers, heroin, and synthetic opioids such as fentanyl—is a serious national crisis that affects public health as well as social and economic welfare. The Centers for Disease Control and Prevention estimates that the total "economic burden" of prescription opioid misuse alone in the United States is $78.5 billion a year, including the costs of healthcare, lost productivity, addiction treatment, and criminal justice involvement.

One way that healthcare providers are working to overcome the opioid crisis is by monitoring the patient cases related to drug and alcohol poisoning that are treated in the emergency department. Statistical reports on drug and alcohol poisonings can be generated by EHR systems and monitored by hospital staff to identify trends. Identified trends can be further analyzed at the individual patient level. See Figure 12.5 for an example of a report of Drug and Alcohol Poisonings Treated in the Emergency Department.

Figure 12.5   Emergency Department, Drug and Alcohol Poisonings Treated

Northstar Medical Center
Emergency Department, Drug/Alcohol Poisonings Treated
12/02/2030

Data Element	Number	Percentage
Total # of Drug/Alcohol Poisoning Visits	1272	
Type of Poisoning		
Non-medical Use of Pharmaceuticals	458	36%
Illicit Drugs	686	54%
Alcohol	128	10%
Age		
0-5	4	<1%
6-14	12	1%
15-19	37	3%
20-29	382	30%
30-39	369	29%
40-49	229	18%
50-59	114	9%

Tutorial 12.6   **EHR**NAVIGAT✚R

Running an Emergency Department Report
Go to your online course to launch Tutorial 12.6. As an admission clerk, practice running and printing an emergency department report using the EHR Navigator.

CHECKP✚INT 12.2

1. An accumulation of relevant data points from a patient's EHR or many patients' EHRs organized for comparison and study is the definition of what term?

2. What is considered the most important use of data analytics in healthcare?

12.6 Disease Surveillance and Monitoring

Disease surveillance and monitoring are important tasks of public health agencies. Because surveillance can directly measure what is going on in the population, it is useful both for measuring the need for interventions and for directly measuring the effects of interventions. The EHR facilitates disease surveillance because

EXPAND YOUR LEARNING

The COVID-19 pandemic is a real-life example of how important disease surveillance and monitoring is to public health. COVID-19 is one of about 120 diseases or conditions health departments voluntarily report to the CDC. More information about this can be found on the CDC website at https://EHR3.ParadigmEducation.com/COVID-19.

diseases are assigned appropriate codes that report to a database. Once the population is identified, researchers can look for trends in the affected population, mortality rates, and so on.

Preventive Medicine

Disease prevention is the goal of preventive medicine, and data analytics can help healthcare providers identify and monitor patients at risk for developing disease. For example, timely immunizations are an important part of preventive medicine. Pediatricians and adult primary care physicians typically administer immunizations and manually track administered immunizations for all of their patients. EHR systems are able to automatically monitor administered immunizations and use data analytics to identify immunizations that are coming due. The physician's office can then contact patients and parents to schedule appointments for immunization administration.

Figure 12.6 is an example of a report of administered immunizations at Northstar Physicians. Note that this report can be generated using specific parameters such as immunization type and dates due. Reports can also be downloaded and analyzed using spreadsheet software as shown in Figure 12.7.

Using data analytics in the prevention of disease caused by the use of tobacco is another way in which patient data in the EHR can be leveraged to improve patient outcomes. Primary care physicians typically address social habits, including tobacco use, at annual physical examination visits. A report with data on self-identified smokers could help physicians identify which patients are at risk for lung cancer and other diseases. Physician offices may also want to use reports to contact patients with smoking cessation information. See Figure 12.8 for an example of a Smoking Cessation Report.

Additional preventive medicine data analytics reports routinely used by primary care physicians include tracking reports for recommended screening tests such as mammograms, colonoscopies, and prostate specific antigen blood tests. HbA1C testing for diabetes control is another routine report that primary care physicians

Figure 12.6 Immunization Rates

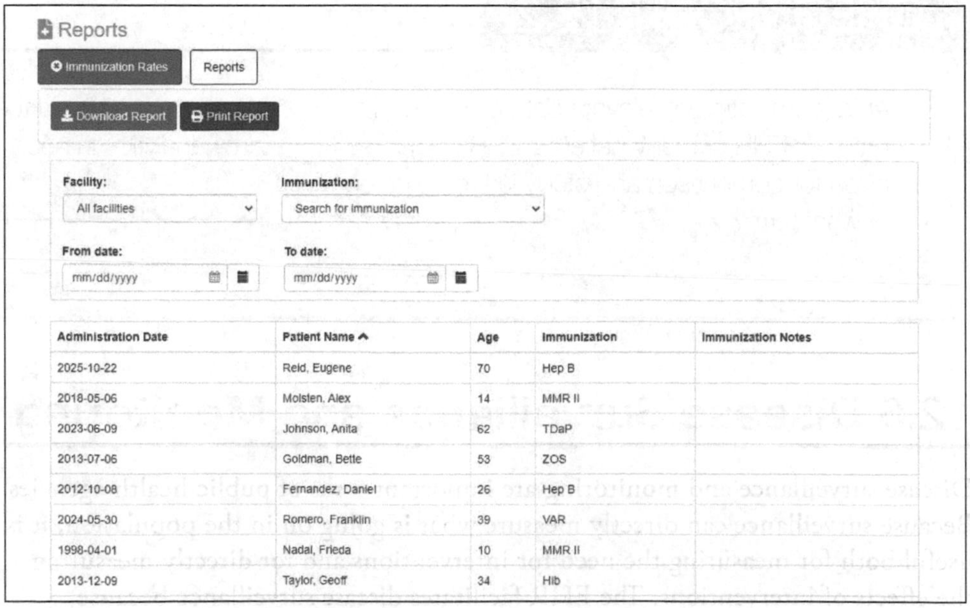

Administration Date	Patient Name	Age	Immunization	Immunization Notes
2025-10-22	Reid, Eugene	70	Hep B	
2018-05-06	Molsten, Alex	14	MMR II	
2023-06-09	Johnson, Anita	62	TDaP	
2013-07-06	Goldman, Bette	53	ZOS	
2012-10-08	Fernandez, Daniel	26	Hep B	
2024-05-30	Romero, Franklin	39	VAR	
1998-04-01	Nadal, Frieda	10	MMR II	
2013-12-09	Taylor, Geoff	34	Hib	

use to ensure that patients are following up with HbA1C blood tests. Refer to Figure 12.9 for an example of a report listing screening tests that are due and Figure 12.10 for a Lab Values Report that lists patients needing to schedule a follow-up HbA1C blood test.

Figure 12.7   Immunization Rates Report Data in Spreadsheet Software

	A	B	C	D	E
1	Administration Date	Patient Name	Age	Immunization	Immunization Notes
2	10/22/2025	Reid, Eugene	75	Hep B	
3	5/6/2018	Molsten, Alex	26	MMR II	
4	6/9/2023	Johnson, Anita	69	TDaP	
5	7/6/2013	Goldman, Bette	70	ZOS	
6	10/8/2012	Fernandez, Daniel	44	Hep B	
7	5/30/2024	Romero, Franklin	45	VAR	
8	4/1/1998	Nadal, Frieda	42	MMR II	
9	12/9/2013	Taylor, Geoff	51	Hib	
10	4/5/2028	Clayton, Heather	38	Hep A	
11	5/16/2018	Oberg, Ingrid	75	TDaP	
12	6/9/2023	Bari, Jennifer	37	HPV	
13	7/6/2013	Wantabe, Kenji	47	MCV4	
14	10/8/2012	Torres, Lourdes	22	Hep B	
15	5/30/2024	Ortiz, Marco	31	PCV13	
16	4/1/1998	Wilkins, Marquita	33	Hib	DECLINED-Due to pain
17	12/9/2013	Fernandez, Mason	7	DTaP-Hib-IPV	
18	6/9/2023	Yang, Sophia	20	HPV	
19	7/6/2013	Wang, Tabitha	52	HPV	
20	10/8/2012	McDowell, Terrence	74	MCV4	
21	5/30/2024	Molsten, Tim	23	PCV13	
22	6/9/2023	Jackson, Todd	46	VAR	
23	7/6/2013	Mulligan, Tyler	26	Vaccinia	
24	10/8/2025	Thomas, William	9	DTaP-Hib-IPV	
25	5/17/1930	Ashfield, John	64	Shingles	
26	5/1/1930	Atwater, Jaiden	5	VARICELLA	DECLINED-Parent Concerned About Side Effects
27	1/15/1930	Bari, Jennifer	37	HPV	
28	3/15/1930	Becker, Jay	54	DTaP	
29	6/22/1930	Binder, Randal	28	Shingles	

Figure 12.8   Smoking Cessation Report

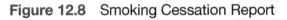

Reports

Smoking Cessation | Reports

Download Report | Print Report

Age	Gender:	Smoking level:
Search by Age	Search by gender	Search by use

RESULTS: Smokers:43 | Male: 40 Female:31 | Heavy:13 Every Day:12 Some Day:18

MRN ^	First Name	Last Name	Age	Sex	Smoker	Level	Years Tobacco-Free
585176	William	Lea	67 years	M	yes	Some Day	
585175	Jami	Stevens	40 years	F	yes	Every Day	
585174	Richard	Owens	30 years	M	yes	Every Day	
585172	Jason	Stallcup	69 years	M	yes	Every Day	
585171	Hallie	Rooney	18 years	F	yes	Some Day	
585169	Marshall	Hammond	63 years	M	yes	Heavy	
585165	Vera	Durante	74 years	F	yes	Every Day	
585164	Arthur	Talley	73 years	M	yes	Heavy	
585163	Carlton	Johnson	17 years	M	yes	Every Day	

Figure 12.9   Needs Annual Test Report

								Preferred Method of			
Patient Last Name ∨	Patient First Name	Gender	MRN#	Date of Birth	Test/Procedure	Date of Last Test/Procedure	Contact	Phone	Cell	Email	

Needs Annual Test
Date of Report: 12/02/2030

Patient Last Name ∨	Patient First Name	Gender	MRN#	Date of Birth	Test/Procedure	Date of Last Test/Procedure	Preferred Method of Contact	Phone	Cell	Email
Durante	Vera	F	585165	4/13/1943	Mammogram	6/5/2030	Cell	513-555-8743	513-555-8744	vdurante@ppi-edu.net
Hubbard	Lorraine	F	585127	10/16/1944	Mammogram	5/24/2029	Cell	513-555-7822	513-555-7282	lrhubbard@ppi-edu.net
Sayler	Olga	F	585157	12/4/1945	Mammogram	9/5/2028	Cell	513-555-7327	513-555-7328	osayler@ppi-edu.net
Capon	Violanda	F	585139	1/22/1946	Mammogram	11/7/2029	Phone	513-555-5703	513-555-5704	vcapon@ppi-edu.net
Goldman	Bette	F	585089	7/30/1947	Mammogram	3/9/2030	Phone	317-555-3232	317-555-4040	bgoldman@ppi-edu.net
Alba	Sally	F	585136	4/22/1948	Mammogram	8/27/2020	Email	859-555-1786	859-555-1787	salba@ppi-edu.net
Johnson	Anita	F	585065	6/14/1948	Mammogram	9/5/2028	Email	859-555-	859-555-	anitapaints@ppi-edu.net

Figure 12.10   Lab Values Report

Reports
Lab Values Report   Reports
Run Report   Print Report

From date:
12/02/2030

No Follow-up HbA1C Test
Date of Report: 12/02/2030

Search

Patient First Name	Patient Last Name ∨	Date of Birth	Date of Last HbA1C Test	HbA1C Value	Preferred Method of Contact	Phone Number	Cell Phone	Email Address
Eugene	Johnson	4/18/1928	4/3/2030	6.4	Phone	513-555-0101	513-555-2013	
Mill	Garrido	1/29/1931	4/3/2030	6.7	Phone	859-555-1195		
Vicki	Remick	2/23/1932	4/4/2030	7.5	Phone	513-555-9395	513=555-9396	vremick@ppi-edu.net
Ethel	Jacobson	8/26/1932	4/5/2030	8.3	Email	513-555-	513-555-	JacobEth@ppi-

Tutorial 12.7

EHRNAVIGAT**⊕**R

Running a Vaccine Effectiveness Report

Go to your online course to launch Tutorial 12.7. As an office manager, practice running and printing a vaccine effectiveness report using the EHR Navigator.

Tutorial 12.8

EHRNAVIGAT✛R

Running a Lab Values Report

Go to your online course to launch Tutorial 12.8. As an office manager, practice running and printing a lab values report using the EHR Navigator.

Research

Clinical researchers benefit significantly from the compilation of patient data generated by EHR systems. The data are more readily available than in the past and data analytics can be used to quickly synthesize the data, freeing up clinicians to focus their time and efforts on clinical research.

There are hundreds of clinical research studies being conducted in the United States and around the world at any given time. Critical research to cure debilitating diseases that often result in death focuses on:

- Diseases that affect all age groups (e.g., cancer, diabetes, and kidney disease)

- Diseases that are experienced more by the elderly (e.g., heart disease, stroke, and high blood pressure)

- Pediatric cancer (the second leading cause of death in children, second only to accidents)

- Suicide (one of the leading causes of death in teenagers)

Clinical research also involves the study of chronic diseases and conditions that do not typically cause death, but make living a quality life, free of pain and distress, difficult, such as:

- Arthritis

- Crohn's disease

- Fibromyalgia

- Mental illness

- Multiple sclerosis

In addition to addressing chronic issues, research is extremely important when it comes to addressing sudden outbreaks of disease, such as the COVID-19 pandemic and the annual rise of infectious diseases such as influenza and pneumonia.

Throughout this chapter we have discussed the important role that EHR systems play in data analytics and how healthcare data analytics is used for patient care, clinical results reporting, required reporting to government agencies and accrediting bodies, disease prevention, quality improvement, and research. The uses of data analytics covered in this chapter just barely scratch the surface of how healthcare data and information can be used. For example, depending on the type of healthcare provider, there may be many reporting requirements, both by accrediting and government entities. Refer to Table 12.1 for examples of required reporting.

Data analytics plays a pivotal role in clinical research, as the availability of timely, accurate data is a tool for clinical researchers to help identify possible cures, immunizations, and other protections.

EXPAND YOUR LEARNING

Johns Hopkins University is a leader in clinical research in the United States. Take a look at some of the topics that they are currently researching at https://EHR3 .ParadigmEducation .com/HopkinsResearch.

Table 12.1 Examples of Required Reporting

Type of Health-care Provider	Name of Report/ Data	Description	Required to Report?	Required by
Acute Care Hospitals	Healthcare Ratings for Acute Care Hospitals	Ratings are based on how well hospitals perform across different areas of quality, such as treating heart attacks, treating pneumonia, readmission rates, and safety of care. Most of the data is derived from submitted claims.	Yes.	CMS
Acute Care Hospitals	Hospital Consumer Assessment of Healthcare Providers and Systems (HCAHPS)	Surveys instrument and data collection methodology for measuring patients' perceptions of their hospital experience	No, but failure to report incurs financial penalties.	CMS
Dialysis Facilities	Clinical and Patient Measures for Dialysis Facilities	Contains data on patient characteristics, treatment patterns, hospitalization, mortality, and transplantation patterns	Yes, Medicare-certified dialysis facilities are required to report.	CMS
Dialysis Facilities	Healthcare Ratings for Dialysis Facilities	The quality rating compares dialysis facilities on important indicators of quality, like how well they avoid unnecessary transfusions and hospital admissions. The quality rating shows how well each dialysis facility delivers care compared to the national average.	Yes.	CMS
Home Health Care	Healthcare Ratings for Home Health Care	The quality rating shows how a home health agency compares to others on measurements of their performance, such as how often the agency began their patient's care in a timely manner or how often a patient got better at walking around. A rating of 3 to 5 stars indicates the agency performed about the same as most agencies.	Yes.	CMS
Long-Term Care Hospitals	Long-term Care Hospital (LTCH) Quality Reporting Program (QRP)	Data pertaining to quality measures, resource use, and other domains, using standardized quality measures and standardized data, e.g., pressure ulcer/injury rates and infections rates.	Yes. Required by the Affordable Care Act and the Medicare Post-Acute Care Transformation Act of 2014	CMS
Nursing Homes	COVID-19 Nursing Home Data	Contains data on staff and resident vaccination rates and other COVID-related data	Yes.	CDC
Nursing Homes	Healthcare Ratings for Nursing Homes	Ratings are based on nursing homes' performance from 3 sources: health inspections, staffing, and quality of resident care measures.	Yes.	CMS

Chapter Summary

Data is valuable to the healthcare industry because data turns into information, and information is priceless when managed and analyzed appropriately. The healthcare industry has experienced an explosion of data due to the implementation of EHR systems.

Data analytics is defined as the practice of exploring and manipulating data for the purposes of identifying new information that can be used to improve the operations of the organization, the delivery of patient care, and patient outcomes; to identify populations and health conditions that are underserved; to identify opportunities to reduce healthcare costs; and to attempt to predict future healthcare needs and trends. Healthcare providers, patients, payers, and other stakeholders are all invested in the goal of providing high-quality health care at the lowest cost. Data analytics is a tool for these interested parties to use to identify opportunities to better achieve this goal.

There are both internal and external users of healthcare data analytics. Internal users include employees working to ensure that the healthcare organization is providing the best care in the most cost-effective manner. External users include government agencies that require reporting from healthcare organizations, accrediting bodies, public health agencies, and interested contracted companies.

The types of healthcare data analytics include descriptive, prescriptive, and predictive analytics. Descriptive analytics uses historical data for the purposes of identifying patterns that could lead to opportunities for improving care, improving the delivery of care, and reducing the costs of care. Predictive analytics in healthcare is the use of historical patient data with the application of statistical algorithms to identify expected future trends in health care. Prescriptive analytics also uses artificial intelligence but takes predictive analytics a step further by identifying the best options for future outcomes.

Data mining is the process of searching for and examining data to organize it into useful patterns and trends. Data mining and reporting structured data can be accomplished quickly and easily using an EHR system because the fixed nature of structured data makes it easy to search, query, and quantify.

Artificial intelligence (AI) is defined as computer systems able to perform tasks that usually require human intelligence. The Internet of Things (IoT) is new terminology used to describe a network of devices that can connect to share data.

A management of information plan is an intentional and strategic plan developed to manage the organization's data and data needs. An organization should implement a data use strategy to develop and implement a useful management of information plan.

EHR systems play an important role in data analytics because they make the patient data more accessible, timely, and accurate. The EHR facilitates the use of healthcare data analytics for patient care, clinical results reporting, required reporting to government agencies and accrediting bodies, disease prevention, quality improvement, and research.

Review and Assessment

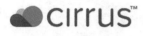

The following Review and Assessment activities are also available online in the Cirrus online course. Your instructor may ask you to complete these activities online. Cirrus also provides access to flash cards, a crossword puzzle, and practice quizzes to help strengthen your understanding of the chapter content.

Acronyms/Initialisms

Study the following acronyms discussed in this chapter. Go to the online course for flash cards of the acronyms and other chapter key terms.

AI: artificial intelligence

CPHA: Commission on Professional and Hospital Activities

HRRP: Hospital Readmissions Reduction Program

IoT: Internet of Things

MIT: management of information team

NPSGs: National Patient Safety Goals of The Joint Commission

Check Your Understanding

To check your understanding of this chapter's key concepts, answer the following questions.

1. Which of the following are included in the definition of *data analytics*?
   a. exploring data
   b. manipulating data
   c. identifying new information
   d. improving operations
   e. All the choices are correct.

2. Internal users of data analytics include all *except* which of the following?
   a. Medical staff
   b. Risk managers
   c. Board of trustees
   d. The Joint Commission

3. Using historical patient data with the application of statistical algorithms to identify future outcomes and trends is the definition of which of the following?
   a. predictive analytics
   b. descriptive analytics
   c. prescriptive analytics
   d. statistical analytics

4. *Data mining* refers to
   a. searching for and examining data to organize it into useful patterns and trends.
   b. interpreting and classifying clinical documentation.

   c.   identifying the best options for achieving future outcomes.

   d.   developing a data use strategy.

5. The management of information plan should take into account all *except* which of the following?

   a.   Patient data

   b.   Financial data

   c.   Human resources data

   d.   Federal aggregate healthcare provider data

6. What is the first step in a good data use strategy?

   a.   Identify the needs of the organization.

   b.   Identify data storage needs.

   c.   Develop a plan.

   d.   Establish a management of information team.

7. Why is the EHR system function of clinical results reporting so important to patient care?

   a.   Healthcare providers are able to view laboratory and diagnostic test results immediately and act upon the results.

   b.   It is one of the National Patient Safety Goals.

   c.   It is the best way to obtain test results.

   d.   It helps prevent adverse drug events.

8. The performance of tasks by computer systems that usually require human intelligence is the definition of which of the following?

   a.   predictive analytics

   b.   artificial intelligence

   c.   data mining

   d.   Internet of Things (IoT)

9. What is the most important use of data analytics in healthcare?

   a.   improving the quality of health care

   b.   reporting required data to federal agencies

   c.   improving clinical documentation

   d.   developing a data use strategy

10. Which of the following should *not* be identified and included in a management of information plan?

   a.   the data generated by the organization

   b.   the users of the data

   c.   the technological systems used by the organization

   d.   the processes used to contribute to the flow of information

Go on the Record

To build on your understanding of the topics in this chapter, complete the following short-answer activities.

1. Discuss the importance of data analytics in improving patient care.

2. Compare and contrast the internal and external users of data analytics.

3. Explain how the EHR supports the use of data analytics in health care.

4. Explain how data analytics contributes to clinical reporting.

Navigate the Field

To gain practice in handling challenging situations in the workplace, consider the following real-world scenarios and identify how you would respond to each.

1. One of your roles at General Hospital is to identify the current Joint Commission National Patient Safety Goals. You notice that The Joint Commission National Patient Safety Goals have not been updated for the current year. Navigate to The Joint Commission National Patient Safety Goals at https://EHR3.ParadigmEducation.com/NPSG. Review each of the eight chapters. Identify one safety goal from each chapter, including the National Patient Safety Goal number (e.g., NPSG 07.01.01), the title (e.g., Prevent Infection), and the ways that the healthcare system can meet the goal (e.g., use the hand-cleaning guidelines from the Centers for Disease Control and Prevention or the World Health Organization, set goals for improving hand cleaning, and use the goals to improve hand cleaning). Prepare a summary of The Joint Commission National Patient Safety Goals in a Word document. Submit your document.

2. You are the Director of HIM for Northstar Medical Center. You have decided that you need to provide an overview of how the HIM professional is involved in data analytics. Research the role of the HIM professional in data analytics. Prepare a short presentation for your next department meeting that covers the five key data analytics roles for HIM professionals.

Think Critically

Continue to think critically about challenging concepts and complete the following activities.

1. You are a data analyst and you have been asked to research three hospitals in your area. Navigate to the American Hospital Director at https://www.ahd.com. Use the search box to look up the hospital profiles. Create a Word document, create a table, and include the following information:

   - Name of the healthcare facility
   - Address of the healthcare facility
   - Total staffed beds
   - Total patient revenue
   - Total discharges
   - Total patient days
   - Total Performance Score (TPS) Quality Score
   - The Joint Commission Status
   - Total revenue
   - Net income (or loss)

Create another table that identifies the three top numbers of patient claims. Include the average charge and the average cost.

After reviewing the data for the three healthcare systems, how does data from the EHR support this information? What does the data tell us about the healthcare system? Submit your tables and explanation in a Word document.

2. In March 2020, the world was hit with a pandemic. Tools were developed to trace the spread of the disease COVID-19. States throughout the US collected data to keep residents informed about a variety of disease data. Go to the State of New Jersey Communicable Disease site at https://EHR3 .ParadigmEducation.com/NJHealth or the State of Massachusetts COVID-19 Response Reporting site at https://EHR3.ParadigmEducation .com/MAHealth. After reviewing the website, identify the data that is available for residents. Prepare a summary of the data available and how the data are used to assist with the prevention and spread of the disease. Submit your summary in a Word document.

Make Your Case

Consider the scenario and then complete the following project.

You are a data analyst at Northstar Health Systems. You serve on the team that is helping to develop health goals for the organization. You have been asked to research the objectives and goals for HealthyPeople 2030. Navigate to https:// EHR3.ParadigmEducation.com/HealthyPeople2030. Create a list of objectives and goals related to following areas:

- Heart Disease and Stroke—General
- Sleep—General
- Health Care Access—Health Insurance

In your report, include the following information for each area:

- Summary
- Status
- Most recent data
- Target
- Baseline
- Desired direction

Include any other information that is important for the team to know for setting the goals and objectives.

Explore the Technology

Complete the EHR Navigator practice assessments that align to each tutorial and the assessments that accompany Chapter 12 located in the online course.

EHRNAVIGAT⊕R

Chapter **13** Clinical Decision Support Systems and Quality Improvement

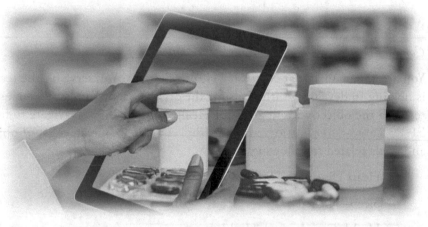

Field Notes

" EHRs have drastically improved communication and continuity for our pulmonary patients. This integrative technology has allowed clinicians to thoroughly review ventilator weaning tolerance from previous facilities and implement achievable goals in improving patient outcomes. "

– Tom Frye, RRT Manager, Respiratory Therapy

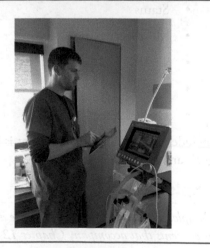

Learning Objectives

13.1 Define *clinical decision support system (CDSS)*.

13.2 Define and discuss the two types of CDSS.

13.3 Discuss the benefits and drawbacks of using a CDSS.

13.4 List and discuss the most common uses of clinical decision support in health care.

13.5 Explain the requirements of the Centers for Medicare & Medicaid Services (CMS) for the clinical decision support rule as part of meaningful use core measures.

13.6 Demonstrate clinical decision support activities in electronic health record (EHR) software, and discuss the role of EHRs in clinical decision support.

13.7 Discuss the role of the EHR in quality improvement.

13.8 Explain the importance of National Quality Measures of The Joint Commission.

13.9 Define and discuss *electronic clinical quality improvement (eCQI)*.

13.10 Define Clinical Documentation Improvement *(CDI)* and discuss its importance in health care.

As you have learned throughout this text, electronic health records (EHRs) improve the quality of patient care in many ways. One of the most significant ways is through the incorporation of clinical decision support systems. A **clinical decision support system (CDSS)** assists healthcare providers with decision-making tasks such as determining diagnoses, choosing the best medications for a patient, and selecting proper diagnostic tests. The CDSS filters EHR data available for a specific patient, producing information based on current healthcare knowledge and interactions among physicians and other healthcare providers to assist them in making decisions that will result in the highest quality of care. This chapter will discuss CDSSs in detail and explore the federal mandates that require healthcare providers to use EHR systems with CDSSs.

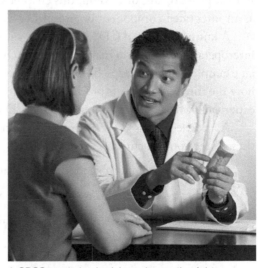

A CDSS can help physicians choose the right medications for a patient.

In addition to a CDSS, the role of EHRs in healthcare quality improvement activities will be discussed. Healthcare providers and organizations constantly strive to improve processes, policies, and procedures that result in higher-quality outcomes. Through data gathering and analysis, EHRs play a significant role in assisting healthcare organizations in these quality improvement activities.

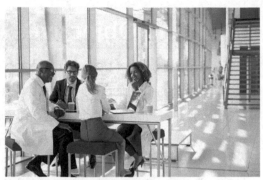
Healthcare organizations work together to improve policies and procedures.

13.1 Clinical Decision Support

The Centers for Medicare & Medicaid Services (CMS) define clinical decision support in relation to the meaningful use standards as "health information technology that builds upon the foundation of an EHR to provide persons involved in care decisions with general and person-specific information, intelligently filtered and organized, at the point of care (POC), to enhance health and health care."

The simplest description of a CDSS is any tool that helps healthcare providers make a better clinical decision. Examples of CDSS tools include computerized alerts and reminders, clinical guidelines, standardized order sets, patient data results and reports, documentation templates, diagnostic support, and clinical workflow tools.

There are two basic types of CDSSs: knowledge based and non–knowledge based. Most CDSSs are **knowledge based** and use inference software and databases containing the most current medical, scientific, and research information. Non–knowledge-based CDSSs utilize artificial intelligence software to study and learn from data and patterns of medical practice, as described in Chapter 12.

CDSSs may also be stand-alone systems or an integrated component of an EHR. For purposes of this discussion, this chapter will focus on the knowledge-based CDSS as an integrated component of an EHR.

A knowledge-based CDSS integrated with an EHR is a good example of semantic interoperability. The data may be shared, exchanged, and interpreted. See Figure 13.1 for an example of a knowledge-based CDSS integrated with an EHR. This figure illustrates how the three components of EHR data, scientific evidence and research, and physician experience work together to make up the CDSS.

A knowledge-based CDSS integrated with an EHR is effective because it utilizes these three components:

1. Subjective and objective clinical patient data from the EHR

2. State-of-the-art scientific evidence and research

3. Physician knowledge, experience, and judgment

Benefits and Drawbacks of Using a CDSS

Using a CDSS has numerous benefits, the most significant of which improve quality of care and healthcare delivery through the following:

- Reduced risk of medication errors

- Reduced risk of misdiagnosis

Figure 13.1   Knowledge-Based CDSS Integrated with EHR

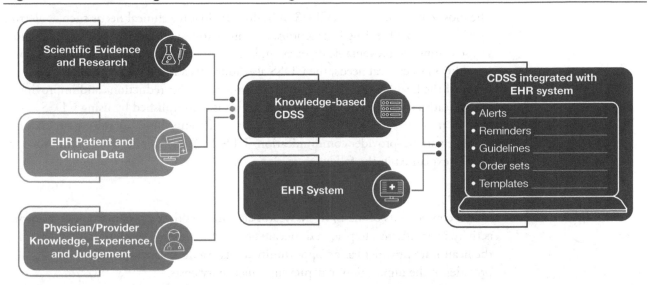

- Increased direct patient care time for healthcare providers

- Access to state-of-the-art data, research, clinical pathways, and guidelines

- Reduction of unnecessary diagnostic tests

- Faster diagnosis, resulting in faster treatment

- Prescriptions for lower-cost medications

However, using a CDSS also has potential drawbacks, including the following:

- High costs of maintaining the CDSS with up-to-date medical research, clinical pathways, guidelines, medication costs, and so forth

- Potential overreliance on computer technology

- Perception by healthcare providers as a threat to clinical knowledge and skills

- Harmful outcomes if software is not thoroughly and continuously updated

ON THE JOB

Strong analytical and technical skills are necessary for a data analyst role in health care. You will need to identify problems or opportunities for improvement, understand cause-and-effect relationships, and present logical solutions.

CHECKP◊INT 13.1

1. Define a clinical decision support system (CDSS).

   _____

   _____

   _____

2. List two types of CDSSs.

   a. _____

   b. _____

3. List three benefits and three potential drawbacks of using a CDSS.

   a. _____

   b. _____

   c. _____

   d. _____

   e. _____

   f. _____

Most Common Uses of a CDSS

The most common uses of a CDSS in health care involve clinical needs such as alerting providers to possible drug interactions, assisting with establishment of correct diagnoses, screening for preventable diseases, and accessing state-of-the-art treatment options. In addition to clinical needs, the CDSS also addresses administrative and financial needs of the healthcare organization by assisting with cost reductions and improving patient satisfaction and provider efficiency. This is accomplished by using CDSS tools to minimize length of hospital stay, alert staff about duplicate testing orders, and increase patient–provider communication. Table 13.1 identifies the common uses of a CDSS, explained in the following sections.

Alerts

CDSS components of the EHR Navigator alert the healthcare provider in the following activity in an attempt to place a duplicate order for computed tomography. Although the healthcare provider has an opportunity to place a duplicate order, alerting the provider to the duplication may prevent unnecessary costs.

Tutorial 13.1   **EHR**NAVIGAT**⊕**R

Adding an Order

Go to the online course to launch Tutorial 13.1. As a physician, practice adding an order using the EHR Navigator.

Table 13.1 Common Uses of a Clinical Decision Support System

Use	Examples
Alerts	• Drug–drug alerts • Drug–food interactions • Duplicate testing alerts • Abnormal laboratory results
Diagnoses	• Suggestions for possible diagnoses that match patient signs and symptoms
Treatment options	• Treatment options and guidelines for specific diagnoses • Medication recommendations
Preventive care	• Immunization due-date alerts • Diagnostic screening • Disease management/prevention
Hospital/provider efficiency	• Care plans and treatment to minimize length of stay • Standardized order sets • Suggestions for lower-cost medications and testing
Cost reductions and improved patient satisfaction	• Duplicate testing alerts • Drug formulary guidelines • Faster diagnosis and treatment

A common use of a CDSS is to prevent adverse drug interactions. For example, a primary care clinic may enter a patient's common prescriptions into the EHR. However, if the patient goes to the hospital and the emergency department does not have access to that list of medications, then the risk for adverse drug interactions increases. The emergency department staff may prescribe a medication that interacts

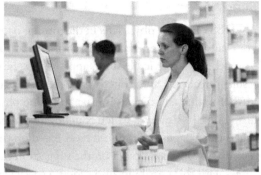

A CDSS alerts prescribers of possible drug interactions.

with the patient's regular prescriptions if the staff is unaware of possible interactions. A CDSS component of an EHR compares the list of the patient's prescriptions with the new prescription, alerting the prescriber if there is a potential interaction. Interoperability of EHR systems can save time, money, and patients' lives.

Consider This

A patient enters an emergency department with shoulder pain and is diagnosed with minor inflammation of his shoulder. The healthcare provider prescribes an anti-inflammatory medication to resolve the inflammation, which eliminates his symptoms of pain. Two months later, the patient returns to the emergency department with gastric bleeding and pain. He is diagnosed with a bleeding ulcer caused by an interaction between the anti-inflammatory medication he took for his shoulder and his regular hypertension medicine. How would a CDSS help prevent this scenario?

Alert Fatigue Are more alerts always better? A phenomenon commonly known as *alert fatigue* has become a significant issue for healthcare organizations following CDSS implementation. Healthcare providers may experience **alert fatigue** after encountering excessive numbers of alerts (e.g., drug–drug, telemetry, and laboratory results outside the normal range) within the EHR system. The provider may ignore such alerts without studying each one because of the large number they encounter in daily practice. The consequences of alert fatigue may be life threatening if a provider inadvertently ignores a serious alert. Therefore, to reduce the chances of alert fatigue, the thresholds of when an alert is triggered in a CDSS must be set at an appropriate level, which can be accomplished by defining policies regarding the types of results (normal, abnormal, and critical) that trigger an alert. Medical staff should be instrumental in determining thresholds to ensure continued buy-in regarding alert delivery from the CDSS. Constant monitoring of these thresholds is imperative to ensure that healthcare providers are alerted when significant or potentially significant care concerns arise. Provider feedback regarding the types of valuable alerts is also important.

WHY YOUR JOB MATTERS

Healthcare providers have the important job of identifying alerts that are serious and require intervention, a task that can be challenging with the high number of alerts that an EHR system might generate.

Tutorial 13.2   EHRNAVIGAT⊕R

Viewing a Drug–Drug Interaction

Go to your online course to launch Tutorial 13.2. As a physician, experience what happens when a drug–drug alert occurs in the EHR Navigator.

Diagnoses

A CDSS can assist physicians in diagnosing patient conditions based on a variety of factors. For example, a college student may present at the emergency department with a high fever, stomach pain, gastric bleeding, appetite loss, headache, and weakness. Routine laboratory results reveal only an elevated white blood cell count. The patient is then admitted for further testing and diagnosis. The attending physician uses the CDSS integrated with the hospital's EHR system, which searches the patient's EHR, filters the information, and suggests a diagnosis of typhoid fever based on the patient's symptoms and a documented recent trip to Kenya. Based on the suggestion from the CDSS, the attending physician agrees with this possibility and orders a special laboratory study for *Salmonella typhi*. The test result is positive for the bacteria, and the physician begins treatment.

Treatment Options

CDSSs can also monitor treatment options and assist healthcare providers in keeping up with the latest advancements in medicine. For example, an oncologist using the CDSS component of the practice's EHR system can review the latest research trials for all types of carcinoma treatments and offer patients choices if traditional treatment options are unsuccessful.

Preventive Care

Good preventive care has a host of benefits. Patients stay healthier when they go to their physicians for routine, preventive care, which in turn can help healthcare facilities save money by catching health issues earlier.

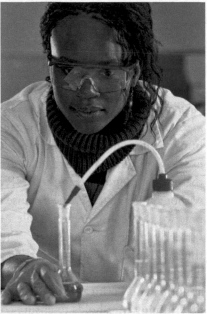

For example, because of the significant health risks associated with undiagnosed diabetes, a physician's practice may routinely use the preventive screening aspect of a CDSS to identify patients at risk for diabetes. According to the American Diabetes Association, anyone with a body mass index above 25 who has additional risk factors, such as high blood pressure and high cholesterol levels, is at risk for diabetes. Therefore, a physician's practice may routinely run reports to identify at-risk patients, sending alerts via their preferred method of contact to ask these patients to make an appointment for diabetes screening. Identifying patients who meet the pattern of certain diseases would be far more complicated without the assistance of a CDSS.

A CDSS allows practitioners to track the latest scientific research.

Tutorial 13.3

Running a Preventive Care Report

Go to your online course to launch Tutorial 13.3. As an office manager, practice running a preventive care report using the EHR Navigator.

Provider Efficiency

A CDSS can contribute to greater efficiencies for providers. The hospital can incorporate the care plans for certain types of diseases in the system, thus making it easier for physicians and other clinicians to follow them and increase compliance with Medicare or accreditation requirements. For example, for patients presenting with a possible diagnosis of pneumonia, the detailed instructions for the care of patients with this diagnosis, also known as the *protocol of care*, includes a chest x-ray and a blood culture within 24 hours of admission to confirm the diagnosis of pneumonia. Such protocols can be programmed in the CDSS, thus contributing to greater compliance with requirements, quicker diagnosis, quicker treatment, and possible decreased length of stay.

Cost Reduction

Another common role a CDSS plays in healthcare support is reducing costs. Patients are becoming increasingly savvier consumers of health care, and often they are invested in keeping costs down. Although many ways exist to help patients and physicians work together to reduce costs, a CDSS plays a key role in achieving cost-effective health care. For example, a family physician who understands how important the cost of medications is to her aging patient population may use the CDSS component of the practice's EHR system to select the best, most cost-effective medications covered by her patients' insurance plans.

13.2 Meaningful Use Requirement

As you learned in Chapter 1, the Health Information Technology for Economic and Clinical Health (HITECH) Act specified criteria for meaningful use of EHRs. Clinical decision support is a requirement of an EHR system that meets specified meaningful use criteria. Each stage (Stages 1, 2, and 3) of meaningful use required an increase in the functionality of the clinical decision support component of the organization's EHR. For example, the Final Rule of Stage 2 required the CDSS to be used to improve performance on high-priority health conditions by using five CDSS interventions related to four or more clinical quality measures (CQMs).

The Final Rule for Stage 3 required the demonstrated use of multiple CDSS interventions that apply to quality measures in at least four of the six National Quality Strategy priorities. The National Quality Strategy priorities include:

1. Preventive care

2. Chronic condition management (e.g., diabetes or coronary artery disease)

3. Appropriateness of lab and radiology orders (e.g., medical appropriateness or cost effectiveness)

4. Advanced medication-related decision support (e.g., renal drug dosing or condition-specific recommendations)

5. Improving the accuracy or completeness of the problem list, medication list, and drug allergies

6. Drug–drug and drug–allergy interaction checks

The National Quality Forum (NQF) is a nonprofit, nonpartisan, membership-based organization that works to bring about improvements in health care. The NQF is responsible for organizing and convening the National Priorities Partnership (NPP).

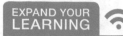
The NPP is a partnership of 52 major national organizations with a shared vision to achieve higher-quality health care that is more cost effective and equitable for all individuals. The NPP provides annual input to the secretary of the US Department of Health and Human Services regarding the National Quality Strategy (NQS) priorities.

Tutorial 13.4 — EHRNAVIGAT✦R

Generating an Attestation Report

Go to your online course and launch Tutorial 13.4. As an IT manager, practice generating an attestation report.

13.3 Role of EHRs in Quality Improvement Activities

EHRs can play a major role in a healthcare organization's quality improvement activities, but the question remains as to whether the healthcare organization is fully utilizing the data available through the use of EHRs. Reporting capabilities in EHR systems provide healthcare organizations with important statistics and can help identify opportunities to improve patient care. A routine review of clinical and outcome data and statistics can assist healthcare providers and administrators to identify potential quality issues.

Typical subject areas of statistical review and monitoring in an inpatient facility include infection rates, ventilator weaning success rates, lengths of stay, fall rates, morbidity and mortality rates, types and frequency of diagnostic tests per diagnosis-related group (DRG), and medication errors. A CDSS integrated with an EHR can provide statistics on many typical functions of an inpatient facility, so physicians, hospital managers, and other stake-holders can take necessary steps to improve areas in which the inpatient facility falls short.

Typical subject areas of statistical review and monitoring in an outpatient facility or physician practice include mammography, diabetes and colorectal screenings, and routine physical examinations. A CDSS integrated with an outpatient EHR system can provide information on that practice's patient population, allowing healthcare staff to send reminders or schedule follow-up procedures.

In our previous discussion of the CDSS requirement in meaningful use, we discussed the NQF, a national initiative to improve health care. There are two other major national initiatives that are important to learn about. These initiatives include the National Quality Measures of The Joint Commission (also known as the *Core Measures*) and the National Quality Measures Clearinghouse (NQMC), which is sponsored by the Agency for Healthcare Research and Quality (AHRQ).

National Quality Measures of The Joint Commission

The Joint Commission took a major role in working toward improving health care in US hospitals as early as 1999 and has continued to roll out more standards and requirements for many providers of health care, with its biggest focus on inpatient acute care hospitals. The Joint Commission's ORYX Program requires hospitals to gather performance data for the purposes of identifying opportunities for improvement in the services they provide. For accreditation purposes, hospitals are required to demonstrate data gathering, data analysis, and steps to improving quality of care. The Joint Commission has worked with CMS to develop a set of common quality measurements, which has resulted in the

Specifications Manual for Hospital Inpatient Quality Measures. This specifications manual contains a data dictionary, measure information forms, algorithms, and other tools to be used by CMS and The Joint Commission. The goal of this common set of quality measures, of course, is to improve quality of care, minimize data collection efforts for these quality measures, and focus efforts on the use of data to improve the delivery and quality of health care in the United States.

For more information regarding the Specifications Manual for Hospital Inpatient Quality Measures, go to https://EHR3.ParadigmEducation.com/Specifications.

National Quality Measures Clearinghouse

The National Quality Measures Clearinghouse (NQMC) is a resource regarding quality measures reported by all types of healthcare settings. These measures are available to the public by accessing the website www.qualitymeasures.ahrq.gov. The NQMC contains two major categories of measures: healthcare delivery measures and population health measures. Healthcare delivery measures are measures of care delivered to individuals and populations defined by their relationship to healthcare providers, organizations, or insurance plans. Population health measures are measures that address health issues of individuals or populations defined by geographic area. Using the search criteria found at the AHRQ quality measures website, healthcare delivery measures and population health measures may be found according to the type of healthcare setting—that is, hospital, ambulatory care, long-term care, or a specific organization such as The Joint Commission or the American Medical Association. It is important to note that the NQMC is a repository for quality measures and measure sets that healthcare organizations may choose to use for research, study, and/or reporting. The NQMC does not, however, gather or report on data from healthcare organizations according to these quality measures.

Electronic Clinical Quality Improvement

The implementation of EHRs has significantly affected the processes of data gathering and data analysis with the goals of improving the quality of health care, reducing the costs of health care, and making health care more accessible to all individuals.

Figure 13.2 demonstrates the process of electronic clinical quality improvement (eCQI). Beginning with the provision of care to patients, patient care and patient

Figure 13.2   eCQI Process

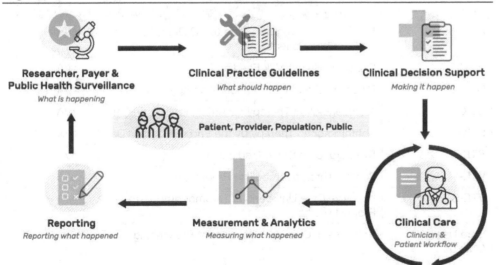

Researcher, Payer & Public Health Surveillance
What is happening

Clinical Practice Guidelines
What should happen

Clinical Decision Support
Making it happen

Patient, Provider, Population, Public

Reporting
Reporting what happened

Measurement & Analytics
Measuring what happened

Clinical Care
Clinician & Patient Workflow

outcomes are then measured using electronic clinical quality measures (eCQMs). These measurements are analyzed, and opportunities for improvement in patient care are identified. Improvements are implemented, patient care is rendered, and the cycle of eCQI is repeated.

CMS and the Office of the National Coordinator for Health Information Technology (ONC) work together to promote eCQI for the monitoring and analysis of the quality of health care provided to patients and the patient outcomes. The use of eCQMs is the primary focus of eCQI. eCQI looks at patient care and outcomes both retrospectively and concurrently with the use of computerized data. The eCQMs use the data from EHRs to measure healthcare quality in the provision of health care and patient outcomes. CMS publishes the annual eCQI reporting requirements for healthcare providers. Healthcare providers must report compliance with these eCQIs to demonstrate that their healthcare system continues to deliver effective, safe, efficient, patient-centered, equitable, and timely care. The reporting requirements for each year may be found on the following CMS website: https://www.cms.gov/Regulations-and-Guidance/Legislation/EHRIncentivePrograms/ClinicalQualityMeasures. An example of the eCQI reporting requirements for hospitals is found in Figure 13.3.

Figure 13.3 2021 eCQI Reporting Requirements for Hospitals

eCQM Reporting Period in 2021

The reporting period for eligible hospitals and CAHs that report eCQMs in the Medicare Promoting Interoperability Program is **two self-selected quarters** of CY 2021 data.

The submission deadline is two months following the close of CY 2021, specifically, **February 28, 2022**.

Reporting Criteria for 2021

Eligible hospitals and CAHs are required to report on at least **four** eCQMs. CMS requires Quality Reporting Document Architecture (QRDA)-I for eCQM submissions for the Medicare Promoting Interoperability Program. For more information on eCQM specifications and CMS's QRDA I Implementation Guide, visit the Electronic Clinical Quality (eCQI) Information Resource Center.

eCQMs for Eligible Hospitals and CAHs for CY 2021		
Short Name	**Measure Name**	**NQF No.**
ED-2	Median Admit Decision Time to ED Departure Time for Admitted Patients	N/A
PC-05	Exclusive Breast Milk Feeding	N/A
STK-2	Discharged on Antithrombotic Therapy	N/A
STK-3	Anticoagulation Therapy for Atrial Fibrillation/Flutter	N/A
STK-5	Antithrombotic Therapy by the End of Hospital Day 2	N/A
STK-6	Discharged on Statin Medication	N/A
VTE-1	Venous Thromboembolism Prophylaxis	N/A
VTE-2	Intensive Care Unit Venous Thromboembolism Prophylaxis	N/A
Safe Use of Opioids	Safe Use of Opioids – Concurrent Prescribing	3316e

In addition to meeting eCQIs required by CMS, hospitals accredited by The Joint Commission are also required to report eCQM data to The Joint Commission to retain accreditation. Many of The Joint Commission eCQMs mirror the eCQIs of CMS; however, The Joint Commission includes eCQMs regarding health topics that they are focused on trying to improve.

Consider This

An interesting eCQM for hospitals to report for 2022 involves the elective delivery of babies before 39 weeks of gestation for nonmedical reasons. The American College of Obstetricians and Gynecologists (ACOG) and the American Academy of Pediatrics (AAP) have had a standard in place requiring 39 completed gestation weeks prior to elective delivery, either vaginal or operative. A survey conducted by the March of Dimes revealed that almost one-third of all babies in the United States are electively delivered, with 5% of all deliveries in this country delivered in a manner that violated the ACOG/AAP guidelines. Most of these were for reasons of convenience and resulted in significant short-term neonatal morbidity. These statistics have led to The Joint Commission focus on elective deliveries. For 2022 deliveries, hospitals will have to report data regarding all deliveries to identify opportunities for improvement in the quality of care both for babies and their mothers.

Future of CDSS and eCQI

Future plans by CMS and ONC include the provision of standards that would require CDSSs to use evidence-based medicine and each patient's personal history, preferences, and data to customize a plan of care for each patient. Evidence-based medicine is the practice of medicine in which the healthcare provider uses the most up-to-date, research-based methods of treating the diagnosis. The use of evidence-based medicine ensures that patients are receiving the benefits of medical breakthroughs and best practices, rather than receiving care from a provider that has "always done it this way."

EXPAND YOUR LEARNING

To stay current with the status of CDSS and eCQI, visit the resource site eCQI Resource Center, managed by HealthIT.gov, and the CDS Connect website, managed by The Agency for Healthcare Research and Quality, at https://EHR3.ParadigmEducation.com/eCQI.

CHECKPOINT 13.2

1. Discuss the role of EHRs in the quality improvement activities of a healthcare organization.

2. List two examples of subject areas of statistical review and monitoring for an inpatient healthcare organization and two examples of subject areas of statistical review and monitoring for an outpatient facility or physician practice.

13.4 Garbage In, Garbage Out

The phrase *garbage in, garbage out* is commonly used in the field of computer science, and it refers to computers that produce faulty output when input data is inaccurate. If the data entered into an EHR system is inaccurate, then the output data is also unreliable, unusable, or, as stated in the previous expression, "garbage."

Members of the healthcare staff must continually review and monitor EHR documentation processes and systems for pertinence and accuracy. Inaccurate and unreliable data residing in a healthcare organization's EHR system is potentially life threatening because healthcare policies, procedures, treatments, and medication decisions are based on this data. Strict procedures must be in place to ensure accurate EHR data and that the correction of any incorrect data is completed in a timely fashion.

Healthcare facilities should create strict documentation policies and guidelines to comply with governmental, regulatory, and industry standards. Facilities should use a standardized format for healthcare documentation, such as SNOMED CT, to record diagnoses and create consistent templates in their EHR systems for documentation.

In addition to standardized documentation, any corrections to EHR data should also be handled consistently. Healthcare facilities should establish policies that outline who may amend records and what guidelines should be followed. For example, as a staff member of the healthcare information team, you may be able to change demographic data, but clinical data can be corrected only by the appropriate clinical staff.

Accurate data is important to patient safety, and it plays an important role in the successful use of a CDSS. The CDSS of an EHR system will not properly function if entered data is not accurate. If a patient's medications are not entered into the EHR system, then the CDSS will not detect drug–drug interactions. If the patient's weight and height are not accurate, then the CDSS cannot accurately assess their risk for diabetes. It is crucial for healthcare facilities to ensure consistent and accurate documentation if they want the CDSS to provide its many benefits.

13.5 Clinical Documentation Improvement

Clinical documentation improvement (CDI) is easily defined because the term describes itself. We know that clinical documentation is the information documented in a health record, and we also know that clinical documentation needs to be accurate, timely, and thorough. A program of CDI is the review and improvement of clinical documentation in a healthcare organization.

Hospitals that implement a formal CDI process typically employ nurses or practitioners certified in documentation improvement. The CDI staff review health records, identifying areas of documentation that are conflicting or incomplete or that require clarification, and then query the physician or provider for documentation to resolve the conflict or deficiency. Physicians and other healthcare providers document in the health record to answer or resolve the query. This has been and continues to be primarily a retrospective process, which is one of the weaknesses of the current state of CDI programs. The best-case scenario, of course, would be for the physicians and providers to document completely at the time services are provided. The next best thing would be to have a CDI program that functions concurrently—in other words, while the patient is still in the hospital. A concurrent CDI program would result in higher-quality care, since documentation conflicts would be resolved quickly, hopefully before the patients receive care based on incorrect documentation that could potentially be harmful. A concurrent CDI program would also result in faster coding and billing time frames after the patient is discharged, because coders would have all the information needed to accurately code the episode of care without having to query physicians and wait for responses.

Implementing Clinical Documentation Improvement Processes

CDI is not a new concept, but with the widespread implementation of EHR systems, CDI processes can be more easily and quickly carried out. For example, with paper health records, the time to locate the record alone can cause a significant delay in the review process. Then there is the manual review and querying of the physician, the physician's location of the paper record, their subsequent clarification documentation, the re-review of the paper record by the CDI and the coder, and other possible steps. You can probably identify many areas in which using an EHR in the CDI process would streamline the processes significantly. The health record is immediately accessible with the EHR, queries can be sent electronically, the physician or provider can add clarifying documentation into the health record immediately, and the coder can be sent an alert that documentation has been added so the coding function can be completed.

CDI has primarily been a process carried out in the hospital setting; however, more physicians' practices are realizing the advantages of implementing a CDI program. They reap the same benefits as a hospital with better documentation, timely billing and coding, and higher quality of care.

As discussed in Chapter 11, information governance is not a new concept, because it has been used in many industries. It is, however, a fairly new buzzword in the healthcare industry, arising primarily with the widespread implementation of EHR systems. Healthcare organizations find themselves faced with more information and documentation than they know what to do with. Implementing a well-organized, successful CDI program should be considered a requirement in all healthcare information governance programs.

Chapter Summary

Clinical decision support is health information technology that builds upon the foundation of an EHR to provide those involved in care decisions with general and patient-specific information. That information is intelligently filtered, organized, and delivered at the point of care to enhance health and health care.

Clinical decision support systems (CDSS) play an important role in EHR systems, elevating the medical record from a stagnant paper chart to an electronic, interactive system that assists with diagnostic decision making and improves quality of care and healthcare delivery. There are two basic types of CDSS: knowledge-based and non–knowledge based. Some of the most common applications of a CDSS are alerts, diagnoses, treatment options, preventive care, hospital and provider efficiencies, cost reductions, and improved patient satisfaction. The benefits of a CDSS include reduced risk of medication errors; reduced risk of misdiagnosis; increased direct patient care time for healthcare providers; access to state-of-the-art data, research, clinical pathways, and guidelines; reduction of unnecessary diagnostic tests; faster diagnosis; faster treatment; and alternative prescriptions for lower-cost medications.

Using a CDSS also has potential drawbacks, including the high costs of maintaining the CDSS, potential overreliance on computer technology, perception by healthcare providers as a threat to clinical knowledge and skills, and harmful outcomes if software is not thoroughly and continuously updated. A CDSS component of an EHR is required as a part of meaningful use standards.

It is imperative that a CDSS is kept up to date with current trends in medical diagnosis and treatment; otherwise, the CDSS may become more of a liability than an asset. EHRs play an important role in a healthcare organization's quality improvement activities, assisting with assessing and monitoring healthcare processes and outcomes. The Joint Commission has required accredited healthcare organizations to participate in quality improvement activities. It has continued working with CMS to develop a set of common quality measurements, which has resulted in the Specifications Manual for Hospital Inpatient Quality Measures. The goal of this common set of quality measures is to improve quality of care, minimize data collection efforts for these quality measures, and focus efforts on the use of data to improve the delivery and quality of health care in the United States.

The implementation of EHRs has significantly affected the processes of data gathering and data analysis, with the goals of improving the quality of health care, reducing the costs of health care, and making health care more accessible to all individuals. The use of electronic clinical quality measures (eCQMs) is the primary focus of electronic clinical quality improvement (eCQI). eCQI looks at both past and current patient care and outcomes with the use of computerized data. eCQMs use the data from EHRs to measure healthcare quality in the provision of health care and patient outcomes. Future plans by CMS and ONC include the provision of standards that would require a CDSS to use evidence-based medicine and each patient's personal history, preferences, and data to customize a plan of care for each patient.

The phrase *garbage in, garbage out* is commonly used in the field of computer science, and it refers to computers that produce faulty output when input data is inaccurate. If the data entered into an EHR system is inaccurate, then the output data is also unreliable and unusable. Healthcare facilities should create strict documentation policies and guidelines to comply with governmental, regulatory, and industry standards. Facilities should use a standardized format for healthcare documentation, such as SNOMED CT, to record diagnoses and create consistent templates in their EHR systems for documentation.

Clinical documentation improvement (CDI) is not a new concept, but with the widespread implementation of EHR systems, CDI processes can be more easily and quickly carried out. CDI has primarily been a process used in the hospital setting; however, more physicians' practices are realizing the advantages of implementing a CDI program. They reap the same benefits as a hospital with better documentation, timely billing and coding, and higher quality of care.

Review and Assessment

The following Review and Assessment activities are also available online in the Cirrus online course. Your instructor may ask you to complete these activities online. Cirrus also provides access to flash cards, a crossword puzzle, and practice quizzes to help strengthen your understanding of the chapter content.

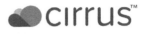

Acronyms/Initialisms

Study the following acronyms discussed in this chapter. Go to the online course for flash cards of the acronyms and other chapter key terms.

CDSS: clinical decision support system

CMS: Centers for Medicare & Medicaid Services

DRG: diagnosis-related group

HITECH: Health Information Technology for Economic and Clinical Health (Act)

ONC: Office of the National Coordinator for Health Information Technology

Check Your Understanding

To check your understanding of this chapter's key concepts, answer the following questions.

1. All of the following are examples of clinical decision support system (CDSS) tools *except*

   a. computerized alerts and reminders.

   b. clinical guidelines.

   c. standardized order sets.

   d. email tools.

2. Which of the following is a benefit of using a CDSS?

   a. It helps eliminate the need for medical research.

   b. It may promote an overreliance on computer technology.

   c. It helps reduce the risk of medication errors.

   d. It may produce alert fatigue.

3. The two basic types of CDSS are

   a. knowledge driven and documentation driven.

   b. knowledge based and documentation based.

   c. knowledge driven and non–knowledge driven.

   d. knowledge based and non–knowledge based.

4. All of the following are drawbacks of a CDSS *except*

   a. the cost of maintenance of the CDSS.

   b. an overreliance on computer technology.

   c. a perceived threat by healthcare providers to their knowledge and skills.

   d. software that does not need updating.

5. Typical subject areas of statistical review and monitoring in an inpatient facility include all of these, *except*

    a. lengths of stay.

    b. ventilation wean rates.

    c. the number of cardiologists on staff.

    d. infection rates.

6. True/False: A 2005 review of 100 studies showed that CDSSs improved practitioner performance in 95% of the studies.

7. True/False: A facility's drug–drug interaction software component meets the requirement for a CDSS as required for meaningful use.

8. True/False: The electronic health record (EHR) can play a major role in a healthcare organization's quality improvement activities.

9. True/False: Corrections to EHR documentation are *never* allowed.

10. True/False: Clinical decision support does *not* play a role in cost-effective health care.

Go on the Record

To build on your understanding of the topics in this chapter, complete the following short-answer activities.

1. Why is the CDSS a necessary component of an EHR system?

2. Describe the two different types of CDSSs.

3. Describe three benefits of CDSSs.

4. List three common uses of CDSSs with examples.

5. Briefly describe how a concurrent CDI program results in higher-quality care.

Navigate the Field

To gain practice in handling challenging situations in the workplace, consider the following real-world scenarios and identify how you would respond to each.

1. As the information technology manager for Northstar Medical Center, you receive a report that physicians have substantially increased their disregard for the clinical decision support system laboratory result alerts. You take this information to the president of the medical staff of the facility. Do you agree that this was the appropriate action to take? If so, what should the president of the medical staff do? If not, what should you, as the IT manager, have done instead?

2. You are the manager of a hospital that has recently incorporated a CDSS. One of your staff members does not want to use the new system, as he feels it makes him overly reliant on technology and does not use his knowledge and experience as a physician. How would you explain the advantages of a CDSS and persuade him to use it in practice?

Think Critically

Continue to think critically about challenging concepts and complete the following activities.

1. Identify *Yes* or *No* if the following are examples of clinical decision support:

   _____ a.   Dr. Smith is alerted to a drug–drug interaction.

   _____ b.   The dietician for Northstar Physicians mails out information about diabetes to patients diagnosed with diabetes mellitus.

   _____ c.   Dr. Jones is an orthopedic surgeon who takes a "time-out" for "right patient, right procedure, right site."

   _____ d.   A pharmacist receives an alert regarding a lower-cost medication to be substituted for a patient's current medication.

   _____ e.   A pharmacist looks up a national drug code number to order a medication.

2. Research and identify the top three clinical decision support systems. Briefly discuss the components of each of these systems and identify the interoperability of each system.

Make Your Case

Consider the scenario and then complete the following project.

You are the office manager for the BayView Physician Group and have been asked to prepare a presentation for the staff regarding the CDSS component of the EHR system that its group uses. The physicians would like you to explain to the staff the following items:

- Definition of a CDSS

- Why a CDSS is important

- Whether or not a CDSS is a requirement

- Three examples of how the staff of the BayView Physician Group will use the CDSS

Prepare the presentation for the BayView Physician Group staff.

Explore the Technology

Complete the EHR Navigator practice assessments that align to each tutorial and the assessments that accompany Chapter 13 located in the online course.

EHRNAVIGAT✚R

Chapter 14 eHealth and Population Health

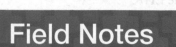

Field Notes

"Implementing an electronic system has simplified the ability to prescribe and transmit prescriptions between prescribers and pharmacies. Electronic prescriptions improve efficiency and decrease transcribing errors, thus improving safety for patients. Technology in the pharmacy setting is evolving. Linking medication therapy management (MTM) into our workflow provides health information—such as vaccine status, gaps in disease state management, and other possible medication adherence concerns—at our fingertips for certain patients. This is helping to maximize patient care at the pharmacy."

– Melanie Fisher, PharmD

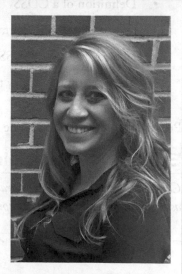

14.1 Define and differentiate *eHealth*, *telemedicine*, and *telehealth*.

14.2 Describe the communication technologies used in eHealth.

14.3 Explain how the advancements in eHealth benefit healthcare providers and patients.

14.4 Identify obstacles to the expansion of eHealth.

14.5 Define and discuss *population health*, including the 6/18 and HI-5 initiatives.

14.6 Discuss the role that EHRs play in population health.

14.7 Define and discuss the content of the personal health record (PHR).

14.8 Identify the types of PHRs along with their advantages and disadvantages.

14.9 Identify and discuss the components of a patient portal.

Consumers today are faced with many decisions regarding their health care. For that reason, they have become better educated about healthcare costs, treatment options, and preventive care. Treatment options have been expanded for most patients to include eHealth options. In addition to becoming more informed, many individuals have taken control of their health care by creating a personal health record (PHR) or participating in a patient portal. Healthcare providers, payers, individuals, and the government have been initiating population health strategies and activities with the goals of improving the health of groups of people, the quality of care, and the outcomes of treatment while managing costs. This chapter examines eHealth, PHRs, and population health and their evolving roles in patient care.

14.1 eHealth

eHealth is an overarching term that encompasses telemedicine, telehealth, and mHealth. **eHealth** specifically refers to the practice of health care using electronic processes and technology such as electronic health records (EHRs), laboratory and radiology systems, and patient scheduling systems. Telemedicine and telehealth, like eHealth, use electronic processes, electronic information, and telecommunications technologies to support and promote healthcare activities. **Telemedicine** is an older term that refers only to the clinical provision of healthcare in a remote manner. **Telehealth** is a broader term that refers not only to the clinical provision of health care in a remote manner but also to patient and professional health-related education, public health, and health administration. **mHealth** is the practice of health care that uses electronic processes conducted on a mobile device.

No matter the term, the primary goal of those using electronic processes, electronic information, and telecommunication in health care is to improve patient health and patient outcomes with cost and time savings as added benefits. Electronic processes in health care give providers improved access to patient health records and communication tools—primarily via the EHR—while providing patients with better access to healthcare services via telehealth. As with any standard healthcare practices, the security of patient information must also be considered in the use of telehealth technologies. Health Insurance Portability and Accountability Act (HIPAA) privacy and security requirements are still enforced when patients and providers use telehealth technologies. The healthcare provider must use technology that ensures that the patient's protected health information (PHI) is secure and cannot be hacked or released without proper authorization.

Communication Technologies

There are four types of communication technologies used in eHealth: synchronous, asynchronous, remote patient monitoring (RPM), and mHealth.

Synchronous Communication

Synchronous describes communication between individuals or groups that is conducted live, in real time. Synchronous communication can be as complex as a video conference or as simple as a telephone conversation. Examples of synchronous communication in eHealth include a video-enabled, real-time visit between a patient and a healthcare provider or a phone conversation between healthcare providers to discuss a patient's case.

Asynchronous Communication

Asynchronous describes communication that is *not* accomplished in real time. Asynchronous visits and consults can be accomplished through a healthcare provider's EHR or a special web portal. For example, you may be familiar with a software program called *MyChart*, a web portal offered by many healthcare providers who use the Epic EHR software. On MyChart, patients can schedule appointments, review lab results, keep track of their medications and immunizations, pay their bills, and email their providers for healthcare advice and services at their convenience. An asynchronous exchange between a patient and a provider is known as an *eVisit*, and an asynchronous consultation between physicians is known as an *eConsult*.

Remote Patient Monitoring

Remote patient monitoring (RPM) involves the use of mobile medical devices and technology to gather patient clinical data such as vital signs and blood pressure, as well as information on the medical device, such as a pacemaker status or glucose meter readings. Recall from Chapter 12 that networked devices that share data are referred to as the *Internet of Things (IoT)*, and in health care, these devices are typically used for RPM. There are a number of benefits to the use of RPM, including:

- Timely identification of potential health issues
- The patient's ability to receive healthcare monitoring within their own home
- The provider's ability to monitor more patients since face-to-face visits do not need to be conducted
- Cost savings for both patients and health insurers
- Comfort provided to patients who know their chronic condition is being monitored

Consider This

Daniel, an 84-year-old with a cardiac pacemaker who lives in a rural area of Ohio, 50 miles from his cardiologist. Daniel is not able to drive himself to the doctor's office for weekly pacemaker checks to ensure that his pacemaker is working correctly and that the battery does not need to be changed. Telehealth has significantly and positively impacted Daniel's life by enabling remote cardiac pacemaker monitoring via the internet, allowing Daniel to receive this healthcare service in his own home. In addition to improving Daniel's care, in this example, both Daniel and his physician save time since Daniel does not have to be seen in an office setting. RPM also reduces Daniel's transportation and health insurance costs, and he gains peace of mind knowing that when his pacemaker needs an adjustment or a new battery, he will be notified by his healthcare provider. This is just one example of how telehealth—specifically RPM—is improving patient care, reducing costs, and saving time.

mHealth

The fourth type of communication technology used in telehealth is mHealth. mHealth is the practice of healthcare that uses electronic processes conducted on a mobile device such as a tablet or smartphone.

CHECKPOINT 14.1

1. Define *eHealth*.

_____

_____

2. List the four types of communication technologies used in eHealth.

a. _____

b. _____

c. _____

d. _____

3. Explain the difference between synchronous and asynchronous communication.

_____

_____

_____

_____

_____

_____

14.2 eHealth: Past, Present, and Future

It may surprise you to learn that telemedicine or telehealth can be traced back to the late 1800s, when a physician used the telephone to care for patients in an effort to reduce office visits. In the 1920s, a radio was used to communicate healthcare information to ships. Today, telehealth has been used to improve access to dental services, ophthalmology services, pharmacy services, and many other specialty services.

Providers of dermatology and psychology services are some of the most prominent users of telehealth. Instead of trying to describe a skin condition over the phone or waiting months for a dermatology appointment, the patient answers questions and uploads an image of the skin condition in an eVisit, and the provider reviews and diagnoses the condition. The provider can even follow the diagnosis with an eprescription if needed. Likewise, a patient or client in need of psychological counseling could use telehealth to receive treatment that would not otherwise be available due to their geographical location, or their reluctance or inability to leave their home.

The combination of technology and convenience makes eHealth a low-cost, timesaving, and overall better patient experience for those who have access and know how to use it. Key research studies on telehealth have demonstrated myriad benefits, such as a reduction in the time patients with cancer wait to receive biopsies and pathology reports. Patients with asthma and diabetes have also benefited from the remote monitoring of their vital signs and adjustment of medications, leading to reduced emergency department visits. When thinking of the potential benefits of eHealth, consider not just the provision of clinical services but also the patient education that can occur with telehealth. With telehealth, individuals and groups of patients receive timely information on a variety of topics, such as the importance of immunizations, how to manage a chronic disease such as diabetes, and what to do in the case of an emergency.

With advancements in technology, many doors are opening for the use of telehealth. In general, the older population is not as receptive to synchronous telehealth, because it involves the real-time use of technology that may be difficult. However, the older patient population embraces asynchronous telehealth and RPM since they can stay at home thanks to the remote monitoring of their condition. The younger population is more receptive to synchronous telehealth as they are typically adept with the technology needed to conduct real-time healthcare services. Younger patients often choose an eVisit over a traditional office visit so that they can schedule their healthcare services at their convenience. As technology continues to evolve and the population continues to drive the need, telehealth will grow and become more common.

Reimbursement for telehealth is one of the obstacles hindering its widespread use. There are federal and state policies regarding the reimbursement of telehealth as well as individual insurance payer policies that influence accessibility for patients and providers. While Medicare, Medicaid, and commercial insurance payers will reimburse providers for some telehealth services, there are many restrictions placed on who can be reimbursed for providing these services, which patients and conditions qualify for them, and which type of telehealth communication technologies can be used to render healthcare services. Expanding reimbursement for services related to chronic conditions could help improve patient outcomes and reduce health costs. Chronic conditions are the leading cause of death and disability and account for the majority of the $3.5 trillion in annual health costs in the United States. According to the Centers for Disease Control and Prevention (CDC), 6 out of 10 adults in the United States have at least one chronic condition, and 4 out of 10 adults have two or more chronic conditions. Telehealth will undoubtedly continue to be used to diagnose and treat these chronic conditions if the reimbursement for telehealth services is improved by payers and state and federal policies.

In an effort to advance the growth and use of telehealth in rural areas, the federal government has made grants available. Healthcare providers can apply for grants to expand telehealth services if they are located in a rural area. To determine whether their practice is in an area that meets the federal government's definition of *rural*, providers

<aside>
WHY YOUR JOB MATTERS

Similar to the EHR, telehealth technology saves both time and money which can be better spent on patient care.
</aside>

can visit https://www.hrsa.gov/rural-health/telehealth/index.html. In addition, the federal government established and now funds Telehealth Resource Centers (TRCs) to provide assistance, education, and information to organizations and individuals who are providing health care at a distance. Information regarding TRCs can be found at https://www.telehealthresourcecenter.org/.

While the primary goal of telehealth is to improve patient care and outcomes, healthcare providers need to be reasonably reimbursed for their services. The COVID-19 pandemic contributed significantly to the expansion of the use and acceptance of telehealth visits and reimbursement for these visits. The Centers for Medicare & Medicaid Services (CMS) established a waiver in March 2020 to allow Medicare to pay for visits provided via telehealth, and insurance companies quickly followed suit. With a wider use of telehealth, many healthcare providers are finding appropriate situations in which telehealth is the best option for providing care.

Emergency departments have found several uses for telehealth, including the following:

- Tele-triage: Tele-triage is like traditional triage but uses technology to supplement or replace elements of the patient interaction. Tele-triage involves screening patients remotely to determine the patient's condition and the care needed.

- Tele-emergency medicine: Tele-emergency medicine connects providers at a central hub emergency department to providers and patients at spoke hospitals (often small, remote, or rural) through video or similar telehealth technology.

- Virtual rounds: Telehealth technology can be used by healthcare providers to virtually check on emergency department patients. This helps limit the number of providers who are physically present and exposed to contagious diseases. It also saves time and conserves personal protective equipment.

- eConsults: eConsults help providers get recommendations from other providers with specialty expertise. eConsults can be used by all healthcare providers to obtain recommendations from specialists all over the world. Consider a child living in a rural area with no direct access to pediatric specialists and how telehealth can provide timely assessment and recommendations for treatment.

- Telehealth for follow-up care: Telehealth technology can also be used to provide follow-up care for patients who were triaged but not sent to the emergency department or for patients after they are discharged from the emergency department.

ON THE JOB

Some may think the medical office staff find the implementation of telehealth a complication to their jobs. According to a 2016 study, the medical office staff found that telehealth actually improved their jobs with increased efficiency, reduced exposure to illness, shorter wait times, less crowded waiting rooms, and more profitable practices.

CHECKPOINT 14.2

1. What is the primary goal of telehealth?

_____

2. What has been one of the obstacles hindering the widespread use of telehealth?

_____

3. How is the federal government helping to advance the growth and use of telehealth in rural areas?

_____

_____

_____

14.3 Population Health

The US healthcare system is structured to focus on the health of every citizen in the treatment of disease and with the encouragement of good health and wellness. Population health focuses on the health of groups of people rather than individuals. People may be grouped in many ways, including by diagnoses, geographic location, race, gender, income, health habits, and so on. The goals of population health are to improve the health of groups of people along with improving the quality of care they receive and the outcomes of treatment while managing costs. Achieving the goals of population health requires the collaborative efforts of healthcare providers, payers, individuals, and the government.

According to the CDC, population health identifies significant health concerns and strategies to allocate resources to overcome the issues that drive poor health conditions in an identified population. The CDC has implemented two major population health initiatives: the 6/18 Initiative and the Health Impact in 5 Years (HI-5) Interventions.

6/18 Initiative

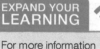

EXPAND YOUR LEARNING

For more information regarding the 6/18 Initiative, review the CDC Factsheet at https://EHR3 .ParadigmEducation .com/6-18Initiative.

The 6/18 Initiative targets 6 common and costly health conditions with 18 proven interventions. Government resources are allocated in order to improve health by providing effective interventions and controlling costs. One of the 6 health conditions is tobacco use, and the goal is to reduce tobacco use by providing education and removing barriers to treatments. Another example is to expand access to the National Diabetes Prevention Program to develop lifestyle changes for preventing type 2 diabetes. Figure 14.1 displays the 6 health conditions addressed by the 6/18 Initiative.

Figure 14.1 6/18 Initiative

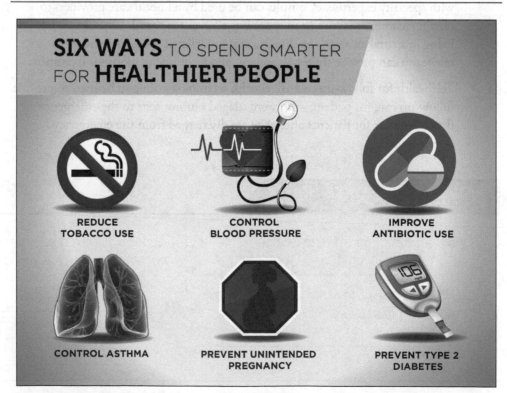

Health Impact in 5 Years (HI-5) Interventions

The Health Impact in 5 Years (HI-5) Interventions is the CDC initiative that addresses **social determinants of health (SDOH)**. The SDOH are conditions in the environments where people are born, live, learn, work, play, worship, and age that affect a wide range of health, functioning, and quality-of-life outcomes and risks. By focusing on SDOH and a community-wide approach, the CDC plans that positive health impacts will be evidenced within 5 years of initiating HI-5 interventions.

The conditions that are addressed by the HI-5 program include:

- Anxiety and depression
- Asthma
- Blood pressure
- Bronchitis
- Cancer
- Cardiovascular disease
- Child abuse and neglect
- Cognitive development
- Dental caries
- Infant mortality

- Liver cirrhosis
- Motor vehicle injuries
- Obesity
- Pneumonia
- Sexually transmittable infections
- Sexual violence
- Teenage pregnancy
- Traumatic brain injury
- Type 2 diabetes
- Youth violence

Figure 14.2 summarizes, in graphic form, the HI-5 Initiative.

EHRs play an important role in population health by making it easier for healthcare organizations to collect standardized, systematic data, improving the organization's reporting capabilities. Efficiently collecting data in a form that can be shared across multiple healthcare organizations allows for quality improvement and prevention activities. EHRs can improve health reporting and surveillance as well as an organization's ability to prevent disease by using reminders to patients for preventive and follow-up care. EHRs also give providers access to clinical protocols.

Figure 14.2 HI-5 Initiative

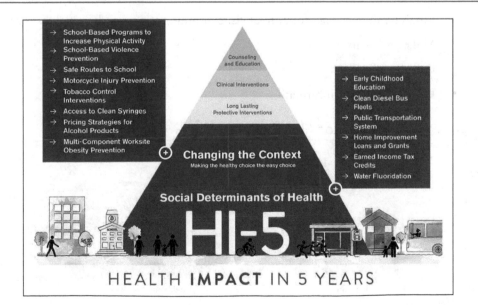

14.4 Personal Health Record

As discussed in this chapter, one of the goals of population health is for individuals to participate more in their own health and treatments. A **personal health record (PHR)** is a paper collection of health information or an electronic application through which patients can maintain and manage their health information (and that of others for whom they are authorized) in a private, secure, and confidential environment. It is a tool that enables individuals to work with practitioners to make more informed decisions, which may contribute to better quality of care.

The concept of the electronic PHR was not introduced until the 21st century, however, patients were encouraged to keep a written PHR as early as the 1950s (see PHR Timeline). Today, EHR systems are required to have a PHR component for patients to use. Most PHRs are initiated for a patient upon contact with a provider organization (e.g., a hospital or physician's practice) and are typically referred to as a *patient portal*. Personal health records and patient portals have two primary goals: (1) to have health information available at the point of care and (2) to help foster enhanced communication between the patient and the healthcare provider. The result is a record that contains a complete overview of the individual's health history and current health status. See Figure 14.3 for an illustration of how the PHR facilitates the flow of information between the patient and the healthcare provider. In addition to forming a complete summary of an individual's health, a PHR may also be used to do the following:

- Track and update healthcare information from any location via a computer, tablet, or smartphone 24 hours a day

- Coordinate care among selected healthcare providers and facilities

- Locate information about diseases and conditions

- Avoid duplication of tests and procedures

- Monitor prescriptions, allergies, wellness, and research

- Share health information with selected providers and healthcare facilities

- Schedule appointments, including face-to-face and telehealth visits

- Communicate with healthcare providers (i.e., via messaging)

- Email reminders (e.g., for annual visits, immunizations, and annual testing)

- Make payments

- Request referrals

- Update insurance information

Figure 14.3 Information Flow with the PHR

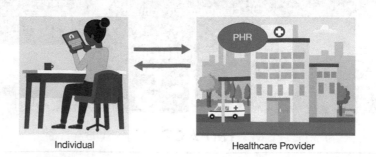

Individual   Healthcare Provider

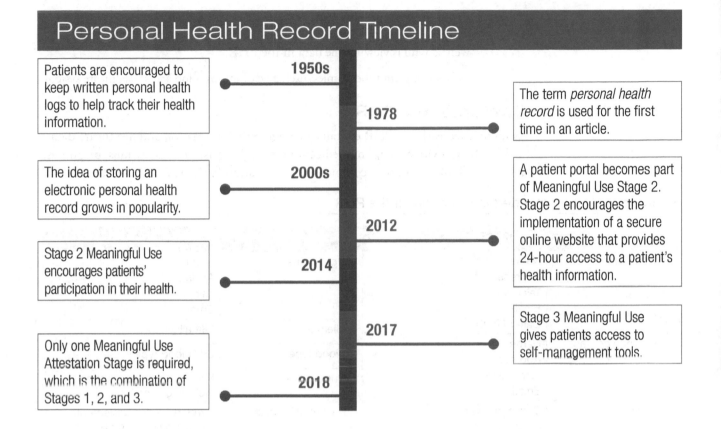

Personal Health Record Timeline

1950s — Patients are encouraged to keep written personal health logs to help track their health information.

1978 — The term *personal health record* is used for the first time in an article.

2000s — The idea of storing an electronic personal health record grows in popularity.

2012 — A patient portal becomes part of Meaningful Use Stage 2. Stage 2 encourages the implementation of a secure online website that provides 24-hour access to a patient's health information.

2014 — Stage 2 Meaningful Use encourages patients' participation in their health.

2017 — Stage 3 Meaningful Use gives patients access to self-management tools.

2018 — Only one Meaningful Use Attestation Stage is required, which is the combination of Stages 1, 2, and 3.

Rise of the PHR

The Markle Foundation, an organization that promotes the use of technology to improve people's lives, created Markle Connecting for Health, a public–private collaboration focused on improving health through the use of information technology. Representatives from more than 100 collaborating organizations were tasked to develop policies that would be shared among patients and healthcare providers. The outcomes of this working group were as follows:

- Accelerate the development of the PHR

- Increase the patient's relationship with a healthcare provider and involvement in their care and safety

- Develop a common data set

- Develop a variety of approaches to creating a PHR

To fulfill these goals, Markle Connecting for Health developed seven best practices for a PHR:

1. Each individual would have their own PHR.

2. PHRs are to provide a complete medical history for an individual from birth to death.

3. PHRs are to contain information from healthcare providers.

4. PHRs are to be accessible from any place at any time.

5. PHRs are to be private and secure.

6. PHRs are to be transparent. An individual can see who entered data, when the data was entered, and where data was imported or transferred from as well as who is viewing the data in the PHR.

7. PHRs will permit the seamless exchange of information across healthcare systems.

Contents of a PHR

As mentioned earlier, a PHR contains demographic information and healthcare data, such as the individual's current medications, allergies, past hospitalizations, diagnoses, and more. Table 14.1 lists recommended information for inclusion in a PHR.

Table 14.1 Recommended Information for the PHR

Category	Data	Category	Data
Demographic	Name Address Telephone Email Date of birth	Optometrist	Name Address Telephone Email
Emergency contact	Name Address Telephone Email	Allergies	List all allergies
		Blood type	List blood type
Insurance information	Company name Address Telephone Group number	Current medications	Every drug or supplement, including vitamins
		Past medications	Every drug or supplement, including vitamins taken in the past
Religious preferences	Name of spiritual leader Address Telephone Email	Immunizations, vaccinations	Flu shots and other vaccinations, including dates
		Illnesses, conditions, treatments	Diagnoses, treatments, dates of occurrence, and failed treatments
Advance directives	Scanned copies of Do Not Resuscitate directive, living will, and healthcare proxy	Hospitalizations	Inpatient and outpatient services
Providers	Name Address Telephone Email Specialty	Pregnancies	All maternity encounters (live, stillbirth, etc.)
		Surgeries	All inpatient and outpatient surgeries
		Additional medical tests	All medical tests
Health issues	List health issues providers are addressing	Permission forms	Release of information and medical procedures
Dentist(s)	Name Address Telephone Email	Imaging	X-rays Magnetic resonance imaging Computed tomography scans
Dental issues	List dental issues providers are addressing	Alternative therapies	Alternative therapies or treatments
Pharmacy	Name Address Telephone Email	Correspondence	Correspondence among health-care providers and facilities

14.5 General Types of PHRs

There are three general types of PHRs: paper, computer based, and web based. Each type of PHR has certain advantages and disadvantages that individuals need to consider.

Paper PHRs

The traditional paper PHR, a collection of medical documents and personal journals of an individual's health history, rose to prominence in the 1950s as families were encouraged to document medical treatments (including drug therapy), procedures, and vaccinations. The goals also included monitoring and improving their overall health status. This type is losing its appeal as electronic recordkeeping becomes the norm.

Advantages

A paper PHR has the advantage of being a low-cost method of recordkeeping. Individuals who continue to use a paper health record also like the privacy and security of keeping the record safe at home rather than out in cyberspace. This type of record is portable and can be carried by a patient to a healthcare visit.

Disadvantages

There are many disadvantages associated with a paper PHR. For a patient, a paper health record may be difficult to assemble, organize, and update. Without an established format, a paper PHR may also lack the necessary details to provide a complete picture of the patient's health status. Lastly, in an emergency, a paper record may be either unavailable for use or difficult to decipher by an attending healthcare provider or emergency facility. The privacy and security of paper PHRs are also drawbacks to this type of record. Unless placed in a secure location, a paper PHR is accessible to others who may invade the privacy of the record's owner.

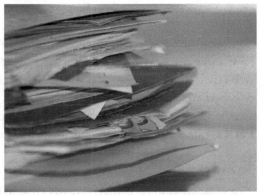
Paper PHR files are difficult to store and organize.

Computer-Based PHRs

Computer- or software-based PHRs are similar to paper PHRs, but they have an electronic format. Patients can purchase or download PHR software and install it on their chosen electronic devices. This type of PHR system is known as a stand-alone or untethered PHR, and it is not designed to share information electronically with other PHR or EHR systems. The patient or a designee is responsible for entering the data into the program as well as attaching any documents or images to accompany the data. Therefore, the patient is in control of an untethered PHR. When the patient visits a healthcare provider or facility, they can print the health information or transfer it to a portable storage device, such as a flash drive, memory card, or CD, so that the data can be transferred to the legal health record.

Advantages

In addition to the portability feature mentioned earlier, computer- or software-based PHRs are often password protected and are not connected to the internet, making these health records more secure than paper PHRs. Computer-based PHRs also allow patients to back up their health information, thus helping to prevent a loss of valuable data.

Disadvantages

Of course, the data contained in computer-based PHRs is only as accurate as the accuracy of the typist. Patients must exercise caution when inputting information into the health record. Another disadvantage of these records is the lack of internet connectivity. Although this feature aids security of data, it also makes patients bear the sole responsibility of updating their health records and maintaining their accuracy. Lastly, not all healthcare providers have computer system compatibility that allows them to accept an external media transfer of information into the EHR. If the system is not compatible, then the healthcare provider or facility cannot read or upload the information.

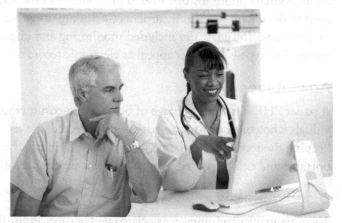

Patients can take their paper or electronic PHRs to their healthcare providers to view.

Web-Based PHRs

To use web-based PHRs, patients must have access to a computer or digital device and have an internet connection. With the expansion of digital and mobile technology, web-based PHRs are the most widely used PHRs. Web-based PHRs are either tethered or untethered. A **web-based tethered PHR** is a system in which health information is attached to a specific organization's health information system. A **web-based untethered PHR** is not attached to a specific organization's health information system.

Tethered PHRs

This web-based PHR may be provided through a patient's health insurance, employer, healthcare facility, or healthcare provider and is stored on a server owned by a third-party organization. To gain access to health data on a tethered PHR, a patient must use a portal. Once access is granted, a patient may make only limited changes to the record, such a change in insurance coverage. Because the PHR is attached to a covered entity, the patient's health information is protected by HIPAA. However, patients should be aware that this type of PHR does not meet the best practices criteria of the Markle Foundation.

Tethered PHRs may be provided by health insurers, healthcare facilities, and employers, as discussed next.

Health Insurer–Provided PHRs Many health insurers offer subscribers the opportunity to participate in their health care with tethered PHRs known as **health insurer–provided PHRs**. A health insurer often populates information about a subscriber, such as insurance claim information, a list of providers, prescriptions, and benefits coverage. However, a subscriber can also enter their own data. Subscribers may also access additional resources, such as wellness information on exercise, nutrition, weight loss, pregnancy, smoking cessation, and other topics that will encourage them to make healthy choices to improve their quality of life as well as reduce costs to the health insurer. Because health insurer–provided PHRs are owned by companies rather than patients, these records are not considered to be "true" PHRs. One advantage of a health insurer–provided PHR is that the health insurer updates the PHR as information becomes available. This way, the patient is not solely responsible for entering health information updates. Information may be extracted, printed, saved, and sent to various healthcare providers or facilities.

Facility-Provided PHRs   Another type of tethered PHR comes from a physician or healthcare facility. This type of PHR, known as a **facility-provided PHR**, links the EHR and the PHR and allows the patient to access the PHR portion online, using a username and access code. This type of technology is relatively new and is increasing in popularity. Many of these types of PHRs are static, meaning that the patient may only view the information. There are several features that a tethered PHR from a physician or healthcare facility may include, such as a messaging feature that provides the patient with the opportunity to email a provider, request an appointment, view test results, request a prescription refill, and view reminders. The section titled "Patient Portal" describes the features of a facility-provided PHR. See Figures 14.4 and 14.5 to view screenshots from this type of portal.

Employer-Provided PHRs   Employers are also getting involved in the area of PHRs. In 2006, several companies, including Intel, BP America, Pitney Bowes, and Walmart, formed an organization called Dossia. In 2008, Dossia offered PHRs to employees of its member companies. This type of PHR, known as an **employer-provided PHR**, contains data from hospitals, physicians' offices, health plans, laboratories, and pharmacies as well as information entered by the employee. The goal of employer-provided PHRs is to enable employees to make better health decisions. Achieving this goal is a win–win situation for both employees and employers: employees improve their health and well-being, and employers reap the benefit of decreased insurance costs and employee absenteeism.

Figure 14.4   Log-In Screen of a Facility-Provided PHR/Patient Portal

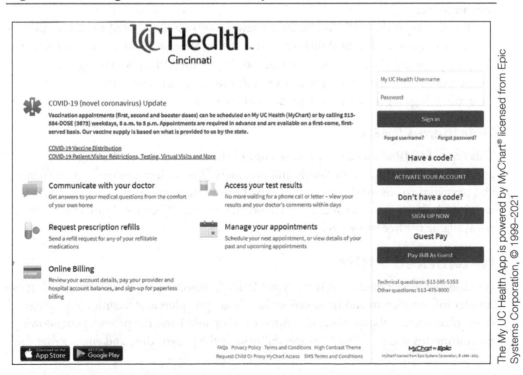

Figure 14.5 Facility-Provided PHR/Patient Portal

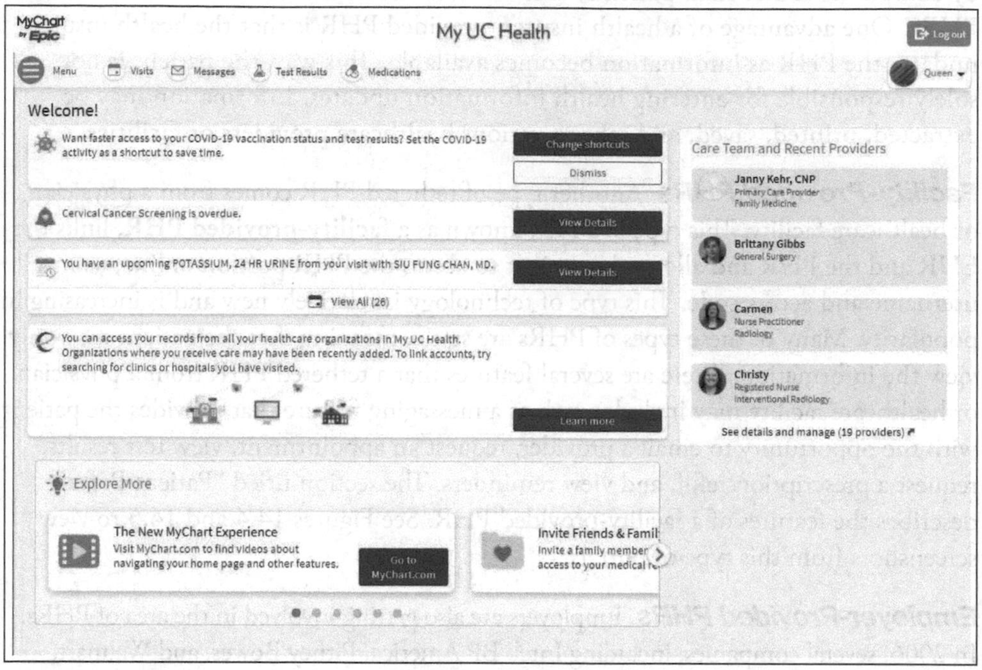

There are several advantages to using an employer-provided PHR. One of the biggest advantages is that this type of PHR is not limited to one healthcare provider or facility. Employees may enter health information from all of their providers and can determine what information can be shared. Another advantage is that, because the PHR is web based, patients can access the content anytime and from anywhere. For example, patients can access their PHRs from providers' offices or healthcare facilities by entering a username and password. Lastly, an employer-provided PHR is available to the employee for life, even if they are no longer employed by one of the organizations.

Employer-provided PHRs also have a few disadvantages. One of the disadvantages is that employees are responsible for entering the information and keeping it current. Another potential disadvantage for an employer-provided PHR is that many employees are not comfortable sharing sensitive health information with their employers or have misgivings regarding how their data will be used.

Untethered PHRs

This type of PHR allows the patient to control the information in the record by customizing access rights for family and providers. The patient can create a username and password to ensure the security of their health information. Because the PHR is web based, the patient can access the record at any time. Web-based untethered PHRs are available for free or by paying a fee.

Networked PHRs

A web-based, networked PHR is the type Markle Connecting for Health imagined. It can transfer information to and from various healthcare providers and facilities (e.g., physicians, pharmacies, laboratories, and insurance companies) and the patient, thus allowing for continuous updates. This interoperability saves the patient time and ensures that the information in the patient's PHR is accurate and current. For example, when a patient visits a dermatologist, the office staff updates the patient's diagnoses and procedures. Then, when that patient goes to the pharmacy to retrieve the prescription the dermatologist just prescribed, the pharmacy staff updates the insurance claim information to the networked PHR.

A networked PHR has several advantages:

- This type of PHR is accessible anytime from anywhere as long as the patient has an internet connection.

- Information is shared among multiple providers and facilities, unlike the other types of PHRs previously discussed.

- Individuals can select the information that is shared with family, healthcare providers, and facilities.

- The PHR is kept more accurate, up to date, and complete because of the input by healthcare staff.

Although the networked PHR offers several advantages, one disadvantage is the issue of privacy and security. The exchange of information over the internet and among multiple healthcare providers and facilities opens the PHR for potential compromise of health information.

CHECKPOINT 14.3

1. What are the advantages and disadvantages of a paper PHR?

   _____

   _____

2. What are the advantages and disadvantages of a computer-based PHR?

   _____

   _____

3. List three types of web-based PHRs.

   a. _____

   b. _____

   c. _____

Overall Challenges of PHRs

Similar to the lack of EHR interoperability that we have discussed previously, PHRs are faced with the same communication challenges. Some networked PHRs can communicate with healthcare provider systems, but many PHRs are not interoperable.

Privacy and security concerns also affect the adoption of PHRs. Those PHRs not offered by HIPAA-covered entities fall under the privacy policies of the PHR vendor, as well as any other applicable laws that govern how information in the PHR is protected. In addition, there is currently no federal law that covers the storage or transmission of PHR content. These privacy and security issues are troubling and must be addressed.

Finally, depending on the type of PHR, the information in the record may not be accurate, up to date, or both. For PHRs to be effective, patients must assume the responsibility of maintaining the record—a task that can be time consuming.

Consider This

American Health Information Management Association (AHIMA) prepared an article to help consumers select a PHR to meet their needs. To access this article, go to https://EHR3 .ParadigmEducation.com/AHIMA-PHR.

Read the article and review the questions to ask when choosing a PHR. Consider how you would answer the questions. How would your answers apply to the type of PHR that would fit your situation?

14.6 The EHR–PHR Connection

As you have already learned, an EHR system stores information about a patient's health. Depending on the type of PHR a patient establishes, their information may be shared and/or integrated. Although an EHR and a PHR have different characteristics, these records share a common goal: to provide a complete picture of a patient's past and current health status. To meet this goal, the two entities must be connected, allowing for the exchange of information.

Healthcare organizations agree that the key to the effective use of PHRs is the linkage to an EHR system. The Office of the National Coordinator for Health Information Technology (ONC) has determined that a PHR plays an important role in the implementation of the EHR and the Nationwide Health Information Network (NHIN).

The Institute of Medicine (IOM) also agrees that a PHR can help providers using an EHR system. In its research, the IOM discovered that patients see many different healthcare providers in a variety of healthcare facilities, and often these providers do not have a complete view of the patient's health history because each provider and facility keeps individual records on patients. A networked PHR, discussed earlier, is the tool that allows complete health record access by all parties.

Consider This

Sally was a 70-year-old woman diagnosed with heart failure five years ago. Since then, she had been taking warfarin, an anticoagulant, to help reduce the risk of stroke. While attending her water aerobics class, she began to feel lightheaded and short of breath. She collapsed and was rushed to the hospital. The aerobics instructor, who was only an acquaintance, knew none of the medications Sally was taking nor how to contact her next of kin. The hospital placed Sally on heparin to reduce her risk of developing blood clots while in the hospital.

Heparin is also an anticoagulant and, when given with warfarin, increases the risk of bleeding. These medications are sometimes used together but only with special monitoring. Because the staff members at the hospital were unaware that Sally was taking warfarin, they were not monitoring her as closely as they should have been. Sally experienced internal bleeding and died while in the hospital. How could this tragedy have been prevented if Sally had a PHR?

14.7 Patient Portal

The concept of patient portals was created out of the growing popularity of PHRs as well as the adoption of EHR technology because they interface with the healthcare facility's EHR system. A patient portal provides a patient access to their medical records, appointments, messages, billing, connection to family records, and administrative information.

During a patient visit, healthcare providers offering patient portal access will invite patients to register for access, ultimately providing them with usernames and access codes. Patients can then create an account and gain access to the portal.

Many facilities have implemented patient portals to help them achieve Stage 2 and 3 meaningful use patient engagement and self-management requirements.

Log In

The Northstar Patient Portal Log-In screen, as shown in Figure 14.6, demonstrates that PHR systems require log in credentials to access a patient's PHR to ensure a patient's privacy and confidentiality of their health information.

Home Page

Many patient portal systems have similar characteristics. The home page of a typical portal includes options for messages, appointments, medical records, family records, billing and insurance, administration, and preferences. There is also an option to link records from multiple healthcare providers. The EHR Navigator has a patient portal integrated with its system, the Northstar Patient Portal. Figure 14.7 illustrates the Northstar Patient Portal home page.

Figure 14.6   Log In

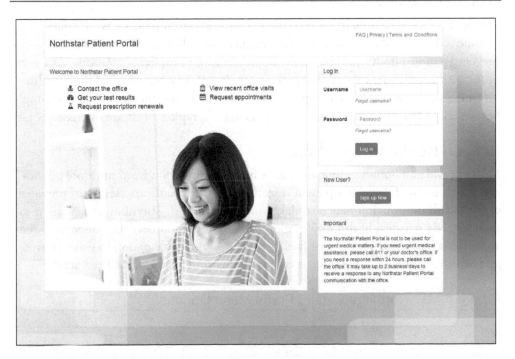

Figure 14.7   Northstar Patient Portal Home Page

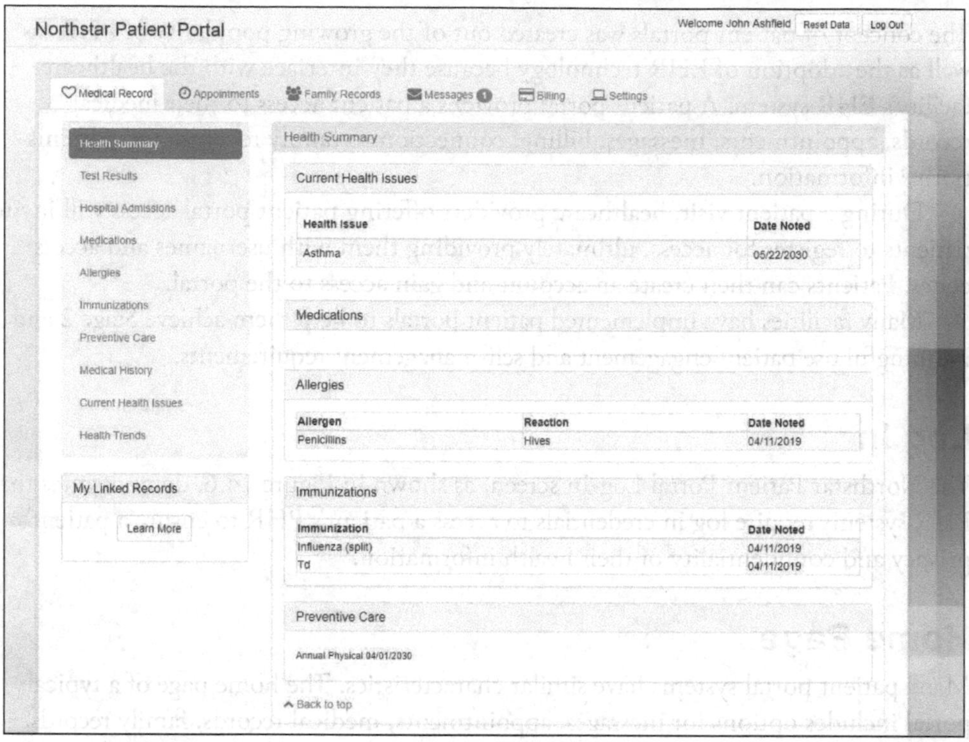

Patient Portal Menu

The Patient Portal Menu provides quick access to the *Medical Record, Appointments, Family Records, Messages, Billing,* and *Settings.* The Northstar Patient Portal menu is shown in Figure 14.8.

Medical Record

The *Medical Record* allows patients to track their health information, which may include test results, current health issues, medications, allergies, immunizations, preventive care, a health summary, medical history, and hospital admissions. As a user of the Northstar Patient Portal, the patient can download a summary of their health information that can be shared with a family member or healthcare provider or simply be available when traveling abroad. Components of a typical PHR are discussed below.

Linking Health Information

PHRs provide an option to link a patient's health information from multiple providers, which is a useful tool if a patient is seen by another healthcare facility or provider, as the health information may be quickly and easily shared. This allows the patient to manage their personal health information from multiple sources. The patient also may authorize a healthcare provider or facility to send health information to other providers and facilities. Linking medical records allows other providers and facilities access to

Figure 14.8   Northstar Patient Portal Menu Options

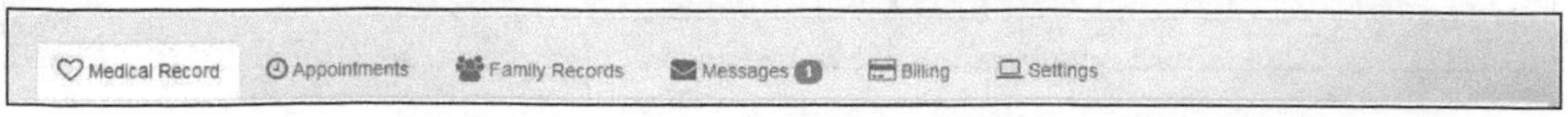

health information such as medications, previous test results, previous procedures, hospital admissions, and any complications experienced. When a healthcare provider has access to a patient's complete health history, the delivery and quality of care improves. The Northstar Patient Portal demonstrates the capability to link records from the Medical Record page as shown in Figure 14.7.

Health Summary

The *Health Summary* feature of the Northstar Patient Portal provides links to current health information, diagnoses, medications, allergies, immunizations, and preventive care information. The *Health Summary* screen is shown in Figure 14.7.

In addition to the health summary, the patient can view diagnostic test results, including laboratory, radiology, and other test results, after the healthcare provider has contacted the patient with any issues with the findings.

A record of the patient's inpatient admissions and outpatient visits, including telehealth visits, are kept in the PHR, as well as a list of the patient's current and past medications. It is imperative that the list of current medications is kept up to date in the event the patient seeks emergency care and is unable to verbally share the names of current medications with the emergency staff.

Wellness and preventive care information is included in a PHR to assist patients and caregivers in the management of recommended exams and testing, such as annual physicals, immunizations, mammography, annual lab tests, tests related to medications such as digoxin levels, and so on.

Appointments

The PHR allows a patient to view upcoming appointments, cancel appointments, or schedule an appointment. To schedule an appointment, the patient selects the healthcare provider they would like to see along with the date and time available on the provider's schedule. In addition, in the *Notes* field, the patient includes a short description of the reason for the appointment and communicates any specific information necessary for the healthcare provider or facility about the requested appointment. Figure 14.9 shows the *Request My Appointment* dialog box. The portal also provides a convenient way for the patient to cancel an appointment. Rather than placing a telephone call, the patient may log in to the patient portal and select the appointment they would like to cancel.

Figure 14.9 Northstar Patient Portal Appointments

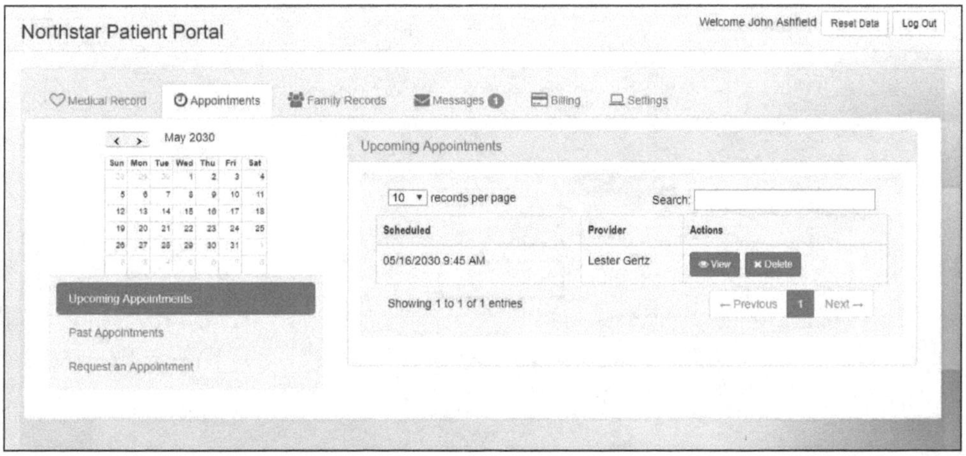

Figure 14.10 Family Records

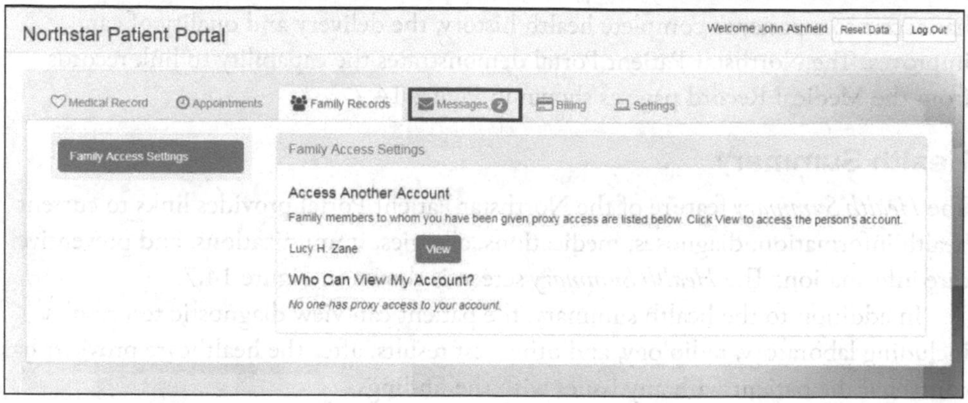

Family Records

Many PHRs have a feature that permits patients to identify family members or friends who may have access to the patient's PHR. The patient may also desire access to the PHRs of their family members, such as a parent who wants to be linked to their child's PHR. In the Northstar Patient Portal, the *Family Records* menu option provides this functionality as shown in Figure 14.10.

Messages

Most PHRs have communication functionality for the patient to request a medication refill, seek medical advice (e.g., ask a non-urgent question), and request a referral to a healthcare specialist. In the Northstar Patient Portal, the communication functionality is accessed from the Messages menu option as shown in Figure 14.11.

Billing

Most PHRs include billing functions such as viewing and updating billing and insurance information and making payments to an account. The patient may track their payments, insurance payments, and outstanding balances through this menu option, as shown in Figure 14.12.

Figure 14.11 Messages

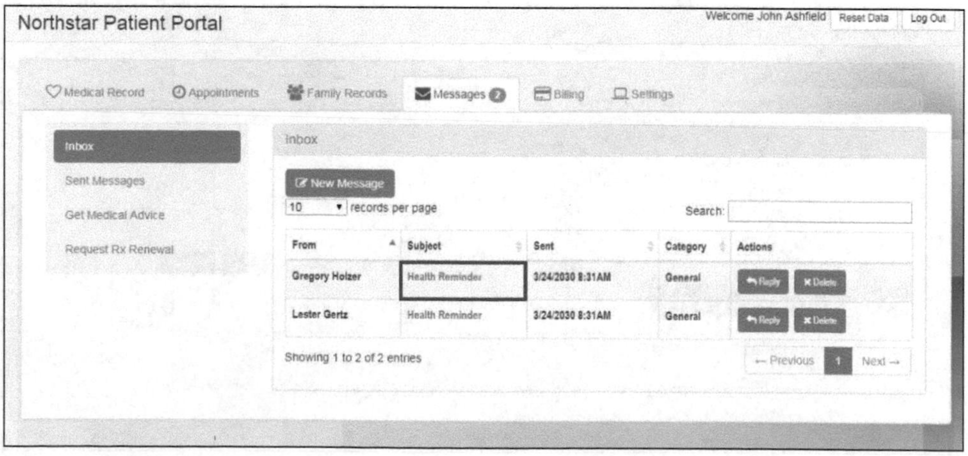

Figure 14.12 Billing

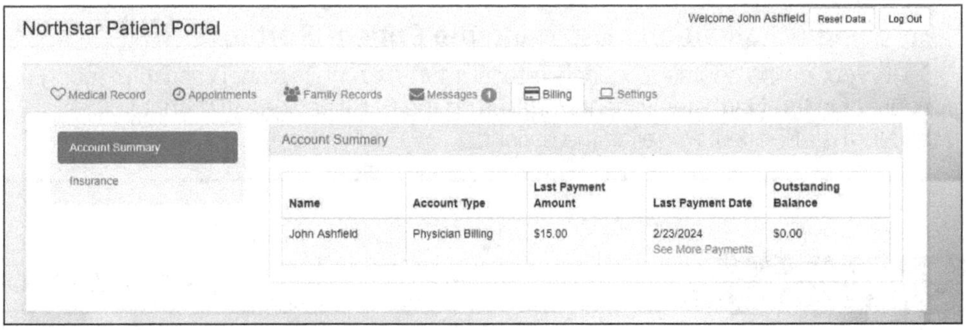

Settings

The *Settings* section of the Northstar Patient Portal (shown in Figure 14.13) includes the patient's *Profile* and *Portable PHR* sections. The *Profile* section includes the patient's address, telephone number, and email address as well as their primary care provider and provider location. The patient may find their PHR identification number, medical record number, or account number for billing purposes in the administrative information. In this section, the patient can edit their demographic information or change their password.

From their PHRs, patients may print or download their health information (e.g., allergies, medications, current health issues, procedures, and test results) to share with others. In the Northstar Patient Portal, this is completed in the *Portable PHR* section of the Settings.

Figure 14.13 Settings

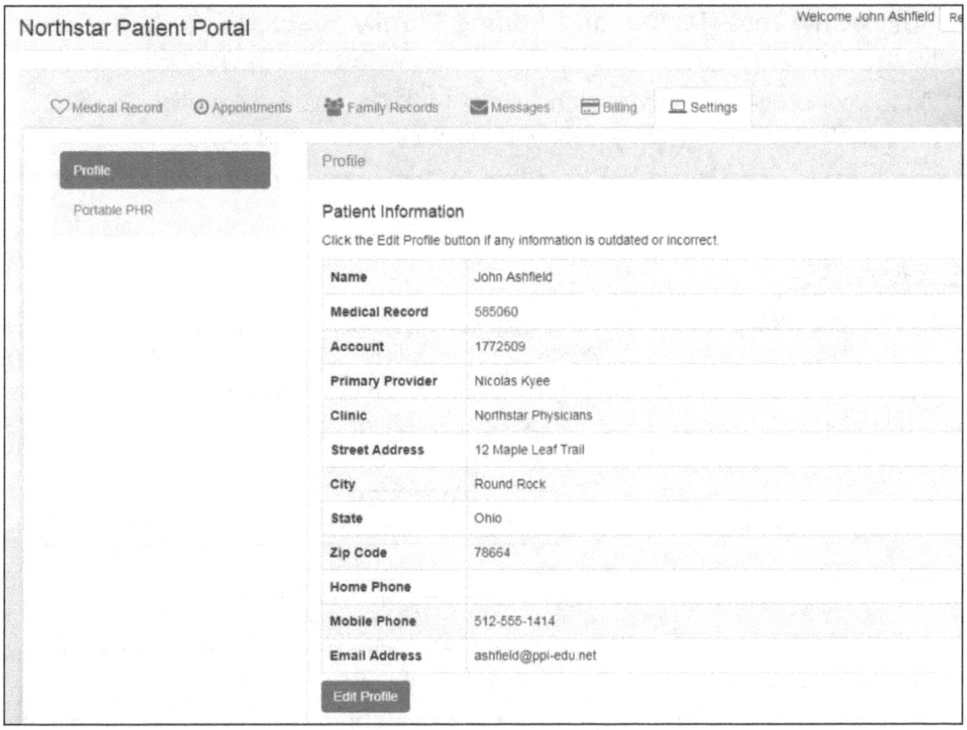

Tutorial 14.1

EHRNAVIGAT❂R

Enrolling a Patient and Exploring the Patient Portal

Go to your online course to launch Tutorial 14.1. As a physician, practice enrolling a patient in the Northstar Patient Portal using the EHR Navigator. Then, explore the Northstar Patient Portal as the patient.

Tutorial 14.2

EHRNAVIGAT❂R

Requesting a Refill and an Appointment in the Patient Portal

Go to your online course to launch Tutorial 14.2. As a patient, practice reviewing a record, requesting a prescription refill, and scheduling an appointment in the Northstar Patient Portal.

Tutorial 14.3

EHRNAVIGAT❂R

Requesting Medical Advice and Printing Information in the Patient Portal

Go to your online course to launch Tutorial 14.3. As a patient, practice requesting medical advice in the Northstar Patient Portal.

Tutorial 14.4

EHRNAVIGAT❂R

Reviewing Test Results and Adding Family History to the Patient Portal

Go to your online course to launch Tutorial 14.4. As a patient, practice viewing test results and adding family history to the Northstar Patient Portal.

CHECKP❂INT 14.4

1. Name four features in a patient portal that you would use to improve monitoring your own health care.

   a. _____

   b. _____

   c. _____

   d. _____

2. Why is it important to link health information together in a patient portal?

   _____

   _____

   _____

   _____

Chapter Summary

Modern healthcare treatment options have been expanded to include eHealth options. *eHealth* is a term that encompasses telemedicine, telehealth, and mHealth. eHealth specifically refers to the practice of health care using electronic processes and technology such as electronic health records (EHRs), laboratory and radiology systems, and patient scheduling systems. *Telemedicine* is an older term that refers only to the clinical provision of healthcare in a remote manner. *Telehealth* is a broader term that refers not only to the clinical provision of health care in a remote manner but also to patient and professional health-related education, public health, and health administration. *mHealth* refers to the practice of health care through electronic processes conducted on a mobile device. There are four types of communication technologies used in eHealth: synchronous, asynchronous, remote patient monitoring (RPM), and mHealth.

Healthcare providers, payers, individuals, and the government have initiated population health strategies and activities with the goals of improving quality of care and the outcomes of treatment while managing costs. Population health focuses on the health of groups of people rather than individuals. The CDC has implemented two major population health initiatives: the 6/18 Initiative and the Health Impact in 5 Years (HI-5) Interventions. The 6/18 Initiative targets 6 common and costly health conditions with 18 proven interventions. Government resources are allocated in order to improve health by providing effective interventions and controlling costs. The HI-5 Interventions addresses social determinants of health (SDOH).

At the individual level, patients are faced with many decisions regarding their care, so they have had to become better educated about healthcare costs, treatment options, and preventive care. Patients can take part in managing their care by creating a personal health record or participating in a patient portal. A personal health record (PHR) is a paper collection of health information or an electronic application through which patients can maintain and manage their health information (and that of others for whom they are authorized) in a private, secure, and confidential environment. PHRs may be paper, computer based, or web based. In addition to the format of PHRs, they can be classified as tethered and untethered. Tethered PHRs are linked to a healthcare provider, facility, or third-party payer. Untethered PHRs are those in which the creator of the PHR enters the health information, and the record is not associated with a healthcare provider, facility, or third-party payer. Many parties play an important role in keeping the PHR up to date, and patients and providers use PHRs to help them make better medical decisions, avoid duplicate tests, reduce adverse drug interactions, and support wellness and preventive care.

As PHRs have grown in popularity, many healthcare providers have created their own patient portals as part of the EHR technology. A typical patient portal includes messaging, scheduling, medical history, billing and insurance, and administrative features. The patient portal, along with the PHR, improves the delivery and quality of health care.

Review and Assessment

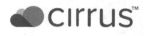

The following Review and Assessment activities are also available online in the Cirrus online course. Your instructor may ask you to complete these activities online. Cirrus also provides access to flash cards, a crossword puzzle, and practice quizzes to help strengthen your understanding of the chapter content.

Acronyms/Initialisms

Study the following acronyms discussed in this chapter. Go to the online course for flash cards of the acronyms and other chapter key terms.

AHIMA: American Health Information Management Association

CMS: Centers for Medicare & Medicaid Services

HHS: US Department of Health and Human Services

HIMSS: Health Information and Management Systems Society

HIPAA: Health Insurance Portability and Accountability Act

IOM: Institute of Medicine

NHIN: Nationwide Health Information Network

ONC: Office of the National Coordinator of Health Information Technology

PHR: personal health record

TRC: Telehealth Resource Center

Check Your Understanding

To check your understanding of this chapter's key concepts, answer the following questions.

1. *eHealth* is an overarching term that encompasses each of the following, *except*

    a. telemedicine.

    b. telehealth.

    c. population health.

    d. mHealth.

2. Which of the following communication technologies involves the use of mobile medical devices and technology to gather patient clinical data, such as vital signs and blood pressure?

    a. synchronous technology

    b. asynchronous technology

    c. mHealth

    d. remote patient monitoring

3. Which of the following is the CDC initiative that addresses social determinants of health?

    a. HI-5

    b. 6/18 Initiative

    c. PHRs

    d. NHIN

4. Which of the following PHR formats is either tethered or untethered?

   a. paper based

   b. computer based

   c. web based

   d. portal based

5. Which of the following refers not only to the clinical provision of health care in a remote manner but also to patient and professional health-related education, public health, and health administration?

   a. telehealth

   b. telemedicine

   c. mHealth

   d. social determinants of health

6. How many common and costly health conditions are targeted by the 6/18 Initiative?

   a. 2

   b. 5

   c. 6

   d. 8

7. Which of the following organizations promotes the use of technology to improve people's lives?

   a. HI-5

   b. Markle Foundation

   c. CDC

   d. RPM

8. The acronym *PHR* stands for

   a. protected health record.

   b. personal health report.

   c. personal health record.

   d. protected health report.

9. Which of the following is one of the primary goals of the PHR?

   a. acting as a substitute for the legal medical record

   b. developing a common data set

   c. promoting more eVisits

   d. fostering communication between providers and healthcare facilities

10. A tethered PHR is personal health information that

    a. is attached to a specific organization's health information system.

    b. is *not* attached to a specific organization's health information system.

    c. the patient enters into the health information system.

    d. is *not* attached to a specific provider's health information system.

Go on the Record

To build on your understanding of the topics in this chapter, complete the following short-answer activities.

1. What are the benefits of having a patient portal?

2. What are the benefits of using telehealth?

3. How do you see the future of mHealth?

4. What is the purpose of the 6/18 Initiative?

5. Explain the difference between tethered and untethered PHR systems.

Navigate the Field

To gain practice in handling challenging situations in the workplace, consider the following real-world scenarios and identify how you would respond to each.

1. You are presenting to your staff on the different types of communication technologies used in eHealth. Research the technologies presented in this chapter and provide an example of each communication technology that your healthcare organization may use in delivering eHealth. Research how these types of communication technologies can improve patient care.

2. Your healthcare organization implemented telehealth visits during the coronavirus pandemic, and now the organization is discussing whether to continue telehealth visits. You have been asked to present the advantages and disadvantages of discontinuing telehealth visits. After careful review, make a recommendation about the future of telehealth visits at your healthcare organization.

Think Critically

Continue to think critically about challenging concepts and complete the following activities.

1. Prepare a pamphlet for patients of South Community Hospital on the Health Impact in 5 years (HI-5) Interventions. Include information about the goal of HI-5, reminders for preventive and follow-up care, and highlight some potential initiatives South Community Hospital is taking in the community.

2. Investigate the patient portal system that accompanies this textbook, and complete a scavenger hunt by answering questions from your instructor.

3. An interactive website is available for providers to determine whether they are located in a rural area and eligible to apply for grants to fund their expansion of telehealth services. Go to https://EHR3.ParadigmEducation.com/telehealth. Using this website and interactive map, compare your area

with two areas near you that are considered rural. Are you located in a rural area? If not, how far are you from the nearest rural area? What telehealth services are available in your area? Organize, compare, and contrast your findings in a graph, table, paper, or presentation.

4. Find the Telehealth Resource Center (TRC) that provides resources in your area by going to https://EHR3.ParadigmEducation.com/TRC and clicking the interactive map. What useful resources are provided by your TRC? Compare the resources provided by your TRC with three other TRCs of your choice. Organize, compare, and contrast your findings in a graph, table, paper, or presentation.

Make Your Case

Consider the scenario and then complete the following project.

You are a member of the CobaltCare insurance company, which is promoting the patient portal for all of its insured members. You are hosting a session on how to begin to access the patient portal, exploring what information should be included and how to keep patients' health information current. Prepare the presentation you will share with the enrollees who attend the information session.

Explore the Technology

Complete the EHR Navigator practice assessments that align to each tutorial and the assessments that accompany Chapter 14 located in the online course.

EHRNAVIGAT✛R

Checkpoint Answer Keys

Checkpoint 1.1

1. An electronic version of patient files within a single organization that allows healthcare providers to place orders, document results, and store patient information for one facility.

2. An electronic health record is a digital version of a patient's paper chart. EHRs are real-time, patient-centered records that make information available instantly and securely to authorized users. The EHR allows for real-time access and the ability to access all of an individual's health records from multiple healthcare providers.

3. a. An EMR belongs to a single healthcare provider or organization whereas an EHR integrates EMRs from multiple providers.

   b. EHRs contain subsets of patient information from each visit.

   c. EHRs are interactive and can share information among multiple healthcare providers.

Checkpoint 1.2

1. The ability of one information system, computer system, or application to communicate with another information system, computer system, or application.

2. Level 2—Structural interoperability

3. Health Level 7 (HL7) Fast Healthcare Interoperability Resources (FHIR) Release 4.0.1

Checkpoint 1.3

1. a. Improved documentation

   b. Streamlined and rapid communication

   c. Immediate and improved access to patient information

2. a. High cost

   b. Privacy and security

   c. Inexperience in implementation and training

   d. Significant daily process changes

Checkpoint 2.1

1. Data includes the descriptive or numeric attributes of one or more variables. Data collected and analyzed becomes information. A record is a collection, usually in writing, of an account or an occurrence.

2. Administrative data includes demographic information; clinical data is information such as admission dates, office visits, laboratory test results, evaluations, or emergency visits; legal data is composed of consents for treatments and authorizations for the release of information; financial data includes the patient's insurance and payment information.

Checkpoint 2.2

1. The source-oriented record is the most common used by healthcare facilities. It organizes the health documents into sections that contain information from a specified department or type of service.

2. S (subjective) O (objective) A (assessment) P (plan)

Checkpoint 2.3

1. Answers may vary and could include five of the following: admission record, history and physical, progress notes, laboratory tests, diagnostic tests, operative notes, pathology reports, physician orders, consents, consultations, emergency department encounters, and discharge summary.

2. Answers may vary and could include five of the following: demographic information, contact information, history and physical, immunization records, problem lists, allergy lists, prescription lists, progress notes, assessment, consultations, referrals, treatment plans, patient instructions, laboratory tests and results, consents, communication, external correspondence, and financial information.

Checkpoint 3.1

1. a. Input
   b. Processing
   c. Output
   d. Storage
2. A LAN is a group of computers connected through a network confined to a single area or small geographic area. The network is secure and reliable. The networked computer system allows computer workstations to work and communicate together.

Checkpoint 3.2

1. The Messages feature allows you to communicate with other system users in your organization using a HIPAA-compliant feature. It improves the collaboration and continuity of patient care.
2. a. Schedules Overview
   b. View Calendar

Checkpoint 3.3

1. Answers may vary and could include four of the following: medical diagnoses, treatments, procedures, allergies, medical history, medications, test results, and reports.
2. An integrated laboratory feature enables healthcare facilities and providers to connect with national and regional laboratories or to maintain an existing laboratory partner. Integrating laboratories with an EHR system gives you the ability to create laboratory orders and view results from any computer at any time, with abnormal results flagged and organized for easy review.

Checkpoint 4.1

1. Answers may vary and could include four of the following: acute care setting such as a hospital;

ambulatory care settings such as surgery centers, physician's offices, clinics, group practices, emergency departments, therapeutic services, dialysis clinics, birthing centers, cancer treatment centers, home care, correctional facilities, and dentist offices; or other healthcare settings, such as long-term care facilities, behavioral health settings, rehabilitation facilities, and hospice care.

2. A patient goes to an ambulatory care facility for a procedure and complications occur, requiring the patient to be admitted to an acute care facility.

Checkpoint 4.2

1. a. Personal/Family
   b. Workers' Compensation
   c. Third-Party Liability
   d. Corporate
   e. Research
2. If two insurance plans cover a child, then the birthday rule is applied. The birthday rule specifies that the insurance of the parent whose birthday falls first in a calendar year will be the primary insurance. It helps to determine which insurance should be used as the primary insurance.

Checkpoint 5.1

1. Meetings, holidays, lunch hours, surgical schedules, physician rounds, or emergencies
2. a. Open Hours
   b. Time Specified
   c. Wave
   d. Modified Wave
   e. Cluster

Checkpoint 5.2

1. Patient portals are available 24 hours a day and allow the patient to view a provider's calendar. The portal allows patients to enter demographic, insurance, medical history, and current health information prior to the first appointment, reducing the resources necessary from the healthcare facility.
2. a. Select Schedule an Appointment
   b. Select Add Appointment

Checkpoint 5.3

1. a. Change in patient condition

   b. Change in isolation status

   c. Patient preference

2. The patient tracker offers a real-time, at-a-glance view of a patient's current status and location. It improves the healthcare facility's workflow and increases patient satisfaction.

Checkpoint 6.1

1. False. There are three types of permitted disclosures: for purposes of treatment, payment, and healthcare operations.

2. False. HIPAA protects health information in any form or medium.

3. Covered entities

Checkpoint 6.2

1. A civil violation is when a person mistakenly obtains or discloses individually identifiable health information in violation of HIPAA. A criminal violation is when a person knowingly obtains or discloses individually identifiable health information in violation of HIPAA.

2. Answers may vary and could include three of the following: impermissible uses and disclosures of PHI, lack of safeguards of PHI, lack of patient access to his or her PHI, uses or disclosures of more than the minimum necessary PHI, and lack of administrative safeguards of electronic PHI.

Checkpoint 6.3

1. a. General Rules

   b. Administrative Safeguards

   c. Physical Safeguards

   d. Technical Safeguards

   e. Organization Requirements

   f. Policies and Procedures and Documentation Requirements

2. Technical Safeguards

3. Administrative Safeguards

Checkpoint 7.1

1. It requires less personnel time, avoids repetitive request of information from patients, and may allow for more consistent data entry.

2. A history and physical examination (H&P) is a part of all inpatient encounters with healthcare providers and is a valuable tool for the healthcare provider in the identification of diagnoses. It is also the first step in developing a plan of care. The H&P consists of two main elements: a subjective element and an objective element.

Checkpoint 7.2

1. Answers may vary but could include three of the following: improved prescribing accuracy and efficiency; a decreased potential for medication errors and prescription forgeries; improved billing; less risk for potential medication errors due to a healthcare provider's handwriting, illegible faxes, or misinterpretation of prescription abbreviations.

2. The ability to order controlled substances electronically.

Checkpoint 8.1

1. Scope of practice is the allowable procedures and functions that healthcare professionals may perform according to their state licensures.

2. b. transfer.

Checkpoint 8.2

1. Pressure injuries affect patient comfort and healing by causing pain and often infection. They can be difficult to heal due to a patient's medical conditions, such as poor circulation, incontinence, and poor nutritional status. Pressure injuries may result in longer hospital stays and increased cost of care, and they may generally contribute to worse patient prognosis and increased risk of death.

2. The pain assessment includes the type of pain, acute or chronic; the location of the pain; the intensity of the pain; and what, if anything, helps to relieve the pain.

Checkpoint 8.3

1. A flowsheet allows the tracking of patient health data over a period of time, which helps healthcare providers identify whether a patient is stable and recovering or getting worse.

2. Right patient, right medication, right dose, right route, right time, right reason, and right documentation

Checkpoint 8.4

1. Medicare- and Medicaid-certified nursing homes
2. The purpose of a nursing discharge assessment is to document the patient's condition and status at the time of discharge.

Checkpoint 9.1

1. Answers may vary and could include three of the following: reimbursement, research, decision making, public health, quality improvement, resource utilization, or healthcare policy and payment.
2. October 1, 2015
3. 2025–2030

Checkpoint 9.2

1. a. Efficient concurrent and final coding
   b. Accuracy in code assignments
   c. Improved access to health records
2. False. Upcoding is illegal. Unintentional upcoding is considered abuse, and intentional upcoding is considered fraud.

Checkpoint 10.1

1. Health Maintenance Organization (HMO)
2. Preferred Provider Organization (PPO)
3. Consolidated Omnibus Budget Reconciliation Act of 1985 (COBRA)

Checkpoint 10.2

1. Medicare, Medicaid, TRICARE, CHAMPVA, workers' compensation
2. Medicare
3. Income replacement benefits, healthcare treatment, mileage reimbursement, and burial and death benefits

Checkpoint 10.3

1. Day-to-day operations of a medical practice
2. CMS-1500
3. The 837 Claim is also known as the HIPAA form. HIPAA regulations require that most claims be processed electronically using the 837 Claim.

Checkpoint 10.4

1. A billing/status report is generated to determine if the practice is receiving the correct monies owed.
2. Production Report (Production by Procedure, Production by Insurance, Production by Provider)
3. A Production by Provider Report may be used for a variety of reasons, including calculating provider salaries based on the number of patients treated, calculating the number of appointment slots for each provider, scheduling staff, and ordering supplies.

Checkpoint 11.1

1. Answers will vary but must include four of the following: date of birth, race, ethnicity, gender, or laboratory test results.
2. A primary data source is the original data found in the health record. A secondary data source is data collected by someone else or derived from another data source such as an index or registry.

Checkpoint 11.2

1. Together, policies and procedures provide an explanation to employees of the healthcare organization of how to handle data operations. Policies and procedures provide a framework to identify the data standards for a healthcare organization and detail the use of data, such as the policies and procedures for privacy and confidentiality.
2. A data dictionary is important to data standards because it provides a way to prevent inconsistencies, define elements and their meaning, provide consistency, and enforce data standards.
3. Data mapping is a method used to connect data from one system to data of another system. Data in the original or source system are analyzed and matched to data in the target system.

Checkpoint 11.3

1. A data set is a structured collection of related data elements. These data elements have

standard definitions to provide consistent data for all users. A database is a collection of data organized in rows, columns, and tables. The data are indexed. A registry is a database focused on a collection of information about a specific condition or disease, and uses clinical information focused on the outcomes of data before analysis. Indexes in a database are used to find data without searching every entry.

2. Accountability, transparency, integrity, protection, compliance, availability, retention, disposition

Checkpoint 12.1

1. Artificial intelligence

2. Answers will vary but may include sleep monitors, smart contact lenses, wearable smart necklaces to identify if medications have been taken as prescribed, vital signs monitors, glucose monitors, or sleep and safety monitors for infants.

Checkpoint 12.2

1. Clinical results reporting or clinical outputs

2. The improvement of the quality of health care

Checkpoint 13.1

1. Health information technology that integrates with the EHR and assists healthcare providers with decision-making tasks such as determining diagnoses, choosing the best medications for the patient, and selecting proper diagnostic tests.

2. a. Knowledge based

   b. Non–knowledge based

3. Answers may vary and may include three of the following benefits: reduced risk of medication errors; reduced risk of misdiagnosis; increased direct patient care time for healthcare providers; access to state-of-the-art data, research, clinical pathways, and guidelines; reduction of unnecessary diagnostic tests; faster diagnosis, resulting in faster treatment; and prescriptions for lower cost medications. The potential drawbacks may include three of the following: costs of maintaining the CDSS with up-to-date medical research, clinical pathways, guidelines, and medication costs; potential overreliance on computer technology; perception by healthcare

providers as a threat to clinical knowledge and skills; and harmful outcomes if software is not thoroughly and continuously updated.

Checkpoint 13.2

1. The reporting capabilities in EHR systems provide healthcare organizations with important statistics and to identify opportunities for improving patient care.

2. Answers may vary but could include three of the following for inpatient facilities: infection rates, ventilation wean success rates, lengths of stay, fall rates, morbidity and mortality rates, types and frequency of diagnostic tests per diagnosis-related group, and medication errors. Examples for outpatient facilities may include three of the following: mammography, diabetes, and colorectal screenings and routine physical examinations.

Checkpoint 14.1

1. *eHealth* is a term that encompasses telemedicine, telehealth, and mHealth.

2. a. Synchronous

   b. Asynchronous

   c. Remote patient monitoring (RPM)

   d. mHealth

3. *Synchronous* describes communication between individuals or groups that is conducted live, in real time. *Asynchronous* describes communication that is *not* accomplished in real time.

Checkpoint 14.2

1. Improve patient care and outcomes

2. Reimbursement for telehealth

3. In an effort to advance the growth and use of telehealth in rural areas, the federal government has made grants available.

Checkpoint 14.3

1. The advantages may vary but could include: low cost, private, secure, and safe. The disadvantages may vary but could include: difficulty in assembling, organizing, and updating; lack of established format and standard and complete entries to provide a complete picture of a patient's health status; accessibility in an emergency; and legibility or clarity.

2. The advantages may vary but could include: portable, password-protected but not connected to the internet (secure), and less susceptible to data loss if backed up. The disadvantages may vary but could include: inaccurate, lack of internet connectivity, and incompatibility with healthcare provider's computer systems.

3. a. Health insurer–provided

   b. Facility-provided

   c. Employer-provided

Checkpoint 14.4

1. Answers will vary but could include four of the following: medical record, health summary, test results, hospital admission, medications, allergies, immunizations, preventive care, medical history, current health issues, health trends, view my appointments, cancel my appointments, request my appointment, my family records, message center, get medical advice, request Rx refill, request a referral, billing and insurance, billing account summary, insurance summary, settings, or portable PHR.

2. Linking medical records is important because other providers and facilities may need access to health information such as medications, previous test results, previous procedures, hospital admissions, and any complications experienced. When a healthcare provider has access to a patient's health history, the delivery and quality of care improve.

Sample Paper Medical Record

A medical record, in any form, is the legal record of the care and treatment provided to a patient. In *Exploring Electronic Health Records*, Third Edition, you have read about and have experienced hands-on activities using the EHR. In these hands-on activities you accessed the EHR Navigator as many different healthcare professionals including a physician, nurse, IT administrator, admissions clerk, front desk clerk, health information management professional.

Now that you have experienced an EHR, consider a review of a sample paper medical record. Paper records are being phased out, however, you may still encounter a patient's historical information in paper form in the workplace. The average medical record is generally more than 200 pages long. The sample paper medical record included in this appendix is significantly smaller and is meant to provide you with exposure to the typical documents found in a paper medical record. The dates within this sample record reflect a time period when paper records were more common.

The paper medical record in this appendix includes:

- Facesheet
- Consent to Treat
- Informed Consent for Invasive, Diagnostic, Medical & Surgical Procedures
- Notice of Acknowledgment of Advance Directive
- Discharge Summary
- Consultation Report
- History and Physical
- Operative Report

- Physician's Orders
- Progress Notes
- Lab Results
- Radiology Report
- Nurse's Notes
- Physical Therapy Evaluation
- Speech Evaluation
- Patient Continuum of Care Transfer Form
- Medication Administration Record

The health care providers involved in the completion of this paper medical record include:

- Admission Clerk
- Attending Physician
- Consulting Physician
- Surgeon
- Laboratory Technician
- Radiologist
- Nurse

- Physical Therapist
- Speech Therapist

NORTHSTAR MEDICAL CENTER

NORTHSTAR
Medical Center

Facesheet

PATIENT INFORMATION

Patient's Last Name	First	Middle Initial	Type of Care:	☒ In Patient	☐ Same Day Surgery
Walker	Marjorie	R	☐ Maternity ☐ Outpatient	☐ Surgery	

Race	Marital Status	Religion	Primary Language	Date of Birth (mm/dd/yyyy)	Date of Scheduled Visit
Caucasian	M	Mormon	English	06/03/1956	

Physician's Last Name	First Name	☒ Female	Social Security No.
Chaplin	Patrick	☐ Male	000-00-0000

Patient's Street Address	Apt. No.	City	State	Zip
3370 Oakwood Ave		Cincinnati	OH	45203

Home Phone	Work Phone	Cell Phone	Visit Reason or Diagnosis	Admission Date
(513) 555-1632	(513) 555-1818	(513) 555-0823	Left Leg Wound	03/18/2012

Temporary Address	Apt. No.	City	State	Zip

Patient's Current Employer Name	Employer Address	City	State	Zip
Rapid Printing	6240 Parkland Drive	Cincinnati	OH	45201

Employer Phone	Patient's Occupation	Employment Status: ☐ Not Employed ☒ Full Time
(513) 555-1818	Pre-Press Operator	☐ Part Time ☐ Student ☐ Retired and Date:

Full Name of Emergency Contact	Relationship	Home Phone	Work Phone
Fulton Walker	Husband	(513) 555-1632	(513) 555-1471

Have you ever been a patient at Northstar Medical Center? ☒ Yes ☐ No	If yes, when was your last visit? 02/06/1980	Under what name? Buehler

Guarantor

Last Name	First	Middle Initial	Relationship	Date of Birth (mm/dd/yyyy)
Walker	Marjorie	R	Self	06/03/1956

Street Address	Apt. No.	☐ Female	Marital Status	Social Security No.
3370 Oakwood Ave		☐ Male	M	000-00-0000

City	State	Zip	Home Phone	Work Phone	Cell Phone
Cincinnati	OH	45203	(513) 555-1632	(513) 555-1818	(513) 555-0823

Employer Name	Employer Address	City	State	Zip
Rapid Printing	6240 Parkland Drive	Cincinnati	OH	45201

Employer Phone	Occupation	Employment Status: ☐ Not Employed ☒ Full Time
(513) 555-1818	Pre-Press Operator	☐ Part Time ☐ Student ☐ Retired and Date:

Insurance Information

Primary Insurance Name	Name of Insured exactly as appears on card
Cobalt Blue	Marjorie Ruth Walker

Insurance Billing Address	City	State	Zip	Phone No.
PO Box 690	Seattle	WA	98119	(800) 475-755X

Policy No.	Group No.	Plan Code	State	Effective Date	Expiration Date
189624733	9985	3	OH	01/01/2012	12/31/2012

Subscriber's Full Name	Subscriber's Soc. Sec. No.	Subscriber's Date of Birth	☒ Female
Marjorie Ruth Walker	000-00-0000	06/03/1956	☐ Male

Subscriber's Employer name (if self-employed, company name)	Relation to Insured	Subscriber's Employment Status: ☐ Not Employed
Rapid Printing	Self	☒ Full Time ☐ Part Time ☐ Student ☐ Retired and Date:

Subscriber's Employer Address	City	State	Zip	Phone No.
6240 Parkland Drive	Cincinnati	OH	45201	(513) 555-1818

Insurance Information

Medicare Number	Patient's name as appears on card	Effective Date (mm/dd/yyyy)	
		_____	□ Part A (Hospital Benefit)
		_____	□ Part B (Medical Benefit)

Medicaid Number	Patient's name as appears on card	Effective Date	State

Secondary Insurance Name NA		Name of Insured exactly as appears on card			

Insurance Billing Address		City	State	Zip	Phone No. ( )

Policy No. (for BCBS, include 3 letter prefix)	Group No.	Plan Code	State	Effective Date	Expiration Date

Subscriber's Full Name	Subscriber's Soc. Sec. No.	Subscriber's Date of Birth (mm/dd/yyyy)	□ Female □ Male

Subscriber's Employer name (if self-employed, company name)	Relation to Insured	Subscriber's Employment Status: □ Not Employed □ Full Time □ Part Time □ Student □ Retired and Date:

Subscriber's Employer Address	City	State	Zip	Phone No. ( )

Worker's Compensation

Is this visit the result of an accident? □ Yes □ No	□ Employment □ Automobile □ Other	Date of Accident: (mm/dd/yyyy)	Claim No.
Letter of Authorization □ Yes □ No	Claim Adjuster / Contact Name	Phone No. ( )	Insurance Name
Insurance Address	City	State	Zip	Phone No. ( )

Advance Directive

Do you have an Advance Directive, such as a Living Will or Durable Power of Attorney for Health Care?   ☒ Yes   □ No
Please specify the type: Living Will _____
*** *If yes, please bring a copy at the time of your admission****

Self-Pay

* If insured but your procedure is not covered or verified by your plan, a deposit is required at the time of admission.

* If you do not have insurance, please call our *Northstar Financial Services at 513-555-122X* before your scheduled arrival date to discuss financial arrangements.

Additional Information

Do you need special accommodations, such as Translation, Visual Aid, etc.?   □ Yes   □ No

*** If yes, please specify so that prior arrangements can be made for the day of your visit. ***

□ Language Interpreter _____   □ Sign Language Interpreter   □ Visual aid   □ Other: _____

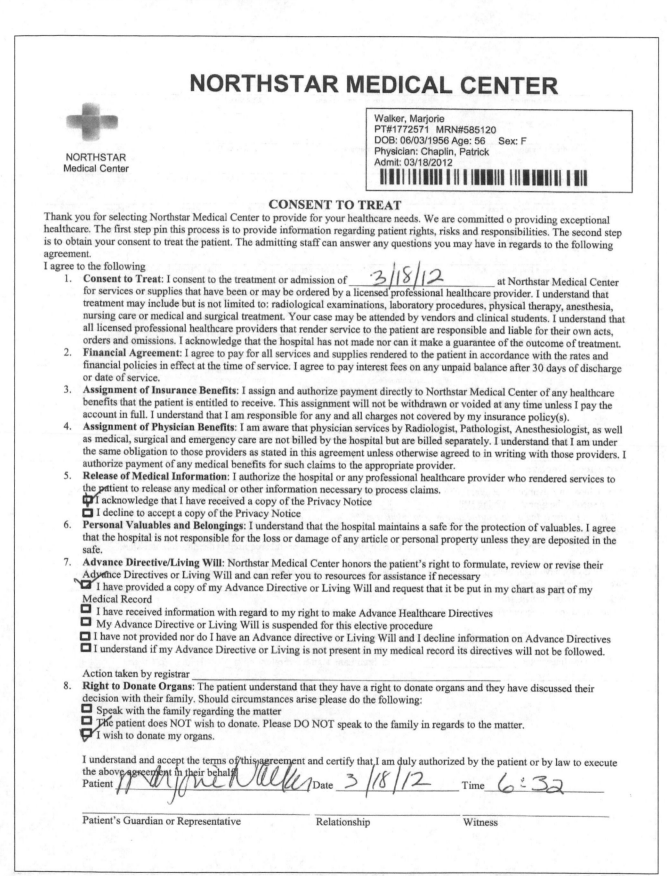

NORTHSTAR MEDICAL CENTER

NORTHSTAR
Medical Center

Walker, Marjorie
PT#1772571 MRN#585120
DOB: 06/03/1956 Age: 56   Sex: F
Physician: Chaplin, Patrick
Admit: 03/18/2012

CONSENT TO TREAT

Thank you for selecting Northstar Medical Center to provide for your healthcare needs. We are committed o providing exceptional healthcare. The first step pin this process is to provide information regarding patient rights, risks and responsibilities. The second step is to obtain your consent to treat the patient. The admitting staff can answer any questions you may have in regards to the following agreement.

I agree to the following

1. **Consent to Treat**: I consent to the treatment or admission of ___3/18/12___ at Northstar Medical Center for services or supplies that have been or may be ordered by a licensed professional healthcare provider. I understand that treatment may include but is not limited to: radiological examinations, laboratory procedures, physical therapy, anesthesia, nursing care or medical and surgical treatment. Your case may be attended by vendors and clinical students. I understand that all licensed professional healthcare providers that render service to the patient are responsible and liable for their own acts, orders and omissions. I acknowledge that the hospital has not made nor can it make a guarantee of the outcome of treatment.

2. **Financial Agreement**: I agree to pay for all services and supplies rendered to the patient in accordance with the rates and financial policies in effect at the time of service. I agree to pay interest fees on any unpaid balance after 30 days of discharge or date of service.

3. **Assignment of Insurance Benefits**: I assign and authorize payment directly to Northstar Medical Center of any healthcare benefits that the patient is entitled to receive. This assignment will not be withdrawn or voided at any time unless I pay the account in full. I understand that I am responsible for any and all charges not covered by my insurance policy(s).

4. **Assignment of Physician Benefits**: I am aware that physician services by Radiologist, Pathologist, Anesthesiologist, as well as medical, surgical and emergency care are not billed by the hospital but are billed separately. I understand that I am under the same obligation to those providers as stated in this agreement unless otherwise agreed to in writing with those providers. I authorize payment of any medical benefits for such claims to the appropriate provider.

5. **Release of Medical Information**: I authorize the hospital or any professional healthcare provider who rendered services to the patient to release any medical or other information necessary to process claims.
    ☑ I acknowledge that I have received a copy of the Privacy Notice
    ☐ I decline to accept a copy of the Privacy Notice

6. **Personal Valuables and Belongings**: I understand that the hospital maintains a safe for the protection of valuables. I agree that the hospital is not responsible for the loss or damage of any article or personal property unless they are deposited in the safe.

7. **Advance Directive/Living Will**: Northstar Medical Center honors the patient's right to formulate, review or revise their Advance Directives or Living Will and can refer you to resources for assistance if necessary
    ☑ I have provided a copy of my Advance Directive or Living Will and request that it be put in my chart as part of my Medical Record
    ☐ I have received information with regard to my right to make Advance Healthcare Directives
    ☐ My Advance Directive or Living Will is suspended for this elective procedure
    ☐ I have not provided nor do I have an Advance directive or Living Will and I decline information on Advance Directives
    ☐ I understand if my Advance Directive or Living is not present in my medical record its directives will not be followed.

    Action taken by registrar _____

8. **Right to Donate Organs**: The patient understand that they have a right to donate organs and they have discussed their decision with their family. Should circumstances arise please do the following:
    ☐ Speak with the family regarding the matter
    ☐ The patient does NOT wish to donate. Please DO NOT speak to the family in regards to the matter.
    ☑ I wish to donate my organs.

I understand and accept the terms of this agreement and certify that I am duly authorized by the patient or by law to execute the above agreement in their behalf

Patient _Marjorie Walker_ Date _3/18/12_ Time _6:32_

_____   _____   _____
Patient's Guardian or Representative   Relationship   Witness

Northstar Medical Center

Informed Consent for Invasive, Diagnostic, Medical & Surgical Procedures

Patient Name ___Walker, Marjorie___

Date of Birth ___6/3/56___

Medical Record # ___585120___

I hereby authorize ___Dr. Stillwater___ and/or ___—___ and/or such assistants and associates as may be selected by him/her/they to perform the following procedure(s)/treatment(s) upon myself/the patient

Procedure(s)/Treatment(s) ___Excisional debridement, Lft leg___

The procedure has been explained to me and I have been told the reasons why I need the procedure. The risks of the procedure have also been explained to me. In addition, I have been told that the procedure may not have the result that I expect. I have also been told about other possible treatments for my condition and what might happen if no treatment is received.

I understand that in addition to the risks describe to me and about this procedure there are risks that may occur with any surgical or medical procedure. I am aware that the practice of medicine and surgery is not an exact science, and that I have not been given any guarantees about the results of this procedure.

I have had enough time to discuss my condition and treatment with my health care providers and all of my questions have been answered to my satisfaction. I believe I have enough information to make an informed decision and I agree to have the procedure. If something unexpected happens and I need additional or different treatment(s) from the treatment I expect, I agree to accept any treatment which is necessary.

I agree to have transfusion of blood and other blood products that may be necessary along with the procedure I am having. The risks, benefits and alternatives have been explained to me and all of my questions have been answered to my satisfaction. If I refuse to have transfusions I will cross out and initial this section and sign a Refusal of Treatment form.

I agree to allow this facility to keep, use or properly dispose of, tissue, and parts of organs that are removed during this procedure.

___Marjorie Walker___   ___3/18/12___

Signature of Patient or Parent/Legal Guardian of Minor Patient   Date

---

If the patient cannot consent for him/herself, the signature of either the health care agent or legal guardian who is acting on behalf of the patient, or the patient's next of kin who is asserting to the treatment for the patient, must be obtained.

_____   _____

Signature of Patient or Parent/Legal Guardian of Minor Patient   Date

_____   _____

Signature and Relationship of Next of Kin   Date

Witness:

I, _____, am a facility employee who is not the patient's physician or authorized health care provider named above and I have witnessed the patient or other appropriate person voluntarily sign this form

_____

Signature and Title of Witness

NORTHSTAR MEDICAL CENTER

NORTHSTAR
Medical Center

Walker, Marjorie
PT#1772571   MRN#585120
DOB: 06/03/1956   Age: 56   Sex: F
Physician: Chaplin, Patrick
Admit: 03/18/2012

NOTICE OF ACKNOWLEDGEMENT ADVANCE DIRECTIVE

PATIENT NAME: _Walker, Marjorie_   DOB: _6/3/56_

An Advance Directive is a legal document allowing a person to give directions about future medical care or to designate another person(s) to make medical decisions if he or she should lose decision making capacity. Advance Directives are the following written instruments: The Living Will and The Durable Power of Attorney for Heath Care. The instrument may be revoked and a notation of the date and time must be made to the patient's medical record.

Do you have an Advance Directive?

A. Directive to Physicians (Living Will)   Yes __✓__ No _____

B. Durable Power of Attorney for Health Care   Yes __✓__ No _____

Is it up to Date?   Yes __✓__   No _____

Where is a copy
located?   _With me_

Principal Agent: _Fulton Walker_

Address: _3370 Oakwood_

Phone #:   _513-555-1632_

Alternate Agent: _Anne Walker_

Address: _1530 Eastland_

Phone #:   _513-555-4445_

Marjorie Walker   _3/18/12_
Signature of Patient or Representative   Date

NORTHSTAR MEDICAL CENTER

NORTHSTAR

Medical Center

Walker, Marjorie
PT#1772571   MRN#585120
DOB: 06/03/1956 Age: 56   Sex: F
Physician: Chaplin, Patrick
Admit: 03/18/2012

Discharge Summary

Date of Discharge: 3/27/2012

Discharge Diagnosis:

1. Left leg wound, S/P MVA, left shin degloving injury
2. Anxiety
3. Hematoma, right thigh
4. Paroxysmal atrial fibrillation

History of Present Illness: This is a 56-year-old white female who on 2/23/12 was involved in a motor vehicle accident when she was driving from Florida to Cincinnati. She was admitted to a Chattanooga, Tennessee hospital and she had suffered multiple rib fractures and also suffered a left nondisplaced fibular fracture and an avulsion and degloving injury on the left shin. She also had possible suprapubic ramus fracture and a fracture of the sternum and a slight laceration of the liver and spleen and she was transfused 19 units of packed red blood cells for acute blood loss anemia. The patient was on Coumadin at the time for atrial fibrillation and she had to be reversed. She also went into a-fib with rapid rate needing Cardizem to reverse it.

She was then transferred to Northstar Medical Center and was pretty stable at the time. She had a lot of pain and then she was seen by Orthopedics for that left tib fib fracture and they said she was okay for weight-bearing and she was see by wound care, physical therapy and occupational therapy. The patient stayed in sinus rhythm throughout. She was maintained on Coumadin and her hemoglobin stayed in the 9 and 10 range and she had later complained of a lot of pain in the right leg and a Doppler had shown some small hematomas, however, the pain and hematomas resolved on their own.

The large wound on her left shin was treated by Dr. Stillwater, Plastic Surgeon. She underwent several debridements of this area and will later likely undergo a skin graft after the wound has healed more.

On the day of discharge, 31 minutes was spent on discharge planning and all medications were discussed with her in detail. Patient is discharged to home with home health care.

Dictated by: Patrick Chaplin, MD

NG
D: 3/27/12 1535
T: 03/28/2012 1124

NORTHSTAR MEDICAL CENTER

NORTHSTAR

Medical Center

Walker, Marjorie
PT#1772571   MRN#585120
DOB: 06/03/1956   Age: 56   Sex: F
Physician: Chaplin, Patrick
Admit: 03/18/2012

CONSULTATION REPORT
PLASTICS AND RECONSTRUCTIVE SURGERY

CHIEF COMPLAINT: Left leg wound

HISTORY OF PRESENT ILLNESS: This is a 56-year-old white female who on 2/23/12 was involved in a motor vehicle accident when she was driving from Florida to Cincinnati. She was admitted to a Chattanooga, Tennessee hospital and she had suffered multiple rib fractures and also suffered a left nondisplaced fibular fracture and an avulsion and degloving injury on the left shin. She also had possible suprapubic ramus fracture and a fracture of the sternum and a slight laceration of the liver and spleen and she was transfused 19 units of packed red blood cells for acute blood loss anemia. The patient was on Coumadin at the time for atrial fibrillation and she had to be reversed. She also went into a-fib with rapid rate needing Cardizem to reverse it.

PAST MEDICAL/SURGICAL HISTORY:
Significant for:
1. Hypertension
2. Rheumatoid arthritis
3. Depression
4. Osteopenia
5. Hyperlipidemia
6. History of perforated diverticulum, for which she required surgery and had a colostomy, and it was reversed.
7. History of hysterectomy
8. Hypothyroidism
9. Bilateral knee replacements
10. The patient does not report that she has congestive heart failure.
11. She does report that she had an angiogram for evaluation of atrial fibrillation, and she does not have any coronary artery disease.

ALLERGIES:
None

MEDICATIONS:
Prior to this accident included:
1. Methotrexate.
2. Misoprostol
3. Remicade
4. Methimazole

CURRENT MEDICATIONS:
That she was on when transferred from a Chattanooga, Tennessee hospital are as follows:
1. Keflex 500 mg every 8 hours for 5 days
2. Ipratropium as needed
3. Coumadin per pharmacy protocol
4. Lovenox 110 mg subcutaneously every twelve hours, to discontinue when INR is more than 2
5. Atenolol 50 mg every 12 hours
6. Vicodin 5/325 mg every four hours as needed for pain.
7. Paxil 20 mg daily

FAMILY HISTORY:
Positive for father dying of leukocytosis at age of 54. Mother had myocardial infarction at the age of 67. Sister has Parkinson disease and another sister died of colon cancer.

PHYSICAL EXAMINATION:

GENERAL:
She is awake, alert and oriented, in no acute distress.

VITAL SIGNS:
Stable. Her blood pressure this morning is 126/64, temperature 98.6, pulse 72.

HEAD, EYES, EARS, NOSE AND THROAT:
Shows pupils equal, round, and reactive to light and accommodation.   Mucous membranes are moist.

NECK:
Shows no thyromegaly.

LUNGS:
Clear to auscultation.

HEART:
Regular rate and rhythm, a few missed beats.

ABDOMEN:
Shows no organomegaly.

EXTREMITIES:
Dorsalis pedis pulses bilaterally are 2+. There is a vacuum-assisted closure on the left upper skin extending to the knee. Large left lower leg wound with fairly well vascularized red granulation tissue in the bulk of the wound. There is a deep cavity on the medial aspect in the area of the recently evacuated hematoma. There are sutures in place which the patient was unaware and fibrin covering necrotic tissue on the lateral aspect of the wound space. There is no purulent discharge or evidence of infection. Remainder of the left lower extremity shows no other clinically significant lesions.

LABORATORY DATA:
From 3/17/12, her albumin was 2.4, total protein was 5.2. Her CBC from 3/16/12 shows a white cell count of 9.6, hemoglogin 9.7, platelets 252,000. INR was 1.4.

ASSESSMENT AND PLAN:
The patient needs protein repletion. She will ultimately need the sutures removed and the fibrinous exudate debrided from the lateral aspect of the wound. Would recommend resuming negative pressure wound therapy including packing, black GranuFoam dressing into the current hematoma cavity. The patient will ultimately require skin graft reconstruction.

It is always a pleasure seeing and treating your patients. We look forward to seeing and treating other patients in the future.

Dictated by Frank Stillwater, MD

KR
D: 03/20/12 1904
T: 03/20/12 23:50

NORTHSTAR MEDICAL CENTER

NORTHSTAR

Medical Center

Walker, Marjorie
PT#1772571   MRN#585120
DOB: 06/03/1956 Age: 56   Sex: F
Physician: Chaplin, Patrick
Admit: 03/18/2012

HISTORY AND PHYSICAL

HISTORY OF PRESENT ILLNESS:

History of Present Illness: This is a 56-year-old white female who on 2/23/12 was involved in a motor vehicle accident when she was driving from Florida to Cincinnati. She was admitted to a Chattanooga, Tennessee hospital and she had suffered multiple rib fractures and also suffered a left nondisplaced fibular fracture and an avulsion and degloving injury on the left shin. She also had possible suprapubic ramus fracture and a fracture of the sternum and a slight laceration of the liver and spleen and she was transfused 19 units of packed red blood cells for acute blood loss anemia. The patient was on Coumadin at the time for atrial fibrillation and she had to be reversed. She also went into a-fib with rapid rate needing Cardizem to reverse it.

She has been transferred to Northstar Medical Center and is stable at this time. Dr. Stillwater from Plastics will be consulted to address her wound on her left shin. PT, OT and Wound Care will be ordered. We will monitor her atrial fibrillation and labs for anemia.

PAST MEDICAL/SURGICAL HISTORY:

Significant for:

1. Hypertension
2. Rheumatoid arthritis
3. Depression
4. Osteopenia
5. Hyperlipidemia
6. History of perforated diverticulum, for which she required surgery and had a colostomy, and it was reversed.
7. History of hysterectomy
8. Hypothyroidism
9. Bilateral knee replacements
10. The patient does not report that she has congestive heart failure.
11. She does report that she had an angiogram for evaluation of atrial fibrillation, and she does not have any coronary artery disease.

ALLERGIES:

None

MEDICATIONS:

Prior to this accident included:

1. Methotrexate.
2. Misoprostol
3. Remicade
4. Methimazole

CURRENT MEDICATIONS:

That she was on when transferred from a Chattanooga, Tennessee hospital are as follows:

1. Keflex 500 mg every 8 hours for 5 days
2. Ipratropium as needed
3. Coumadin per pharmacy protocol
4. Lovenox 110 mg subcutaneously every twelve hours, to discontinue when INR is more than 2
5. Atenolol 50 mg every 12 hours
6. Vicodin 5/325 mg every four hours as needed for pain.
7. Paxil 20 mg daily

FAMILY HISTORY:

Positive for father dying of leukocytosis at age of 54. Mother had myocardial infarction at the age of 67. Sister has Parkinson disease and another sister died of colon cancer.

PHYSICAL EXAMINATION:

GENERAL:
She is awake, alert and oriented, in no acute distress.

VITAL SIGNS:
Stable. Her blood pressure this morning is 126/64, temperature 98.6, pulse 72.

HEAD, EYES, EARS, NOSE AND THROAT:
Sclerae are anicteric. Mucous membranes are moist.

NECK:
There is no carotid bruit.

LUNGS:
Clear to auscultation.

HEART:
Regular rate and rhythm, a few missed beats.

ABDOMEN:
Soft, nontender.

EXTREMITIES:
Dorsalis pedis pulses bilaterally are 2+. There is a vacuum-assisted closure on the left upper skin extending to the knee.

LABORATORY DATA:
From 3/17/12, her albumin was 2.4, total protein was 5.2. Her CBC from 3/16/12 shows a white cell count of 9.6, hemoglogin 9.7, platelets 252,000. INR was 1.4.

ASSESSMENT AND PLAN:
1. Status post MVA with multiple injuries. Pain control is an issue. Patient will be scheduled for PT and OT Therapy
2. Avulsion/degloving injury of the left shin with large wound. Plastic surgery will be consulted.
3. History of paroxysmal atrial fibrillation. Will follow and monitor.

_____
Patrick Chaplin, MD

KK
Dictated: 3/18/12 14:45
Trans: 3/18/12 18:30

NORTHSTAR MEDICAL CENTER

NORTHSTAR

Medical Center

Walker, Marjorie
PT#1772571   MRN#585120
DOB: 06/03/1956   Age: 56   Sex: F
Physician: Chaplin, Patrick
Admit: 03/18/2012

OPERATIVE REPORT

DATE OF OPERATION: 03/23/12

PREOPERATIVE DIAGNOSIS: Left leg wound

POSTOPERATIVE DIAGNOSIS: Left leg wound

PROCEDURE PERFORMED: Excision, necrotic tissue, left leg wound, 3.0 cm in length. Application of a Kerlix stack and less than 50 sq. cm negative pressure wound therapy dressing.

SURGEON: Frank Stillwater, MD

ASSISTANT: Karen Tweedle, MD

OPERATIVE PROCEDURE: The patient was properly prepped and draped under local sedation. A 0.25% Marcaine was injected circumferentially around the necrotic wound. A wide excision and debridement of the necrotic tissue taken down to the presacral fascia and all necrotic tissue was electrocauterized and removed. All bleeding was cauterized with electrocautery and then a Kerlix stack was then placed and a pressure dressing applied. The patient was sent to recovery in satisfactory condition.

Dictated by Frank Stillwater, MD

GR
D: 3/23/12 11:14
T: 3/23/12 15:10

NORTHSTAR MEDICAL CENTER

NORTHSTAR
Medical Center

Walker, Marjorie
PT#1772571 MRN#585120
DOB: 06/03/1956 Age: 56 Sex: F
Physician: Chaplin, Patrick
Admit: 03/18/2012

PHYSICIAN"S ORDERS

Date/Time		Nurse's Initials
3/18/12 930AM	CBC, BMP in am PT/INR c̄ a.m. labs *Patrick Chaplin MD*	
3/19/12 8AM	U/A, c+s today *Patrick Chaplin MD*	
3/19/12 9AM	D/C oxycontin Vicodin 5/500mg ī po q̄ 4-6° prn pain. *Patrick Chaplin MD*	

NORTHSTAR MEDICAL CENTER

NORTHSTAR
Medical Center

Walker, Marjorie
PT#1772571   MRN#585120
DOB: 06/03/1956   Age: 56 Sex: F
Physician: Chaplin, Patrick
Admit: 03/18/2012

Date/Time	Progress Notes
3/18/12 9:15 AM	FP / Feels better today less N/V. Appetite better. Up to hallway c̄ assistance.

VSS AF
Lys - CTAB
heart - reg rate no murm.
Abd - soft NT NABS
Ext - ø c/c/e
   wound vac in place ⊖ log.

labs pending

A/P - ① wound left leg
       consult surgery
     ② PAF
       coumadin / PT protocol
     ③ High protein diet

               Ann Turnell MD |

NORTHSTAR MEDICAL CENTER

NORTHSTAR

Medical Center

Walker, Marjorie	
PT#1772571	MRN#585120
DOB: 06/03/1956 Age: 56	Sex: F
Physician: Chaplin, Patrick	
Admit: 03/18/2012	

*******************************COMPLETE BLOOD COUNT***

TEST:	WBC	WBC	HGB	HBG	HCT	HCT	PLATELET	PLT	RBC
UNITS:	THOU/mcL	THOU/mcL	g/dl	g/dl	%	%	THOU/mcL	THOU/mcL	THOU/mcL
REF RANGE:	3.9-10.5	3.6-10.5	12.0-15.5	12.0-15.2	36-47	36-46	140-375	140-375	3.80-5.20

Date / Time	WBC	WBC	HGB	HBG	HCT	HCT	PLATELET	PLT	RBC
03/25/2012 0530		6.0 CBCR [NS]		9.7L [NS]		29L [NS]	302 [NS]		
03/24/2012 1115		7.4 CBCR [NS]		9.9L [NS]		30L [NS]	323 [NS}		
03/23/2012		7.8 CBCR [NS}		10.1L [NS]		30L [NS]	311 [NS]		
03/22/2012		7.1 [NS]		8.4L [NS]		27L [NS]		**331** [NS]	
03/21/2012	9.4 [NS]		**9.8L** [NS]		31L [NS]		370 [NS]		3.32L [NS]
03/20/2012	7.9 [NS]		**10.0L** [NS]		32L [NS]		**397H** [NS]		3.32L [NS]

---FOOTNOTES---
[NS]   Tested at Northstar Medical Center

End of Report

NORTHSTAR MEDICAL CENTER

NORTHSTAR

Medical Center

Walker, Marjorie
PT#1772571   MRN#585120
DOB: 06/03/1956   Age: 56   Sex: F
Physician: Chaplin, Patrick
Admit: 03/18/2012

*****************************COAGULATION***

TEST:	PROTIME	INR
UNITS:	Seconds	
REF RANGE:	9.0-11.4	0.8-1.2

03/18/2012

+ 0615   16.9 H 1.6   H
              [NS]   (a)
                      (b)
                      (c)
                      [NS]

---FOOTNOTES---
(a)   INR Therapeutic Ranges:
(b)   Routine Anticoagulation: 2.0 to 3.0
(c)   Aggressive Anticoagulation: 2.5 to 3.5
[NS]   Tested at Northstar Medical Center

End of Report

NORTHSTAR MEDICAL CENTER

NORTHSTAR

Medical Center

Walker, Marjorie	
PT#1772571 MRN#585120	
DOB: 06/03/1956 Age: 56 Sex: F	
Physician: Chaplin, Patrick	
Admit: 03/18/2012	

Ordered by: Patrick Chaplin, MD
*All clinical times shown on this page are in
Knee 2 Views – Right 32017251
Site: Northstar Medical Center Radiology
Rad# X081134773
Unit# M000048880
Location: NSMC14CD
Account#: V10307G7G32B
Req#11-4104931
Order# RAD20120318-0349
Primary Insurance:
Procedure: Knee 2 views – Right 32017251
Admitting Diagnosis: Left Lower Extremity Wound
Reason for exam: Change in Status
Impression
Impression/Conclusion below

Report
Two Views Right Knee 3/20/12

Indication: Motor Vehicle Accident

Comparison: None

Findings: Right total knee arthroplasty is in place. The lateral view was somewhat oblique. No large joint effusion or fracture. There is mild soft tissue swelling

Impression:

No evidence of fracture or gross complication with right total knee arthroplasty in place

Dictated by: Michael Zuckerman MD
Signed by: Michael Zuckerman MD 3/21/2012

End of Report

NORTHSTAR MEDICAL CENTER

NORTHSTAR
Medical Center

Walker, Marjorie
PT#1772571   MRN#585120
DOB: 06/03/1956   Age: 56 Sex: F
Physician: Chaplin, Patrick
Admit: 03/18/2012

Nurse's Notes (Include observations, medications, and treatment when indicated.)

Date/Time	
3/19/12 0816	Assessment complete as noted, sitting up in bed, IVPB infusing s̄ difficulty, dsg dry and intact, foley draining clear yellow urine, denies pain or SOB @ this time will continue to monitor wound care — B. Cullars, RN —
3/19/12 1930	pt resting in bed. A+O X3 VSS LSCTA per nurse assess. Foley draining clear yellow urine. Denies any further issues @ this time. SOB noted previously currently subsided. will cont to monitor. Call light in reach ——— J. Kennedy, RN
3/20/12 0730	VSS. Denies any pain or discomfort at this time. Assessment completed per flow sheet - no changes noted from previous shift. Able to make needs known. Call light in reach. Will monitor ——— J. Smedler, RN

NORTHSTAR MEDICAL CENTER

NORTHSTAR
Medical Center

Walker, Marjorie
PT#1772571   MRN#585120
DOB: 06/03/1956   Age: 56 Sex: F
Physician: Chaplin, Patrick
Admit: 03/18/2012

Nurse's Notes (include observations, medications, and treatment when indicated.)

Date/Time	
3/18/2012 @ 1300	Received pt via ACLS transport. Pt transferred from stretcher to bed. Pt did not bring any personal belongings. Admission assessment completed. VSS & WNL. Dr. Chaplin notified of pt's arrival - orders received. Pt informed of POC & instructed on safety. To include use of call light & bed side controls. Will continue to Monitor S. Schmidt RN.
3/18/2012 2015	Assessment complete & charted. Pt is A+O x4, lungs CTA, +BS x4, no noted edema, heart sounds regular in rhythm. Pt has #20 @ FA dated 3/17 c̄ a dsg that is CD&I. VSS & hardly unchanged from admit. Pt has no needs or questions at this time & denies any pain. Call light left within reach, will continue to monitor. ———————————— S. Salathn RN

NORTHSTAR MEDICAL CENTER

NORTHSTAR
Medical Center

Walker, Marjorie
PT#1772571 MRN#585120
DOB: 06/03/1956 Age: 56 Sex: F
Physician: Chaplin, Patrick
Admit: 03/18/2012

Physical Therapy Ankle Evaluation

DX (L) leg wound, s/p mva, wound care   Date 3/19/12

PMH Rib fx, fibular fx, degloving injury (L) shin, sternum fx, anemia, anxiety, paroxysmal A Fib,

Physician Patrick Chaplin   Onset 2/23/12

Initial Evaluation X   Re-Evaluation_____   Pain Rating_____   Funct. Rating_____   Involved: R L

SUBJECTIVE: Pain with X squatting X walking_____ sitting NA running NA stairs
Pt reports 5/10 (L) leg pain. Pt reports ↑ pain 7/10 c̄ amb c̄ RW c̄ squatting. Pt states she lives c̄ husband + receives his help to get in + out of care. Currently able to live on 1st floor. Reports she is unable to climb 10 steps c̄ 1HR upstairs to her bedroom. Currently has transport w/c, RW, cane (spc.)

Occupation/Social Hx: Pt is a 3rd grade math teacher

Work Duties: standing, walking, bending, squatting, sitting on floor,

Pt. Goals: Pt reports she would like to amb ↑↓ 10 steps 1HR to bedroom, + be able to squat down to floor for return to work

OBJECTIVE:
Gait: _____antalgic Trendelenburg R L _____Crutches X Walker_____Cane_____No AD ☐
_____FWB_____PWB_____TTWB_____NWB X WBAT
Other_____

Observation: (In Standing) (WNL) R L
Knee: _____
Effusion: **R** none ☒ min ☐ mod ☐ severe ☐   **L** none ☒ min ☐ mod ☐ severe ☐
Foot: Pes Cavus R L   Pes Planus (R) (L)   Hallux Valgus R L

Other_____

ROM/ Strength:

	Active			Passive			Strength	
	R	L		R	L		R	L
DF.	4/5 P	3+/5 P		WFL P	WFL P		_____ P	P
PF	4/5 P	4/5 P		P	P		_____ P	P
INV	NT P	NT P		P	P		_____ P	P
EV	P	P		P	P		_____ P	P
1st MTP Ext	P	P		P	P		_____ P	P
				P	P			

Girth Measurements: (From mid-patella)   WNL   ~~Bruising~~   Temp. (WNL) Warm
(L) leg
(B) thigh

	R	L
Around Malleoli	NT	NT
Figure 8		

Palpation: R thigh tenderness anterior L anterior shin tenderness

Resting BP: 124 / 76   **Resting HR:** 71

Name: Marjorie, Walker   **DOB:** 6/3/56

Flexibility: (NT= normal, T= tight, VT= very tight): very tight BLE hamstring

Special Tests: (+ or —)

	R	L		R	L
Anterior Drawer	NT	NT	Eversion Stress Test	NT	NT
Spring Test	+	+	Inversion Stress Test	+	+

Unilateral Stance Time: R __3__ Sec. L __0__ Sec.

Unilat. Heel

Raise X 5:	R WNL ☐	painful ☐	weakness/↓ control ☒	Unable to perform ☐
	L WNL ☐	painful ☒	weakness/↓ control ☐	Unable to perform ☒
6" step test:	R WNL ☐	painful ☐	weakness/↓ control ☐	Unable to perform ☒
	L WNL ☐	painful ☐	weakness/↓ control ☐	Unable to perform ☒
Single leg squat.	R WNL ☐	painful ☐	weakness/↓ control ☐	Unable to perform ☒
	L WNL ☐	painful ☐	weakness/↓ control ☐	Unable to perform ☒

Treatment: Pt perf BLE therex SLR, ABD/ADD, heel slide 2×15. amb 100' x2 c̄ RW ↓ stance time LLE. Pt amb ↑↓ 1 6" step BHR RLE lead c̄ minA.

ASSESSMENT: _____ See Initial Eval Summary/ Plan of Care
Pt demos ↓ BLE strength, ↓ balance ↓ safety awareness. Pt demos ↓ (I) c̄ amb ↓ step length RLE, ↓ stance time LLE, forward head & shoulders. Pt reports ↑ pain c̄ squatting & walking. Pt will benefit from skilled PT to ↓ pain ↑ ability to squat to floor (I) ↑ amb ↑↓ 10 steps IHR to bedroom.

Rehabilitation Potential: (Excellent) Good Fair Poor

STG/LTG: X See Initial Eval Summary/ Plan of Care

PLAN: (Circle)   # Rx/ wk_____ ~ # wks_____

☒ Strengthening ☒ Stretching   ☐ Joint Mobs   ☒ Moist Heat/ Cold Pack
☐ Bracing/ Taping ☐ Ultrasound   ☐ EStim   ☐ PROM   ☒ Gait Training
☒ Other: ___neuro re-ed___

Avg. Pain Rating 6/10   **Self Reported Functional Rating** _____   **Foot Function Index:** _____

Therapist Signature: Josie Thomas PT   **Date:** 3/19/12 **Time:** 4:05pm
Allim Summerly PT

2

NORTHSTAR MEDICAL CENTER

NORTHSTAR
Medical Center

Walker, Marjorie
PT#1772571   MRN#585120
DOB: 06/03/1956   Age: 56   Sex: F
Physician: Chaplin, Patrick
Admit: 03/18/2012

SPEECH EVALUATION FORM

Nature of the communication problem: <u>Speech consulted 2° "slurred speech"</u>
<u>per RN report</u>

Speech/language therapy in the past?   YES___   NO _✓_

Where? <u>N/A</u>   For what reason? <u>N/A</u>

Brief description of problem:
<u>Pt initially admitted to OSH 3-9-12 following MVA, transferred to Northstar</u>
<u>Medical Center for continued wound care, nutritional support and therapy</u>

Any pain associated with this problem? YES___ NO _✓_
Description:
<u>Pt denies pain.</u>

Was this onset gradual or sudden? Describe:
<u>Sudden, following brain trauma sustained in MVA</u>

Mental Status (check all that apply):
       _✓_ alert
       _✓_ responsive
       _✓_ cooperative
       _✓_ confused
       ____ lethargic
       _✓_ impulsive
       ____ uncooperative
       ____ combative
       ____ unresponsive

Oral Motor, Respiration, and Phonation
Lips
       WNL, mild, mode severe impairment
       Observation at rest (WNL, Edema, Erythema, Lesion): <u>Ⓡ - droop, drooling</u>
       Symmetry, range, speed, strength, tone:
              Pucker   <u>reduced</u>
              Retraction   <u>reduced</u>
              Alternating pucker/retraction   <u>reduced speed/coordination</u>

Involuntary movement (e.g., chorea, dystonia, fasciculation, myoclonus, spasms, tremor):

not observed

Tongue
WNL, mild, (mode) severe impairment
Observation at rest (WNL, Edema, Erythema, Lesion): lingual fasciculations
Symmetry, range, speed, strength, tone:
    Protrusion   reduced range + strength
    Retraction   reduced strength
    Lateralization   reduced range + speed
Involuntary movement   as noted above

Jaw
WNL, (mild), mode severe impairment
Observation at rest: rests in slightly open position
    Symmetry, range, speed, strength, tone:
    Opening   reduced oral aperture
    Closing   reduced strength
    Lateralization   reduced ROM
    Protrusion   NT
    Retraction   NT
Involuntary movement   not observed

Soft Palate
WNL, mild, (mode) severe impairment
Observation at rest (WNL, Edema, Erythema, Lesion): WNL
Symmetry, range, speed, strength, tone: ↓ speed, ∅ asymmetry
Elevation   reduced upon phonation
Sustained elevation   reduced upon phonation
Alternating elevation/relaxation   reduced range + speed
Involuntary movement   not present

Respiration/Phonation
Observations/formal measures administered: _____

Activity	Stimulus	Quality	Duration	Loudness	Steadiness
Phonation		WNL ~~Breathy~~ (circled) Hoarse Harsh Strained-Strangled	2 secs WNL Mildly impaired Moderately impaired Severely impaired (circled)	WNL Monoloudness (circled) Excessive loudness Variable loudness	
Oral reading		WNL Breathy (circled) Hoarse Harsh Strained-Strangled	WNL Mildly impaired Moderately impaired Severely impaired (circled)	WNL Monoloudness (circled) Excessive loudness Variable loudness	
Conversation		WNL Breathy (circled) Hoarse Harsh Strained-Strangled	WNL Mildly impaired Moderately impaired Severely impaired (circled)	WNL Monoloudness (circled) Excessive loudness Variable loudness	

Findings
_____Motor speech within normal limits
_____(Mild, mild-moderate, moderate, moderate-severe, severe)apraxia characterized by:

_____
__✓__(Mild, mild-moderate, moderate, moderate-severe, severe) dysarthria characterized by:
    moderate dysarthria 2° breathy vocal quality (suspect vocal
cord involvement), reduced strength + range of motion for oral
Recommendations: (check all that apply) structures, and hypernasality during
    all speech tasks.
        __✓__ Speech-language pathology treatment
            Frequency: 3-5 x/week Duration: 4 weeks
        _____ Augmentative-Alternative Communication or Speech Generating Device evaluation
        _____ Other suggested referrals:
            _____Neurology
            __✓__Otolaryngology
            _____Pulmonology
            _____Other

            X Allison Bing MA.CCC-SLP

NORTHSTAR MEDICAL CENTER

Patient Continuum of Care Transfer Form

Walker, Marjorie
PT#1772571   MRN#585120
DOB: 06/03/1956   Age: 56   Sex: F
Physician: Chaplin, Patrick
Admit: 03/18/2012

Patient Last Name: Walker	Patient First Name: Marjorie
Transfer to: Spring Care	Attending Physician: Chaplin
Reason for Transfer: Wound Care	DATE/TIME: 3/18/12 650

☐ Attempted Treatment in SNF unsuccessful?

☒ Please list ALLERGIES (meds, dyes, food): Latex, Demerol

☐ NKA

Relative / Guardian Notified: Yes ☒ No ☐ Phone Number:

Name of Relative Notified: Jennifer DeCapua

Transfer Ambulance: Life Care

ATTACHMENTS (Please check)
- ☒ Face Sheet
- ☒ History & Physical
- ☐ Discharge Summary
- ☒ MAR
- ☐ Wound Assessment & Tx Sheet
- ☒ Labs
- ☐ Code Status
- ☐ MD Orders
- ☒ X-rays
- ☐ MD Progress Notes
- ☐ Nurse's Notes (last 5 days)
- ☐ Other:
- ☐ Other:

VITAL SIGNS TAKEN Yes ☒ No ☐   Time Taken: 1230 AM ☐ PM ☒

Respirations: 24	Blood glucose: 118 Time: 1210
O2 Sat: 96%	VRE: Yes ☐ No ☒ Hx of ☐
Pulse: 84	MRSA: Yes ☐ No ☒ Hx of ☐
BP: 118/82	C. Diff: Yes ☐ No ☒ Hx of ☐
Temp: 99.2 (A)	ANY pending cultures? Yes ☐ No ☒
Height: 5' 10"	If Yes, what?
Weight: 163 Lbs ☒ Kg ☐	MDRO?

ISOLATION PRECAUTIONS? Yes ☐ No ☒   **TYPE:** Contact ☐ Droplet ☐ Airborne ☐ Other: ☐

VACCINATION HISTORY	SKIN OR PRESSURE ULCER CONCERNS
Pneumococcal Vaccine: Yes ☒ DATE: 3-16-12 Refused ☐	HIGH risk for skin breakdown **PLEASE TURN** Yes ☐ No ☐
Flu Vaccine: Yes ☒ DATE: 11-7-10 Refused ☐	Current Skin Breakdown: Yes ☐ No ☐
Tetanus: Yes ☐ DATE: Refused ☐	Most Recent Treatment Time: AM ☐ PM ☐
TB Skin Test: Negative ☐ Positive ☐ DATE:	Please Treat at (time): AM ☐ PM ☐
OR Chest X-ray ☒ Result Date: /	Treat with (product name): Dakins Solution orig B LE
Comments:	To (what area): (B) LE

MEDICATION INFORMATION	SAFETY CONCERNS	
See Attached Medication Reconciliation	History of Falls Yes ☐ No ☒	Risk for Falls Yes ☐ No ☒
Prefers meds with: Applesauce	Behavior Issues Yes ☐ No ☒	Explain:
Pain Meds in past 24 hours Yes ☒ No ☐	RESTRAINT Use: Yes ☐ No ☒	
Level on **Pain Scale** at time of transfer : (Please circle level) 1 2 3 (4) 5 6 7 8 9 10	Type of Restraint Used:	
	When Used:	

DIET & FEEDING	ELIMINATION	
Current Diet: Diabetic 2000 kcal ADA	Bladder Incontinence ☐	DATE of UTI (within 14 days):
Needs Assistance ☐ Feeds Self ☐ Feeding Tube ☐	Catheter: Yes ☐ No ☐	Date Inserted or Last Changed:
Thickened Liquid ☐ Consistency?	Bowel Incontinence: Yes ☐ No ☐	Colostomy: Yes ☐ No ☐
Supplement ☐ If so, name:	Date of Last BM:	

IMPAIRMENTS/DISABILITIES: (Please check all that apply)	PATIENT EQUIPMENT/BELONGINGS: (Check all sent with resident)	
Speech ☐ Contractures ☐ Mental Confusion ☐ Vision ☒ Hearing ☐ Amputation ☐ Paralysis ☐ Language Barrier ☐	None ☐ Right Hearing Aid ☐ Left Hearing Aid ☐ Glasses ☐ Upper Denture ☐ Lower Denture ☐	
COMMENTS: wears glasses	Jewelry ☐ Please list:	
Report Called to: Jane Elson RN	Other (i.e., prosthesis):	

Nurse Name (Print): Karen Scheitlin RN	Nurse Signature: Karen Scheitlin RN	Phone #: 862-4444	Date/Time: 3/18/12 7:00

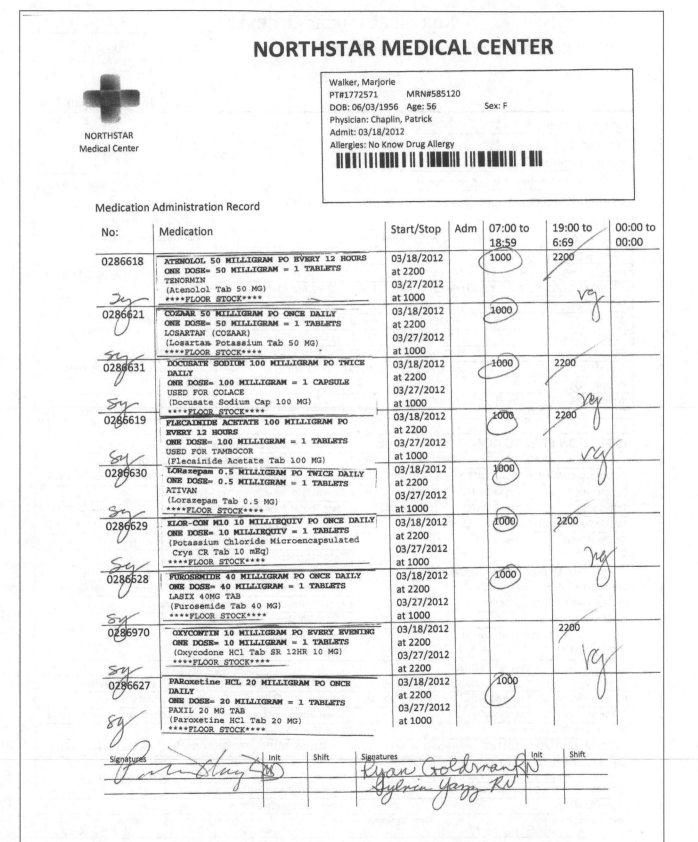

NORTHSTAR MEDICAL CENTER

NORTHSTAR
Medical Center

Walker, Marjorie
PT#1772571   MRN#585120
DOB: 06/03/1956   Age: 56   Sex: F
Physician: Chaplin, Patrick
Admit: 03/18/2012
Allergies: No Know Drug Allergy

Medication Administration Record

No:	Medication	Start/Stop	Adm	07:00 to 18:59	19:00 to 6:69	00:00 to 00:00
0286618	ATENOLOL 50 MILLIGRAM PO EVERY 12 HOURS ONE DOSE= 50 MILLIGRAM = 1 TABLETS TENORMIN (Atenolol Tab 50 MG) ****FLOOR STOCK****	03/18/2012 at 2200 03/27/2012 at 1000		1000	2200	
0286621	COZAAR 50 MILLIGRAM PO ONCE DAILY ONE DOSE= 50 MILLIGRAM = 1 TABLETS LOSARTAN (COZAAR) (Losartan Potassium Tab 50 MG) ****FLOOR STOCK****	03/18/2012 at 2200 03/27/2012 at 1000		1000		
0286631	DOCUSATE SODIUM 100 MILLIGRAM PO TWICE DAILY ONE DOSE= 100 MILLIGRAM = 1 CAPSULE USED FOR COLACE (Docusate Sodium Cap 100 MG) ****FLOOR STOCK****	03/18/2012 at 2200 03/27/2012 at 1000		1000	2200	
0286619	FLECAINIDE ACETATE 100 MILLIGRAM PO EVERY 12 HOURS ONE DOSE= 100 MILLIGRAM = 1 TABLETS USED FOR TAMBOCOR (Flecainide Acetate Tab 100 MG)	03/18/2012 at 2200 03/27/2012 at 1000		1000	2200	
0286630	LORazepam 0.5 MILLIGRAM PO TWICE DAILY ONE DOSE= 0.5 MILLIGRAM = 1 TABLETS ATIVAN (Lorazepam Tab 0.5 MG) ****FLOOR STOCK****	03/18/2012 at 2200 03/27/2012 at 1000		1000		
0286629	KLOR-CON M10 10 MILLIEQUIV PO ONCE DAILY ONE DOSE= 10 MILLIEQUIV = 1 TABLETS (Potassium Chloride Microencapsulated Crys CR Tab 10 mEq) ****FLOOR STOCK****	03/18/2012 at 2200 03/27/2012 at 1000		1000	2200	
0286628	FUROSEMIDE 40 MILLIGRAM PO ONCE DAILY ONE DOSE= 40 MILLIGRAM = 1 TABLETS LASIX 40MG TAB (Furosemide Tab 40 MG) ****FLOOR STOCK****	03/18/2012 at 2200 03/27/2012 at 1000		1000		
0286970	OXYCONTIN 10 MILLIGRAM PO EVERY EVENING ONE DOSE= 10 MILLIGRAM = 1 TABLETS (Oxycodone HCl Tab SR 12HR 10 MG) ****FLOOR STOCK****	03/18/2012 at 2200 03/27/2012 at 2200			2200	
0286627	PARoxetine HCL 20 MILLIGRAM PO ONCE DAILY ONE DOSE= 20 MILLIGRAM = 1 TABLETS PAXIL 20 MG TAB (Paroxetine HCl Tab 20 MG) ****FLOOR STOCK****	03/18/2012 at 2200 03/27/2012 at 1000		1000		

Signatures		Init	Shift	Signatures		Init	Shift
				Ryan Goldman RN			
				Sylvia Yazy RN			

CEHRS Correlation Guide

The following Correlation Guide maps the NHA Certified Electronic Health Record Specialist (CEHRS) Test Plan based on the 2019 Practice Analysis Study to Paradigm's *Exploring Electronic Health Records*, Third Edition, courseware. The CEHRS Summary Examination Outline contains domains that are covered on the examinations and the number of test items per domain. The CEHRS Detailed Examination Outline below includes tasks and knowledge statements associated with each domain on the test plan. Task statements reflect the duties that a candidate will need to know how to properly perform. Knowledge statements reflect information that a candidate will need to know and are in support of task statements. Items on the examination might require recall and critical thinking pertaining to a knowledge statement, a task statement, or both.

NHA (National Healthcareer Association) is a national professional certification organization that offers comprehensive certification and preparation resources for healthcare workers.

NHA had no participation in Paradigm's Correlation Guide.

CEHRS Detailed Examination Outline

Domain 1: Non-Clinical Operations

Domain 1 Task Statements	Exploring EHR3e
1.A. Verify patient identifiers before documenting in the EHR to ensure information is recorded in the correct chart.	Ch 4
1.B. Collect, record, and continuously update patient information (e.g., demographic information, clinical data, coverages/financial/insurance, guarantors, patient preferences).	Ch 4
1.C. Generate encounter documentation (e.g., admission/face sheet, labels, armbands).	Ch 4
1.D. Retrieve patient information from internal databases (e.g., provider database, financial database) to integrate into a patient's EHR.	Ch 4
1.E. Acquire patient data from external sources (e.g., diagnostic laboratories, ancillary facilities, other health care providers, other EHR systems).	Ch 3
1.F. Import information into the EHR from integrated devices (e.g., scanners, fax machines, e-signature pads, cameras).	Ch 3, Ch 7
1.G. Maintain inventory of EHR-related hardware (e.g., e-signature pads, cameras, tablets, mobile devices).	Ch 3
1.H. Coordinate patient flow within the facility (e.g., scheduling, patient registration and verification, check-in/check-out, patient referrals).	Ch 5

1.I. Provide initial and ongoing end-user training of EHR software to maintain competency (e.g., for new hires, upgrades and deployments).	Ch 13
1.J. Share information about updates to EHR software and the implications for workflow.	Ch 13
1.K. Identify data discrepancies within and among multiple EHRs, practice management systems, and other software systems.	Ch 11
1.L. Report or reconcile data discrepancies within and among multiple EHRs, practice management systems, and other software systems.	Ch 11
1.M. Provide support to patients regarding their use of patient portals (e.g., basic introduction, explain utility, grant access, navigation help).	Ch 14
Domain 1: Associated Knowledge Statements	
1.K1. Categories of patient information to be included in the EHR (e.g., demographic information, clinical data, coverages/financial/insurance, guarantors, patient preferences)	Ch 4
1.K2. Patient identifiers (e.g., Medical Record Number [MRN], EHR number, billing number)	Ch 3, Ch 4
1.K3. Search techniques to prevent duplicate Medical Record Numbers (MRNs)	Ch 4
1.K4. External information sources (e.g., diagnostic laboratories, ancillary facilities, other health care providers, other EHR systems)	Ch 3
1.K5. General office skills (e.g., copying, faxing, scanning, data entry)	N/A
1K6. Basic computer knowledge (e.g., word processing, hardware and software concepts, spreadsheets, basic networking)	N/A
1.K7. Procedures to transmit (e.g., import/export) data between devices	Ch 12
1.K8. Methods to inventory EHR-related hardware (e.g., e-signature pads, cameras, tablets, mobile devices) and implications for accurate and inaccurate inventory lists	N/A
1.K9. Provider schedules	Ch 5
1.K10. Scheduling templates and techniques	Ch 5
1.K11. Check-in/check-out procedures	Ch 4, Ch 5
1.K12. Credit card charging procedures	Ch4, Ch 5
1.K13. Acceptable forms of identification	Ch 4, Ch 5
1.K14. Considerations for remote/virtual training and support	Ch 14
1.K15. Coaching and mentoring techniques	N/A
1.K16. EHR training documentation requirements (e.g., who needs training, scheduling needed training, training performed)	Ch 13
1.K17. Available EHR training material	N/A
1.K18 Resources for developing new EHR training materials (e.g., frequently asked questions [FAQs], curriculum)	N/A
1.K19. Procedures to disseminate updated information to staff and others	N/A
1.K20. Basic IT troubleshooting techniques (e.g., making sure components are connected, where to find computer name/IP address, screenshot capture)	Ch 3
1.K21. IT escalation procedures	N/A

Continues

1.K22. EHR software reference library	N/A
1.K23. Data validation techniques and procedures	Ch 11
1.K24. Provider databases, specialties, and National Provider Identifiers (NPIs)	Ch 3
1.K25. Patient portal support (e.g., basic introduction, explain utility, grant access, navigation help)	Ch 14

Domain 2: Clinical Operations

Domain 2 Task Statements	Exploring EHR3e
2.A. Develop clinical templates for data capture (e.g., by diagnosis, by procedure, by practice).	Ch 7
2.B. Securely transmit and exchange patient data internally and externally (e.g., to pharmacies, other health care providers, other agencies) for research, analytics, and continuity of care.	Ch 1, Ch 3
2.C. Review and monitor clinical documentation to ensure completeness and accuracy (e.g., self-review, peer-to-peer).	Ch 7
2.D. Provide point-of-care EHR support (e.g., at-the-elbow, remote) for clinical documentation.	Ch 8
2.E. Input real-time clinical data into the EHR.	Ch 3–Ch 10
2.F. Document patient historic clinical data in the EHR (e.g., medications, immunizations, surgeries).	Ch 7
2.G. Provide support for computerized provider order entry (CPOE).	Ch 3
2.H. Locate and provide patient education materials available within the EHR.	N/A
2.I. Navigate the EHR system to retrieve requested patient data.	Ch 3–Ch 10
Domain 2: Associated Knowledge Statements	
2.K1. Content included in clinical templates (e.g., diagnoses, procedures)	Ch 7
2.K2. Types of information required for specific templates	Ch 7
2.K3. Common uses of clinical templates	Ch 7
2.K4. Telehealth/telemedicine workflows	Ch 14
2.K5. Requirements and procedures to securely transmit data	Ch 6
2.K6. Types of data that must be encrypted and the encryption processes	N/A
2.K7. Types of information that can be shared externally	Ch 2, Ch 6
2.K8. Considerations (e.g., purpose, audience) for transmitting data	Ch 2, Ch 6
2.K9. Common errors in documentation (e.g., directional terms, misspelling of names, conflicting information, duplicate charting)	Ch 7
2.K10. Charting requirements (e.g., primary and secondary diagnosis codes)	Ch 2, Ch 7
2.K11. Charting formats and methods (e.g., problem-oriented medical records [POMR], Subjective, Objective, Assessment, Plan [SOAP], Subjective, Objective, Assessment, Planning, Implementing, Evaluating, Reassessing [SOAPIER]	Ch 2, Ch 7
2.K12. Patient alerts and quality indicators	Ch 13
2.K13. Types of clinical data to be entered during a patient visit	Ch 3–Ch 10
2.K14. Procedures and treatments performed by health care professionals	Ch 9

Continues

2.K15. Types of historic data that must be entered into the EHR (e.g., medications, immunizations, allergies, surgeries)	Ch 7
2.K16. Scope of practice regarding computerized provider order entry (CPOE)	Ch 3
2.K17. Patient education materials available in the EHR (e.g., smoking cessation, wound care, prenatal care) and how to access them (e.g., applicable search terms, how to navigate)	N/A
2.K18. Scope of practice regarding patient education	Ch 8
2.K19. Location of specific patient data in the medical record (e.g., vital signs, medication list, lot number, blood glucose)	Ch 3, Ch 7

Domain 3: Revenue Cycle/Finance

Domain 3 Task Statements	Exploring EHR3e
3.A. Find codes in databases (e.g., International Statistical Classification of Diseases and Related Health Problems [ICD], Current Procedural Terminology [CPT], and Healthcare Common Procedure Coding System [HCPCS]).	Ch 9
3.B. Navigate the EHR to create a superbill, encounter forms, fee slips, or charge forms.	Ch 10
3.C. Enter the diagnosis and procedure codes billing information (e.g., from a superbill) into the EHR system for claims processing.	Ch 9
3.D. Verify that all diagnoses and procedural descriptions for reimbursement are accurately documented in he EHR.	Ch 9, Ch 10
3.E. Verify insurance and eligibility in the EHR.	Ch 4
3.F. Obtain and document authorizations in the EHR.	Ch 6
3.G. Provide estimated patient costs.	Ch 10
3.H. Navigate the EHR to provide patient statements.	Ch 10
3.I. Collect and post payments to a patient's account.	Ch 4, Ch 10
Domain 3: Associated Knowledge Statements	
3.K1. The link between documentation accuracy and reimbursement	Ch 7, Ch 10
3.K2. Types of codes (e.g., Current Procedure Terminology [CPT], International Classification of Diseases [ICD], Healthcare Common Procedure Coding System [HCPCS])	Ch 9
3.K3. Search and look-up procedures within classification codes	Ch 9
3.K4. The structure of coding and classification systems	Ch 9
3.K5. Clinical vocabularies associated with various classification systems	Ch 9
3.K6. Structure of a patient chart	Ch 2
3.K7. Medical necessity and code linkage	Ch 9
3.K8. Methods and procedures to optimize reimbursement	Ch 10
3.K9. National Correct Coding Initiative (NCCI) standards	N/A
3.K10. Real-time eligibility for services and supplies	Ch 4
3.K11. Reimbursement systems and processes (e.g., Medicare, Medicaid, workers' compensation, third-party payer insurance)	Ch 10

Continues

3.K12. Guarantors	Ch 4, Ch 10
3.K13. Fee schedules	Ch 10
3.K14. Explanation of Benefits (EOB) and Remittance Advice (RA)	Ch 10
3.K15. Procedures to obtain and document prior authorizations and pre-authorizations (e.g., pharmacological, referral, medical equipment, health care services)	N/A
3.K16. Payers' policies regarding authorizations	Ch 10
3.K17. Procedures to obtain estimated costs	Ch 10
3.K18. Payment methods (e.g., credit card charging procedures, cash application)	Ch 5
3.K19. Balance reconciliation (e.g., between the EHR and receipts)	Ch 10
3.K20. Documentation for both payment and non-payment	Ch 10
3.K21. Health insurance terminology	Ch 10
3.K22. Health care revenue cycle	Ch 10
3.K23. Claims submission procedures	Ch 10
3.K24. Electronic Data Interchange (EDI)	Ch 1

Domain 4: Regulatory Compliance

Domain 4 Task Statements	Exploring EHR3e
4.A. Adhere to professional standards of care as they pertain to health records.	Ch 2
4.B. Maintain confidentiality and security of protected health information (PHI) in compliance with the HIPAA Privacy Rule, the Health Information Technology for Economic and Clinical Health (HITECH) Act, and facility policy.	Ch 6
4.C. Educate others regarding compliance with best practices to safeguard electronic information and assist with enforcement of compliant behaviors.	Ch 6
4.D. Identify non-compliant behaviors (e.g., sharing passwords, unlocked room) that represent threats to the security of electronic information.	Ch 3
4.E. Allocate access controls within the EHR system based on user roles and predetermined privileges.	Ch 3
4.F. Verify and assist with compliance of access controls (i.e., privileges) within the EHR system.	Ch 3
4.G. De-identify protected health information (PHI).	Ch 6
4.H. Release protected health information (PHI) in accordance with the HIPAA Privacy Rule and facility policy.	Ch 6
4.I. Participate in internal audits of the EHR (e.g., consent forms, release of information forms, signature on file).	Ch 4
4.J. Comply with regulations regarding the use of abbreviations in the EHR system.	Ch 3
4.K. Initiate down-time procedures related to the EHR (e.g., data recovery).	N/A
4.L. Comply with the requirements of EHR incentive programs.	Ch 1

Continues

Domain 4: Associated Knowledge Statements	
4.K1. Types of data considered protected health information (PHI) (e.g., email addresses, next of kin, phone numbers, social security numbers)	Ch 6
4.K2. Methods and procedures used to de-identify protected health information (PHI)	Ch 6
4.K3. HIPAA requirements	Ch 6
4.K4. Best practices to maintain the security of electronic information	Ch 6
4.K5. Legal ramifications related to inaccuracies in the EHR	Ch 6
4.K6. Legal requirements for sharing or transmitting data externally	Ch 6
4.K7. Potential security breaches	Ch 6
4.K8. Escalation procedures	N/A
4.K9. Federal guidelines on reporting breaches	Ch 6
4.K10. Procedures to safeguard data (e.g., screen savers, password rules, screen visors)	Ch 3
4.K11. Adult learning and education techniques	N/A
4.K12. Required IT controls	N/A
4.K13. Role-based privileges	Ch 3
4.K14. Acceptable abbreviation practices and policies	Ch 2
4.K15. Data backup and recovery methods	Ch 3
4.K16. Data storage guidelines	N/A
4.K17. Consequences of noncompliance to regulations (e.g., penalties, non-payment, sanctions)	Ch 6
4.K18. EHR incentive programs and their requirements	Ch 1

Domain 5: Reporting

Domain 5 Task Statements	Exploring EHR3e
5.A. Run and execute standardized financial reports (e.g., aging, carriers, financial guarantor, relative value, cost of procedures, prospective payment systems).	Ch 7
5.B. Run and execute standardized clinical reports to track patient outcomes (e.g., by diagnosis, by procedure, by provider) for the support of continuity of care.	Ch 7
5.C. Generate ad hoc financial reports using fields in the EHR system.	Ch 7
5.D. Generate ad hoc clinical reports using fields in the EHR system.	Ch 7
5.E. Generate statistical reports for quality improvement (QI) measures, productivity, metrics, and research.	Ch 7
5.F. Compile data from the EHR for external reporting (e.g., for Meaningful Use/Quality Payment Program [QPP]).	Ch 13
5.G. Verify the accuracy of generated reports prior to distribution (e.g., check for errors).	N/A

Continues

Domain 5: Associated Knowledge Statements	
5.K1. Methods to generate reports (e.g., running queries, executing standardized reports, creating custom reports)	Ch 7
5.K2. Provider, diagnosis, and procedures reports	Ch 7
5.K3. Types and requirements of financial reports	Ch 7
5.K4. Types and requirements of clinical reports	Ch 7
5.K5. Data mining and extraction methods	Ch 11
5.K6. Quality improvement measures (e.g., average length of stay, patient outcomes, diagnoses, infection rates)	Ch 13
5.K7. Common reporting errors (e.g., missing fields, too much data on report)	Ch 12

Glossary

A

abuse unintentional upcoding

Accreditation Association for Ambulatory Health Care (AAAHC) a specialty accrediting organization

activities of daily living (ADLs) the fundamental skills that an individual needs to be able to perform so they can independently care for themselves; these skills include eating, bathing, dressing, and toileting as well as mobility

addressable standard a standard that should be met if it is a reasonable and appropriate safeguard in the entity's environment

administrative data includes demographic information about the patient such as the patient's name, address, date of birth, race, primary language, religion, and marital status

admission assessment a detailed assessment of the patient upon admission, typically assigned to the admitting nurse, who welcomes the patient to the nursing unit, obtains admission orders, conducts all admission documentation, and schedules all of the initial care and treatment of the patient

admission date the day and time the patient is admitted to the acute care facility

admission orders the order(s) provided upon admission of an inpatient; must include instructions for the patient's diet, medications, activities, diagnostic testing, laboratory and radiology tests, and monitoring orders

admission/registration clerks staff members generally responsible for entering insurance information into the electronic health record system at the time the patient is admitted to an inpatient hospital or scheduled for treatment at an outpatient facility or physician's office; also known as *patient access specialists*

advance directive a document that provides information about how the patient would like to be treated if they are no longer able to make their own medical decisions

adverse drug event (ADE) occurs when a patient is negatively affected upon the administration of a medication; this may result in a minor condition such as indigestion or a rash or could be serious enough to result in a patient's death

Affordable Care Act (ACA) enacted in March 2010 with the goal of providing quality, affordable health care for all Americans; enacted in two parts: the Patient Protection and Affordable Care Act and the Health Care and Education Reconciliation Act

Agency for Healthcare Research and Quality (AHRQ) an organization that focuses on improving the safety and quality of health care; their core competencies are focused on data, analytics, health system research, and practice improvement

alert fatigue a condition that arises when excessive numbers of alerts cause healthcare providers to disregard them

allowed amount the average or maximum amount that may be reimbursed per service, procedure, or item to the provider from the insurance payer

American College of Surgeons (ACS) an organization that developed a hospital standardization program establishing the minimum standards for reporting care and treatment

American Health Information Management Association (AHIMA) a professional organization that provides resources, education, and networking with other professionals, focusing on the quality of health information used in the delivery of health care

American Recovery and Reinvestment Act of 2009 (ARRA) an economic stimulus package signed into law by President Barack Obama

annual limit a cap on the benefits the insurance company will pay in a year

artificial intelligence (AI) computer systems able to perform tasks that usually require human intelligence

assessment the evaluation of subjective and objective information, resulting in patient risk values, diagnoses, and conditions; varies depending on the focus of the assessment

assignment of benefits a patient authorization form that allows their health insurance or third-party provider to reimburse the healthcare provider or facility directly

Association for Healthcare Documentation Integrity (AHDI) a professional organization that sets and upholds standards for education and practice in the field of clinical documentation that ensure the highest level of accuracy, privacy, and security for the US healthcare systems in order to protect public health, increase patient safety, and improve quality of care for healthcare customers

asynchronous describes communication that is not accomplished in real time, such as visits and consults accomplished through a healthcare provider's electronic health record or a special web portal

automated data collection when the data from the initial patient encounter is automatically copied over to each new patient encounter

automatic method the entry of results that allows those results to be immediately available

B

bar-coded medication administration (BCMA) a process to record medication administration using a barcode to identify and confirm that the correct patient receives the correct medication; a function paired with the eMAR to reduce medication errors

behavioral health setting a facility that provides care to patients with psychiatric diagnoses

benefit year the year of insurance benefits coverage under an individual health insurance plan

big data large data sets that are analyzed to reveal trends and patterns

billing/payment status report lists the status of every patient account, allowing the billing staff to identify claims that need to be billed or rebilled and insurance payers that need to be contacted regarding lack of payment

birthday rule a rule that specifies that the insurance of the parent whose birthday falls first in a calendar year will be the primary insurance for a child

breach an impermissible use or disclosure under the Privacy Rule that compromises the security or privacy of protected health information such that the use or disclosure poses a significant risk of financial, reputational, or other harm to the affected individual

burial and death benefits workers' compensation paid to the dependent(s) of an employee who died from a work-related illness or injury; death benefits are typically a percentage of the employee's average wages; burial benefits may be paid to the person who paid for burial expenses

C

cancer registry a collection of data focusing on cancer and tumor diseases

care plan a patient's road map to better health, developed by the entire clinical team in conjunction with the patient; also known as a *treatment plan* or *plan of care*

Centers for Medicare & Medicaid Services (CMS) a federal agency that oversees federal healthcare programs, including Medicare Conditions of Participation (CoPs)

Certified Health Data Analyst (CHDA®) a certification that demonstrates an individual's expertise in data analysis to include acquiring, managing, analyzing, interpreting, and transforming data into accurate, consistent, and timely information while balancing the organization's strategic vision with daily operations

certified nursing assistants (CNAs) certified professionals who work in a variety of healthcare settings, including hospitals, long-term care facilities, home health care, rehabilitation hospitals, and psychiatric facilities; also known as *state-tested nursing assistants (STNAs), state-registered nursing assistants (SRNAs), geriatric nursing assistants (GNAs)*, and *licensed nursing assistants (LNAs)*

CHAMPVA a comprehensive healthcare benefits program in which the Department of Veterans Affairs shares the cost of covered healthcare services and supplies with eligible beneficiaries

charge entry the process of entering medical codes into the billing system

checking out the procedure for a patient leaving an outpatient facility

chief complaint a narrative articulated by the patient as their reason for seeking health services

claim scrubbing the process of checking claims for errors prior to transmitting them to insurance companies

classification system a standardized coding method that organizes diagnoses and procedures into related groups to facilitate reimbursement, reporting, and clinical research

clean claims claims without errors

clearinghouse a company that accepts electronic claims from healthcare providers, scrubs the claims, transmits the clean claims to the appropriate payer, and returns the claims that have errors to the healthcare provider

clinical coders professionals who assign or validate diagnostic and procedural codes to represent the patient's diseases or conditions and the treatment rendered

clinical data information such as admission dates, office visits, laboratory test results, evaluations, or emergency visits

clinical decision support system (CDSS) a computer system, usually integrated with the EHR system, that assists healthcare providers with decision-making tasks such as determining diagnoses, choosing the best medications to order for a patient, and selecting proper diagnostic tests

clinical documentation contains data related to the patient's clinical status that is entered into the patient's EHR or paper record; also known as *clinical inputs*

clinical documentation cycle a cycle of assessment, care plan, progress notes, and reassessment; the cycle begins with a clinician's first encounter with a patient and continues with each subsequent encounter

clinical encoder a software program that helps coding professionals navigate coding pathways with the end result of assigning codes

clinical inputs the data entered into the patient record related to the patient's clinical status; data may be structured or unstructured; also known as *clinical documentation*

clinical results reporting an electronic health record system function that allows healthcare providers to view laboratory and diagnostic test results immediately, provided there is an interface between the clinical results system and the EHR

ClinicalTrials.gov a registry that provides access to information on publicly and privately funded clinical studies

cloned progress note an identical note resulting from copying and pasting from one encounter or visit to another; also known as *copycat charting*

cloud storage refers to virtual servers where data and the EHR system are backed up

cluster a type of schedule in which similar appointments are scheduled together at specific times of the day

CMS Medicare Physician Fee Schedule (MPFS) a standardized fee-paying schedule

CMS-1500 a universal claim form accepted by Medicare, Medicaid, and most insurance payers

coinsurance the insured person's share of the costs of a covered healthcare service, calculated as a percentage of the allowed amount for the service

Commission for Accreditation of Rehabilitation Facilities (CARF) an independent, nonprofit organization that focuses on aging services, behavioral health, child and youth services, employment and community services, medical rehabilitation, and opioid treatment programs

Community Health Accreditation Program (CHAP) a specialty accrediting organization

computer-assisted coding (CAC) programs that automatically assign diagnosis and procedure codes based on electronic documentation, which can increase the productivity of a coder by up to 20%

computer protocol a standardized method of communicating or transmitting data between two computer systems

concurrent coding the process of coding while a patient is still receiving treatment in a hospital

Consolidated Omnibus Budget Reconciliation Act (COBRA) a federal law that may allow individuals to temporarily keep health coverage after their employment ends, after they lose coverage as a dependent of the covered employee, or after another qualifying event

controlled substance a drug declared by US federal or state law to be illegal for sale or use but may be dispensed under a healthcare provider's prescription

Controlled Substances Act of 1970 legislation that placed tight controls on the pharmaceutical and healthcare industries and outlined the five schedules of controlled substances based on potential for harm

conversion factor (CF) a fiscal-year monetary amount arrived at by a formula set by US Congress to convert GPCI into a dollar amount that reflects several elements

copayment the amount that an insured individual must pay for healthcare services received, typically office visits, urgent care visits, or emergency department encounters

core data elements the data elements that are necessary for the master patient index and include patient identification number, patient name, date of birth, Social Security number, address, etc.

covered dependents the spouse and children who are included in an individual's health insurance coverage

covered entities entities that have to comply with HIPAA Privacy and Security Rules; these include healthcare providers, health plans, and healthcare clearinghouses transmitting health information in an electronic format

crosswalking the process of translating a code in one code set to a code in another code set

Current Dental Terminology (CDT®) a classification system used to code dental procedures

Current Procedural Terminology (CPT®) one of the most widely used classification systems in the United States used to code outpatient procedures for facility coding, as well as all physician services rendered

D

data descriptive or numeric attributes of one or more variables

data analytics the practice of exploring and manipulating data for the purposes of identifying new information that can be used to improve the operations of the organization

data collection both manual and automated collection of information

data dictionary a document that describes the content, format, and structure of data elements within a database

Data Elements for Emergency Department Systems (DEEDS) uniform specifications for data entered into emergency department patient records

data integrity the accuracy, completeness, and reliability of data in the electronic health record

data mapping a method that is used to connect data from one system to data of another system, may use data dictionary or data sets

data mining the process of searching and examining data to organize and reorganize it into useful information, patterns, and trends

data set a structured collection of related data elements

data sort arranging data in a particular sequence, from high to low or low to high

data standards agreed-upon definitions and formats of data

data stewardship the authority and responsibility associated with collecting, using, and disclosing health information in its identifiable and aggregate forms

data warehouse a database that accesses data from multiple databases that are integrated to be used for analytic purposes

database a collection of data that is organized in rows, columns, and tables

day sheet a report of practice activity for a 24-hour period that is used to reconcile patient accounts on a daily basis to ensure that no fraud, abuse, or theft is occurring

deductible the amount an insured individual must pay out of pocket before the insurance will pay

deficiencies publicly available survey results for each nursing facility that list the regulations that are not being followed

deidentified health information health information that neither identifies an individual nor provides a reasonable basis to identify an individual

demographic information information provided by the patient that includes name, date of birth, address, phone number, email address, etc.

deposit report generated daily, weekly, monthly, and yearly for the deposits made from insurance payers and from patient payments

descriptive analytics refers to using historical data to identify patterns and study trends in historical events

diagnosis a statement or conclusion that describes a patient's illness, disease, or health problem

diagnosis-related group (DRG) a patient classification system that groups hospital patients of similar age, sex, diagnoses, and treatments

***Diagnostic and Statistical Manual of Mental Disorders*, Fifth Edition (DSM-5)** a classification system used to classify psychiatric disorders

discharge date the day and time the patient is discharged from the facility

discharge disposition the patient's destination following a stay in the hospital

discharged the procedure for a patient leaving an inpatient facility

discharged not final billed (DNFB) describes patient accounts that are not able to be final billed to the insurance company or responsible party due to a lack of final coding, insurance verification, or other data errors

E

eHealth refers to the practice of health care using electronic processes and technology such as electronic health records, laboratory and radiology systems, and patient scheduling systems

electronic health record (EHR) a digital version of a patient's paper chart with patient health information gathered from multiple healthcare providers; also a computer system used to improve healthcare delivery

Electronic Health Record Modernization (EHRM) a program that allows the US Department of Veterans Affairs (VA) and the Department of Defense (DOD) to use the same EHR vendor

electronic medical record (EMR) an electronic version of patient files within a single organization that allows healthcare providers to place orders, document results, and store patient information

electronic medication administration record (eMAR) the electronic documentation of medications administered to patients by nurses and other qualified healthcare staff

electronic patient tracking (EPT) function of an EHR system that tracks a patient's location from the time of their arrival at the healthcare organization to their discharge (for inpatients) or checkout (for outpatients)

electronic protected health information (ePHI) protected health information in electronic format

electronic superbill an itemized form that allows charges to be captured from a patient visit

electronic treatment administration record (eTAR) the electronic documentation of patient treatments

employer-provided PHR a personal health record (PHR) offered by an employer containing data from hospitals, physicians' offices, health plans, laboratories, and pharmacies as well as information entered by the employee, all of which is meant to enable employees to make better health decisions

enterprise data storage a centralized system (online or offline) that businesses use for managing and protecting data

enterprise identification number (EIN) an identifier used by an organization to identify a patient across various healthcare settings

enterprise master patient index (EMPI) a database that maintains patient identifier information across an EHR system for all healthcare settings, allowing a healthcare organization to compile the patient's information into one index using registration, scheduling, financial, and clinical information

e-prescribing a process that allows a physician, nurse practitioner, or physician assistant to electronically transmit a new prescription or renewal authorization to a pharmacy; also known as *electronic prescribing*

established patient a patient who has received professional services from a healthcare provider or a provider in the same group and/or specialty within the past three years

external data data from outside the organization

F

facility identifier an identifier that indicates the healthcare setting where the patient is seeking care

facility-provided PHR a type of tethered personal health record (PHR) that comes from a physician or healthcare facility

fall risk assessment an evaluation that includes scoring the presence or absence of fall risk factors, resulting in a cumulative score that indicates the degree to which a patient is at risk for falling

fee-for-service a reimbursement method that requests payment for each service or procedure

fee schedule a price list of services and procedures

financial data information that includes the patient's insurance and payment information for healthcare services

flowsheet a type of documentation tool used to record patient-related values over time; a flowsheet displays a patient's progress regarding anything that a provider needs to monitor, such as weight, fluid input, lab values, and blood glucose levels

format the organizing principle for health documents from all departments in a healthcare facility

foundational interoperability a level of communication infrastructure that allows systems to securely exchange data without any ability to interpret the shared data, also Level 1 interoperability

fraud intentional upcoding

functionality the ability to create and manage EHRs for all patients in a healthcare facility and automate workflow

G

general consent for treatment a form used in acute care facilities that gives the healthcare provider the right to treat a patient

geographic practice cost indices (GPCI) adjustments applied to the relative value units to account for variations in the costs of practicing medicine in specific geographic regions

geriatric nursing assistants (GNAs) See entry for *certified nursing assistants (CNAs)*

group health insurance plan an insurance plan that provides healthcare coverage to a specific group of people, typically based on an employer

guarantor the person or financial entity that guarantees payment on any unpaid balances on an account

guarantor account a record that saves the information about the guarantor, including the guarantor's name and address

H

Health Care and Education Reconciliation Act an amendment to the Affordable Care Act

health coverage legal entitlement to payment or reimbursement for healthcare costs, generally under a contract with a health insurance company, a group health plan offered in connection with employment, or a government program like Medicare, Medicaid, or the Children's Health Insurance Program (CHIP)

health information management (HIM) the practice of planning information systems, developing health policy, identifying current and future information needs, and practicing the maintenance and care of health records

Health Information Technology for Economic and Clinical Health (HITECH) Act an act enacted in February 2009 as part of the ARRA that promoted the nationwide implementation of EHR technology

health insurance a type of insurance that pays for healthcare services that are incurred by the insured person(s)

Health Insurance Portability and Accountability Act of 1996 (HIPAA) a comprehensive federal law passed in 1996 to protect all patient-identifiable medical information

health insurer–provided PHRs personal health record (PHR) systems owned by a health insurance company where the insurer populates information about a subscriber, such as insurance claim information, a list of providers, prescriptions, and benefits coverage

health IT ecosystem a collection of individuals and groups that are interested in health information technology

Health Level 7 (HL7) the most common healthcare communication protocol that focuses on the exchange of clinical and administrative data

health maintenance organization (HMO) a type of health insurance plan that usually limits coverage to include care only from providers who work for or contract with the HMO

Health Maintenance Organization (HMO) Act an act that provided grants to employers who set up HMOs

health record an accumulation of information about a patient's past and present health

Health Resources and Services Administration (HRSA) an agency of the US Department of Health and Human Services; focuses on improving health and health equity through innovative programs and a skilled health workforce and providing access to services to those who are economically or medically vulnerable

Healthcare Common Procedure Coding System (HCPCS) a classification system used to code ancillary services and procedures

Healthcare Cost and Utilization Project (HCUP) a collection of databases that is sponsored by the Agency for Healthcare Research and Quality

healthcare delivery (HCD) system a healthcare facility; also the owner of the electronic medical record

healthcare facility an organization, such as a hospital, clinic, dental office, outpatient surgery center, birthing center, or nursing home, that performs healthcare services

healthcare informatics the study of managing health information

Healthcare Information and Management Systems Society (HIMSS) an organization that focuses on using information technology and management systems to improve the quality and delivery of health care

healthcare treatment covered workers' compensation reimbursement to the medical provider who treats the work-related injury or illness, paid directly by the patient's employer's insurer

healthcare-associated infections (HAIs) infections contracted by a patient during a stay in a medical facility

HealthData.gov provides access to health data with the hope of improving healthcare quality

hibernation mode a privacy feature in an EHR system that prevents disclosure of PHI

HIPAA Eligibility Transaction System (HETS) a Medicare eligibility database application

HIPAA X12 837 Healthcare Claim electronic claim generated by software and then transmitted to appropriate insurance payers, also known as the *837 Claim* or the *HIPAA Claim*

Hippocrates considered one of the most important figures in medical history; among the first to describe and document many diseases and medical conditions

history the subjective element of the history and physical examination report that includes history of present illness, past medical history, allergies, medications currently prescribed to the patient, and family and social histories

history and physical examination (H&P) a report that helps identify and treat patient diagnoses; consists of two main elements: a subjective element and an objective element

hospice care short-term, palliative care provided to terminally ill patients within acute care or home care settings

hospice services care for those who are at the end of life

hospital acquired describes diagnoses and conditions that developed when the patient was an inpatient in the hospital

hospital chargemaster a computer database that compiles all procedures, services, supplies, and drugs that are billed to insurance payers

Hospital Compare part of the CMS's Hospital Quality Initiative; meant to provide data to examine how well a hospital delivers quality care and how healthcare organizations can improve

hybrid health record a patient record that is stored on paper and electronically

I

immunization registry includes patient data for various immunizations

indexes in a database, these are used to find data without searching every row

individual health insurance plan an insurance plan that an individual purchases for themselves and/or their family

individually identifiable health information information, including demographic data, that identifies an individual

informatics the science of processing data for storage and retrieval

information data collected and analyzed

information blocking a practice by a health IT developer of certified health IT, health information network, health information exchange, or healthcare provider that, except as required by law or specified by the Secretary of the US Department of Health and Human Services as a reasonable and necessary activity, is likely to interfere with the access, exchange, or use of electronic protected health information

information governance an effective framework for the access and use of healthcare data including the policies, procedures, and processes for data and information creation, storage, access, use, analysis, archival, and deletion

information processing cycle the sequence of events that provide the building blocks for the EHR system, including four components: input, processing, output, and storage

in-network describes providers or healthcare facilities that are part of a health plan's group of providers with which it has negotiated a discount

inpatient a patient who occupies a hospital bed for at least one night in the course of treatment, examination, or observation

inpatient prospective payment system (IPPS) the first diagnosis-related group (DRG) system that was implemented in 1983 to reimburse acute care hospitals for the treatment of Medicare patients

input the first component of the information processing cycle; data entered by the user of the EHR system (e.g., the patient's first name, last name, identification number, and test results)

input device a device used to enter data into an EHR system; includes keyboard, mouse, scanner, microphone, camera, stylus, and touchscreen

insurance audits reviews conducted by insurance companies or auditing companies hired to review coding assignments on behalf of insurance companies

insurance verifier the person who confirms the patient's insurance coverage with the insurance company

intake fluids taken by mouth, feeding tubes, and intravenous catheters

intake and output (I&O) monitoring the measurement and recording of a patient's intake and output of fluids for assessing and controlling patient hydration and fluid balance, sometimes recorded via flowsheet

integrated care the systematic coordination of health care

integrated health record a health record format that is organized either in chronologic or reverse chronologic order

interface provides communication flow between two or more computer systems

internal data data accessed from within the healthcare organization

International Classification of Diseases (ICD) one of the most widely used classification systems used to code diagnoses and procedures for inpatients and diagnoses for all healthcare providers

Internet of Things (IoT) describes networks of devices that can connect to share data; in health care, it is a network of patient data devices

interoperability the ability of an EHR system to exchange data with other sources of health information, including pharmacies, laboratories, and other healthcare providers

isolation status the precautions that must be taken by healthcare staff and visitors to avoid the spread of bacterial or viral infections

K

knowledge based describes a clinical decision support system that utilizes inference software and databases containing the most current medical, scientific, and research information

L

legal data information composed of consents for treatment and authorizations for the release of information

licensed nursing assistants (LNAs) See entry for *certified nursing assistants (CNAs)*

licensed practical nurses (LPNs) licensed professionals who perform basic nursing functions such as taking blood pressure readings and other vital signs, catheter care, and wound care; also known as *licensed vocational nurses (LVNs)* in California and Texas

licensed vocational nurses (LVNs) licensed practical nurses are known as LVNs in California and Texas

lifetime limit a cap on the total lifetime benefits one may receive from an insurance company

limited data set protected health information from which certain specified direct identifiers of individuals and their relatives, household members, and employers have been removed

local area network (LAN) a group of computers connected through a network confined to a single area or small geographic area such as a building or hospital campus

longitudinal describes a patient's record that will continue to develop over the course of care

long-term care care that is more custodial in nature, such as treatment of chronic conditions and assistance with activities of daily living that are primarily provided by patient care assistants with oversight by nursing staff and an attending physician

long-term care facility a facility in which patients typically reside for more than 30 days

long-term care nursing discharge assessment similar to a nursing discharge assessment from the hospital, this report includes the choices of discharge disposition from a long-term care facility

M

management of information plan encompasses all technological systems used by the organization; all the data generated, used, and stored; and all the processes used to contribute to the flow of information

manual data collection a process initiated by a staff member upon initial patient contact with a healthcare facility, done without the aid of an automatic system

manual method the process of clinical results reporting in which a printed report is faxed and then scanned into the electronic health record for access

master patient index (MPI) a database created by a healthcare organization to assign a unique medical record number to each patient served, thus allowing easy retrieval and maintenance of patient information; also known as a *patient list*

meaningful use the set of standards that governs the use of EHRs and allows eligible providers and hospitals to earn incentive payments by meeting specific criteria

MEDCIN a system of common clinical and medical terms primarily used in physicians' offices

Medicaid a state-administered health insurance program for low-income families and children, pregnant women, the elderly, people with disabilities, and in some states, other qualified adults

medical coder a professional who plays a key role in the billing process by coding diagnoses and procedures in preparation for billing claims

medical coding the process of assigning and validating standardized alphanumeric identifiers to the diagnoses and procedures documented in a health record

medical procedure an activity performed on an individual to improve health, treat disease or injury, or identify a diagnosis

Medicare a federal health insurance program for people who are age 65 or older and certain younger people with disabilities

Medicare Part A hospital insurance; covers inpatient care in hospitals, including critical access hospitals and skilled nursing facilities (not custodial or long-term care)

Medicare Part B medical insurance; covers physicians' services and outpatient care

Medicare Part C a program that gave more coverage options in the private insurance market and added options such as prescription drug coverage for Medicare subscribers who wished to pay for additional coverage; also known as *Medicare Advantage*

Medicare Part D a program that helps pay for prescription drugs for Medicare beneficiaries who have a plan that includes Medicare prescription drug coverage

Medicare Prescription Drug Improvement and Modernization Act of 2003 the law that added an optional prescription drug benefit to Medicare recipients

Medicare Provider Analysis and Review (MEDPAR) a database that contains inpatient hospital and skilled nursing facility records for all Medicare beneficiaries

Medigap Medicare supplemental insurance

mHealth the practice of health care that uses electronic processes conducted on a mobile device

mileage reimbursement workers' compensation paid by employers for the mileage costs and for some of the wages employees lose while in transit to and from and during their medical appointments

Minimum Data Set (MDS) a standardized, primary screening and assessment tool of health status for all residents of Medicare- and Medicaid-certified nursing homes

minimum necessary a concept required by the Privacy Rule that states that covered entities must make reasonable efforts to limit the use, disclosure of, and requests for the minimum amount of protected health information necessary to accomplish the intended purpose

minimum standards a set of requirements for reporting care and treatment

modified wave a type of schedule in which patients arrive at planned intervals in the first half hour; then, in the second half hour, the healthcare provider catches up

morbidity the rates of diseases in a population; illness statistics

mortality the rate of death in a population; death statistics

N

National Committee for Quality Assurance (NCQA) an independent, nonprofit organization that focuses on healthcare quality

National Committee on Vital and Health Statistics (NCVHS) an advisory body to the US Department of Health and Human Services; the NCVHS completed a review of core health data elements and developed a list and definitions of the 42 core elements that can be used in a variety of healthcare settings

National Practitioner Data Bank (NPDB) a database that contains information on medical malpractice payments and actions against healthcare practitioners, providers, and suppliers

Nationwide Health Information Network (NHIN) a set of standards that enables the secure exchange of health information over the internet

new patient a patient who has not received any services from a healthcare provider or a provider in the group in the same specialty within the past three years

no interoperability describes a stand-alone system that does not communicate with other computer systems, also Level 0 interoperability

nomenclature a common system of naming things

noncovered entities entities that do not have to comply with HIPAA Privacy and Security Rules; these include workers' compensation carriers, employers, marketing firms, life insurance companies, pharmaceutical manufacturers, casualty insurance carriers, pharmacy benefit management companies, and crime victim compensation programs

no-shows patients who do not show for their scheduled appointments

nursing discharge assessment an assessment completed upon the discharge of a patient from an inpatient facility to document the patient's condition and status at the time of discharge

nursing plan of care a working communication tool for nurses to share nursing diagnoses, desired patient outcomes related to the diagnoses, the interventions that the nursing staff will perform or direct, and evaluation indicating if the outcome was achieved

O

objective element the portion of the history and physical examination report that includes the physical examination by the nursing or medical staff

Office for Civil Rights (OCR) the agency responsible for enforcing the HIPAA Privacy and Security Rules

Office of the National Coordinator for Health Information Technology (ONC) the US federal body that recommends policies, procedures, protocols, and standards for interoperability; part of the US Department of Health and Human Services

Omnibus Reconciliation Act of 1980 the act that expanded home health services and also brought Medigap under federal oversight

open hours a type of schedule typically used in an urgent care setting in which patients are seen throughout certain time frames or on a first-come, first-served basis

operative report a form of clinical documentation that contains the details of a particular surgery or procedure performed on a patient

optional data elements the data elements that are optional for the master patient index, including marital status, telephone number, mother's maiden name, place of birth, advance directive decision making, organ donor status, emergency contact, allergies, and problem list

organization interoperability level a level of communication where the policies of data sharing both within and between organizations and individuals are created and maintained; also Level 4 interoperability

Outcome and Assessment Information Set (OASIS) a group of data elements that represent core items of a comprehensive assessment for an adult home care patient

out-of-network describes physicians, hospitals, or other healthcare providers who are considered nonparticipants in an insurance plan (usually an HMO or PPO)

out-of-pocket amount expenses for medical care that are not reimbursed by the insurance company; these include deductibles, coinsurance, and copayments for covered services plus all costs for services that are not covered

outpatient a patient who does not spend more than 24 hours in a healthcare facility

output fluid that is measured from the kidneys, the gastrointestinal tract, drainage tubes, and wounds

output the third component of the information processing cycle; processed and organized data that provides meaningful information for the user

output device a device that displays the results from EHRs; includes computer monitor, digital device screen, and printer

P

pain assessment an assessment of a patient's type of pain, acute or chronic; the location of the pain; the intensity of the pain; and what, if anything, helps to relieve the pain

patient aging report an accounts receivable report that shows how long patients have owed money to the practice

patient day sheet a daily reconciliation or balancing sheet used to prevent fraud

patient identification number a unique patient or medical record number

patient ledger a report that reflects the patient's financial status in summary and/or in detail

patient portal a secure website that gives patients access to their health records and facilitates communication and scheduling

Patient Protection and Affordable Care Act the law that expanded health insurance coverage for Americans

payment day sheet similar to the patient day sheet, except that it lists only payments made during the 24-hour period

permanent partial disability (PPD) benefits income replacement benefit paid when medical maximum improvement has been achieved and a worker may be able to work in some capacity, but their injury has caused damage for an indefinite period and they cannot return to their old occupation

permanent total disability (PTD) benefits income replacement benefit paid when the worker's injury permanently prevents them from returning to their former occupation

personal health record (PHR) an emerging health information technology initiative that gives patients a tool to improve the quality of their healthcare; these records are updated and maintained by the patient

physical examination the objective element of the history and physical examination report; this procedure is conducted by the nursing or medical staff and consists of a physical examination of body systems, an assessment of the patient and their condition, and a treatment plan

physician query a request, typically from a coder or a case manager, to add documentation to the health record that clarifies a diagnosis or procedure performed

pilot a test run of the EHR system

point of service (POS) plan a hybrid of HMO and PPO health plans

policies principles or guidelines that are agreed upon by the organization

practice management the day-to-day operations of a medical practice

predictive analytics the use of historical patient data with the application of statistical algorithms to identify expected future outcomes and trends in health care

preferred provider organization (PPO) a type of health plan that contracts with medical providers, such as hospitals and physicians, to create a network of participating providers

premium a specified number of consistent payments for any type of insurance

prescriptive analytics the use of artificial intelligence to present "what if" options to give decision makers the opportunity to select the best option for the desired outcome

present on admission (POA) indicates diagnoses and conditions that the patient already had when they were admitted to the healthcare organization

pressure injuries localized damage to the skin and underlying soft tissue usually over a bony prominence or related to a medical or other device; formerly called *pressure ulcers*

primary data source data and information from the patient's electronic health record

Privacy Rule the standards developed with the intent to define protected health information and the entities and circumstances in which it may be used or disclosed by covered entities

Problem-Oriented Medical Information System (PROMIS) a software program developed at the University of Vermont under a federal grant in the 1970s

problem-oriented medical record (POMR) a medical record format that takes a systematic approach to documentation

problem-oriented record (POR) a health record format that focuses on assessment of the clinical documentation by healthcare providers and the creation of a plan that addresses the patient's health concerns

procedure day sheet similar to a patient day sheet, except that this report lists only the procedures charged during the 24-hour period

procedures methods used to put policies in action within the healthcare organization

processing the second component of the information processing cycle; the steps of analyzing or comparing data to make it usable within the system

production by insurance report reflects the amount of revenue generated by each insurance carrier

production by procedure report reflects the number of procedures performed during a specific period along with the associated revenue

production by provider report shows how many patients are treated within a specified period by each provider in a practice, along with the revenue generated

production reports assists the practice manager with budgeting and revenue management

progress notes the portion of the health record in which healthcare providers of all disciplines document the patient's progress or lack thereof in relation to the established goals of the care plan

protected health information (PHI) all individually identifiable health information held or transmitted by a covered entity or its business associate, in any form or media, whether electronic, paper, or oral

Q

qualifying stay a hospital stay of at least 3 days during the 30 days before admission to the skilled nursing facility

Quality Improvement Organization (QIO) a group of health experts, providers, and consumers who are dedicated to improving the quality of care for people with Medicare

R

rapid response teams (RRTs) an interdisciplinary group of hospital staff that are called to quickly assess a patient who has been observed by a nurse of other healthcare worker as declining and potentially headed toward a critical situation, such as cardiac arrest

record a collection, usually in writing, of an account or an occurrence

registered health information administrator (RHIA) a professional who works as a liaison between healthcare providers, organization staff, payers, and patients; an expert in managing health information and the professional responsible for managing health information

registered health information technician (RHIT) a professional who performs the technical procedures related to the management of health information, frequently working in positions of medical coding, billing, and data management

registered nurses (RNs) state board-certified nurses typically assigned a group of patients in a healthcare setting and responsible for the overall assessment, care planning, and treatment of those patients and supervising LPNs and CNAs; require an associate or bachelor's degree from an approved nursing school

registrar the healthcare personnel at the admission or registration desk who is the initial contact for a patient responsible for collecting demographic and administrative data

rehabilitation facility a facility that offers acute care and ambulatory care, typically serving patients recovering from accidents, injuries, or surgeries

reimbursement the act of compensating a person for services rendered

relative value units (RVUs) used to calculate the value of a service or procedure; calculated for work RVUs, practice expense RVUs, and malpractice RVUs

remittance advice (RA) report lists the patient's information and amount paid by Medicare or another payer to the physician's practice

remote patient monitoring (RPM) involves the use of mobile medical devices and technology to gather patient clinical data such as vital signs and blood pressure, as well as information on the medical device, such as a pacemaker status or glucose meter readings

required standard the portions of the standards with which each covered entity must comply

resident the preferred term for patient in a long-term care facility

resolution agreement a contract signed by the federal government and a covered entity in which the covered entity agrees to perform certain obligations (e.g., staff training regarding privacy and confidentiality or audits of all releases of health information to ensure compliance) and to send reports to the federal government for a certain period (typically three years)

resource-based relative value scale (RBRVS) used to create the CMS Medicare Physician Fee Schedule

revenue cycle management all administrative and clinical functions that contribute to the capture, management, and collection of patient service revenue

review of systems (ROS) an examination of each body system that includes physical assessment of general appearance; vital signs; head, ears, eyes, nose, and throat (HEENT); respiratory; cardiovascular; gastrointestinal; genitourinary; musculoskeletal; and neurologic

rollout the process of introducing an EHR to a facility that occurs in three phases: organizational, training, and operational

S

scope of practice the allowable procedures and functions that healthcare professionals may perform according to their state licensures

secondary data source data and information from indexes and registries and any other non-primary source

security the standard that prevents data loss and ensures that patient health information is private

Security Rule the standards developed to address the security provisions of HIPAA; also known as *Security Standards for the Protection of Electronic Protected Health Information*

Security Standards for the Protection of Electronic Protected Health Information the standards developed to address the security provisions of HIPAA; also known as the *Security Rule*

self-pay patients patients who do not have any type of insurance coverage and must pay for healthcare services themselves

semantic interoperability level a high level of interoperability that allows the meaning of the data to be shared; the data and information may also be interpreted, allowing EHR systems to function; also Level 3 interoperability

situation, background, assessment, recommendation (SBAR) a communication tool typically used when patient's status must be shared quickly and succinctly as well as during shift handoffs

skilled care skilled nursing or rehabilitation services that are provided by licensed health professionals such as nurses and physical therapists and are ordered by a doctor

skilled nursing facility an inpatient setting with the staff and equipment available to provide skilled nursing care and, in most cases, skilled rehabilitative (physical, occupational, speech, and respiratory) services

skin assessment an assessment of any and all skin injuries and conditions (e.g., skin tears, bruises, scabs, rashes, or pressure injuries) that must be carefully identified and documented upon admission of a patient to ensure that all injuries and conditions are known and appropriately treated

SNOMED CT a standardized vocabulary of clinical terminology used by healthcare providers for clinical documentation and reporting; considered the most comprehensive healthcare terminology in the world

SOAP note a popular form of nursing note that contains the subjective, objective, assessment, and plan components all in one note

social determinants of health (SDOH) conditions in the environments where people are born, live, learn, work, play, worship, and age that affect a wide range of health, functioning, and quality-of-life outcomes and risks

source-oriented record (SOR) a health record format used most by healthcare facilities; organizes health documents into sections that contain information collected from a specific department or type of service

standard precautions CDC guidelines for preventing the transmission of infections in all healthcare settings

state registered nursing assistants (SRNAs) See entry for *certified nursing assistants (CNAs)*

state tested nursing assistants (STNAs) See entry for *certified nursing assistants (CNAs)*

storage the fourth component of the information processing cycle; patient information is stored so that it can be retrieved, added to, or modified for later use

storage device a device where data for the EHR may be stored, such as on a dedicated server at the healthcare facility or on a server provided by a vendor; if an EHR system is networked, then the storage may exist on the healthcare system's server

strategic plan an organization's process of defining its direction by including goals or objectives and a sequence of steps to achieve each goal and objective

structural interoperability level a level of communication that provides a common data format, syntax, and organization for data exchange; the data can be interpreted, but the meaning of the data may not be understood; also Level 2 interoperability

subjective element the portion of the history and physical examination report that relies on patient narrative

subscriber the person whose insurance coverage is used for acute or ambulatory care

synchronous describes communication between individuals or groups that is conducted live, in real time, such as via a video conference or a telephone conversation

T

telehealth refers not only to the clinical provision of health care in a remote manner but also to patient and professional health-related education, public health, and health administration

telemedicine refers to the clinical provision of health care in a remote manner

template a preformatted file that provides prompts to obtain specific, consistent information

temporary partial disability (TPD) benefits income replacement benefit paid when an employee works in a reduced capacity but cannot work to the same extent as they could before their injury or illness

temporary total disability (TTD) benefits income replacement benefit paid when an employee has been injured at work and cannot perform their work duties

The Joint Commission an independent, not-for-profit organization that accredits and certifies a variety of healthcare organizations; formerly known as the Joint Commission on Accreditation of Healthcare Organizations (JCAHO)

third-party payer an entity other than the patient that is financially responsible for payment of the medical bill

time specified a type of schedule used in an acute care setting in which patients are given a specific date and time to arrive at a facility

transfer form similar to a nursing discharge assessment, this form indicates the status and condition of the patient upon discharge, such as prognosis, advance directives in place, follow-up appointments scheduled, and diagnoses

transfer orders a type of admission order generated when a patient transfers settings; must be approved by the admitting physician

transmission-based precautions CDC guidelines for preventing the transmission of infections specifically when a patient is known or suspected to be infected or colonized with infectious agents; divided into three categories: contract precautions, droplet precautions, and airborne precautions

trauma registry includes the collection, storage, and reporting of patient trauma data

treatment plan a plan a healthcare practitioner decides on to treat a patient's diagnoses

treatment, payment, healthcare operations (TPO) three types of permitted disclosures referred to collectively

TRICARE a Department of Defense regionally managed healthcare program for active duty and retired members of the uniformed services, their families, and survivors

U

UHDDS core data elements a set of patient-specific data elements outlined by the Uniform Hospital Discharge Data Set (UHDDS) committee

Uniform Ambulatory Care Data Set (UACDS) data set used for reporting outpatient data in ambulatory care settings, used to ensure that all healthcare settings and providers gather identical patient data in a consistent manner

Uniform Hospital Discharge Data Set (UHDDS) data set used for reporting inpatient data in acute care hospitals

unstructured data a format in which data is stored in a free-form format rather than in a database; examples include progress notes, test interpretations, and operative reports

upcoding the illegal act of assigning inaccurate codes for the purpose of claiming a higher-paying diagnosis-related group (DRG) and therefore increased reimbursement

W

wave a type of schedule in which patients are scheduled to arrive at the beginning of the hour, and the number of appointments is determined by dividing the hour by the length of an average visit or procedure

web-based tethered PHR a personal health record (PHR) system in which health information is attached to a specific organization's health information system

web-based untethered PHR a personal health record (PHR) system that is not attached to a specific organization's health information system

wide area network (WAN) a network that covers a broader area than a LAN, spanning regions, countries, or the world

Work Plan an annual report created by the Office of the Inspector General that establishes areas of healthcare documentation and billing practices to be addressed and audited during the year

workers' compensation an insurance plan that employers are required to have to cover employees who get sick or injured on the job

workflow analysis a review of how an organization currently functions and how paper records are used to care for patients

work-list reports reports that present the patient accounts for coding in a priority order, beginning with the oldest accounts with the highest balances

workstation a computer paired with input and output devices

Index

Note: Page numbers followed by *f* and *t* represent figures and tables respectively.

Photo Credits

Front Matter

Page xiii: top photo: © Chaay_Tee/Shutterstock.com, bottom photo: © Brian Eagan; Page xv: clockwise from top left: Source: HealthIT.gov, Source: HHS.gov, © Sarah Foltz, Source: Office of OCR, center: © Paradigm Education Solutions; Page xvii: © Paradigm Education Solutions; Page xviii: top: © Paradigm Education Solutions, bottom: © Paradigm Education Solutions; Page xix: top: © Darline Foltz, bottom: © Karen Lankisch

Chapter 1

Page 1: top: © TarikVision/Shutterstock.com, bottom: © Patrick Gruesser; Page 2: © iStockphoto/dra_schwartz; Page 3: © Paradigm Education Solutions; Page 4: © Monkey Business Images/Shutterstock.com; Page 5: © Paradigm Education Solutions; Page 7: © Paradigm Education Solutions; Page 8: Source: HealthIT.gov; Page 9: © Paradigm Education Solutions; Page 12: © Paradigm Education Solutions; Page 13: © Paradigm Education Solutions; Page 14: © Paradigm Education Solutions; Page 15: © iStockphoto/Pamela Moore

Chapter 2

Page 28: top: © Tero Vesalainen/Shutterstock.com, bottom: © Elizabeth Zimmerly; Page 29: © Rohane Hamilton/Shutterstock.com; Page 30: top: © iStockphoto/imagestock, bottom: © Smart7/Shutterstock.com; Page 31: top: © SPb photo maker/Shutterstock.com, bottom: © Marc Dietrich/Shutterstock.com; Page 33: © Makistock/Shutterstock.com; Page 34: © Paradigm Education Solutions; Page 35: top: © Bob Pool/Shutterstock.com, bottom: © Paradigm Education Solutions; Page 36: © Paradigm Education Solutions; Page 37: © Paradigm Education Solutions; Page 38: top: © yanugkelid/Shutterstock.com, bottom: © Paradigm Education Solutions; Page 45: © iStockphoto/babyblueut; Page 46: © Paul Vinten/Shutterstock.com; Page 48: © Zmaster/Shutterstock.com, computer screen © Paradigm Education Solutions; Page 50: © Paradigm Education Solutions; Page 51: © The Joint Commission, 2021. Reprinted with permission; Page 54: © Paradigm Education Solutions; Page 55: © iStockphoto/joeynick; Page 56: © iStockphoto/macrovector; Page 57: © Paradigm Education Solutions; Page 58: © iStockphoto/macrovector

Chapter 3

Page 65: top: © Interior Design/Shutterstock.com, bottom: © Michelle Watters; Page 66: © Paradigm Education Solutions; Page 67: © Paradigm Education Solutions; Page 68: © O n E Studio/Shutterstock.com; Page 69: © Ohmega1982/Shutterstock.com; Page 70: © Can Yesil/Shutterstock.com; Pages 72-97: all screen captures and icons © Paradigm Education Solutions

Chapter 4

Page 101: top: © ideyweb/Shutterstock.com, bottom: © Tracy Clyburn; Page 103: © wavebreakmedia/Shutterstock.com; Page 104: © Monkey Business Images/Shutterstock.com; Page 105: © iStockphoto/101dalmatians; Page 106: © iStockphoto/SolStock; Page 107: © Paradigm Education Solutions; Page 108: © Paradigm Education Solutions; Page 109: © Paradigm Education Solutions; Page 112: © Tyler Olson/Shutterstock.com; Pages 114-126: all screen captures and images © Paradigm Education Solutions

Chapter 5

Page 128: top: © iStockphoto/exdez, bottom: © Collette Eisen; Page 129: © iStockphoto/DenGuy; Page 130: top: © Paradigm Education Solutions, bottom: © Paradigm Education Solutions; Page 131: © Paradigm Education Solutions; Page 132: © Paradigm Education Solutions; Page 133: © iStockphoto/Mark Bowden; Page 134: © Monkey Business Images/Shutterstock.com; Page 135: © Paradigm Education Solutions; Page 136: top:

© Paradigm Education Solutions, bottom: © Paradigm Education Solutions; Page 137: top: © iStockphoto/annedde, bottom: © Paradigm Education Solutions; Page 139: © Paradigm Education Solutions; Page 141: © Monkey Business Images/Shutterstock.com; Page 142: © iStockphoto/vn; Page 143: top: © Paradigm Education Solutions, bottom: © Paradigm Education Solutions

Chapter 6

Page 148: top: © Nata-Lia/Shutterstock.com, bottom: © Kim Shearer; Page 150: © Paradigm Education Solutions; Page 153: © zimmytws/Shutterstock.com; Page 155: © iStockphoto/leezsnow; Page 158: © Paradigm Education Solutions; Page 160: Source: Office of OCR; Page 161: © Joanna Dorota/Shutterstock.com; Page 163: © Roman Arbuzov/Shutterstock.com; Page 165: © Robert A. Levy Photography, LLC/Shutterstock.com; Page 166: © Tero Vesalainen/Shutterstock.com; Page 167: Source: HHS.gov; Page 171: Source: HealthIT.gov

Chapter 7

Page 178: top: © ProStockStudio/Shutterstock.com, bottom: © Sarah Foltz; Page 180: © iStockphoto/Sportstock; Page 181: © Paradigm Education Solutions; Page 182: © Rocketclips, Inc./Shutterstock.com; Page 183: © Paradigm Education Solutions; Page 184: © Paradigm Education Solutions; Page 186: Source: HealthIT.gov; Page 188: top: © Paradigm Education Solutions, bottom: © Paradigm Education Solutions/George Brainard; Page 189: © Scott Rothstein/Shutterstock.com; Page 195: © Paradigm Education Solutions

Chapter 8

Page 201: top: © Chaay_Tee/Shutterstock.com, bottom: © Brian Eagan; Page 203: © Rawpixel.com/Shutterstock.com; Page 204: © Gorodenkoff/Shutterstock.com; Page 207: © Paradigm Education Solutions; Page 209: top: © Paradigm Education Solutions, bottom: © Angela Schmidt/Shutterstock.com; Page 210: © Paradigm Education Solutions; Page 211: top: © Anna Rassadnikova/Shutterstock.com, bottom: © Paradigm Education Solutions; Pages 212-219: © Paradigm Education Solutions; Page 220: top: © Paradigm Education Solutions, bottom: © Jodi Jacobson/iStockphoto.com; Pages 221-226: © Paradigm Education Solutions; Page 228: top: © Paradigm Education Solutions, bottom: © michaeljung/Shutterstock.com; Page 229: top: © Paradigm Education Solutions, bottom: © andresr/Getty Images; Page 230: © Paradigm Education Solutions; Page 231: © Paradigm Education Solutions; Page 232: © Paradigm Education Solutions; Page 233: top: © Paradigm Education Solutions, bottom: © Monkey Business Images/Shutterstock.com; Page 234: © Paradigm Education Solutions; Page 235: © Paradigm Education Solutions

Chapter 9

Page 240: top: © Andrey_Popov/Shutterstock.com, bottom: © Jody Pruss; Page 241: © BAZA Production/Shutterstock.com; Page 247: © iStockphoto/bjones27; Page 249: © Keith Bell/Shutterstock.com; Page 251: © Paradigm Education Solutions; Page 252: © Paradigm Education Solutions; Page 254: © Paradigm Education Solutions

Chapter 10

Page 261: © iStock.com/PeopleImages; Page 263: © Paradigm Education Solutions; Page 264: © iStock.com/Weekend Images Inc.; Page 266: © iStock.com/uschools; Page 268: © Valeri Potapova/Shutterstock.com; Page 272: © YAKOBCHUKVIACHESLAV/Shutterstock.com; Page 273: © ALPAPROD/Shutterstock.com; Page 275: © Paradigm Education Solutions; Page 276: top: Source: CMS.gov, bottom: © Paradigm Education Solutions; Page 278: © Paradigm Education Solutions; Page 279: Source: CMS.gov; Page 280: Source: CMS.gov; Page 282: © iStock.com/rowlbodvar; Pages 283-296: © Paradigm Education Solutions

Chapter 11

Page 302: top: © iStock.com/Hilch, bottom: © Ryan Jeska; Page 304: © Andrey_Popov/Shutterstock.com; Page 305: top: Source: Alissa Eckert, MSMI, Dan Higgins, MAMS, bottom: © iStock.com/kali9; Page 309: © Paradigm Education Solutions; Page 312: Source: HealthData.gov; Page 313: © iStock.com/KatarzynaBialasiewicz; Page 315: © iStock.com/simonkr

Chapter 12

Page 324: top: © Billion Photos/Shutterstock.com, bottom: © Linette Kallaos; Page 326: © Spectral-Design/Shutterstock.com; Page 328: © Andrey_Popov/Shutterstock.com; Page 329: © Paradigm Education Solutions; Page 331: © Rocketclips, Inc./Shutterstock.com; Page 332: © Gorodenkoff/Shutterstock.com, lab results screen © Paradigm Education Solutions; Page 334: Source: The Joint Commission; Pages 335-340: © Paradigm Education Solutions

Chapter 13

Page 348: top: © vectorfusionart/Shutterstock.com, bottom: © Tom Frye; Page 349: © iofoto/Shutterstock.com; Page 350: © Monkey Business Images/Shutterstock.com; Page 351: © Paradigm Education Solutions; Page 353: © iStock.com/stevecoleimages; Page 354: © iStock.com/Sproetniek; Page 357: Source: HealthIT.gov; Page 358: Source: CMS

Chapter 14

Page 366: top: © ArtemisDiana/Shutterstock.com, bottom: © Melanie Fisher; Page 372: Source: CDC; Page 373: Source: CDC; Page 374: © Paradigm Education Solutions; Page 377: © iStock.com/andhedesigns; Page 378: © iStock.com/Christopher Futcher; Page 379: © Epic Systems Corporation; Page 380: © Epic Systems Corporation; Pages 383-387: © Paradigm Education Solutions

Appendix B

All images © Paradigm Education Solutions